HOW FOOD WORKS

DK

HOW
FOOD
WORKS

Editorial consultant
Dr. Sarah Brewer

Contributors
Joel Levy, Ginny Smith

Project Art Editors
Duncan Turner
Francis Wong
Steve Woosnam-Savage

Senior Editor
Rob Houston

Editors
Lili Bryant
Wendy Horobin
Janet Mohun
Martyn Page
Francesco Piscitelli

Designers
Gregory McCarthy

Illustrators
Mark Clifton
Phil Gamble
Mike Garland

US Editor
Margaret Parrish

Managing Art Editor
Michael Duffy

Jacket Editor
Claire Gell

Senior Jacket Designer
Mark Cavanagh

Managing Editor
Angeles Gavira Guerrero

Jackets Design Development Manager
Sophia MTT

Producer, Pre-production
Catherine Williams

Producer
Anna Vallarino

Publisher
Liz Wheeler

Art Director
Karen Self

Publishing Director
Jonathan Metcalf

First American Edition, 2017
Published in the United States by DK Publishing
345 Hudson Street, New York, New York 10014

READER NOTICE

How Food Works provides information on a wide range of food science and nutritional topics and every effort has been made to ensure that the information is accurate. The book is not a substitute for expert nutritional advice, however, and you are advised always to consult a professional for specific information on personal nutritional matters. The authors, contributors, consultants, and publisher do not accept any legal responsibility for any personal injury or other damage or loss arising from any use or misuse of the information in this book.

A catalog record for this book is available from the Library of Congress.
ISBN: 978-1-4654-6119-3

DK books are available at special discounts when purchased in bulk for sales promotions, premiums, fund-raising, or educational use. For details, contact: DK Publishing Special Markets, 345 Hudson Street, New York, New York 10014
SpecialSales@dk.com

Printed in USA

A WORLD OF IDEAS:
SEE ALL THERE IS TO KNOW

www.dk.com

CONTENTS

TYPES OF FOOD

DRINKS

DIETS

FOOD AND ENVIRONMENT

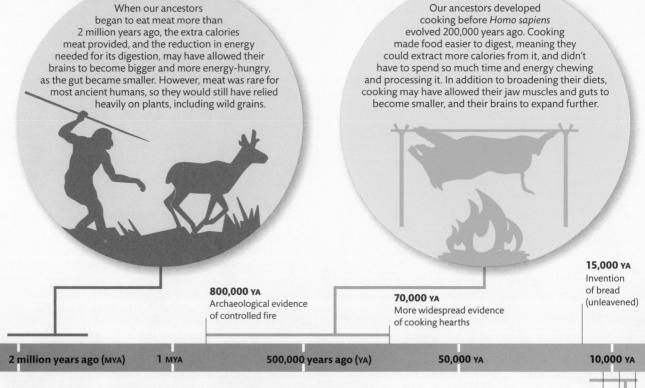

MEAT EATING

When our ancestors began to eat meat more than 2 million years ago, the extra calories meat provided, and the reduction in energy needed for its digestion, may have allowed their brains to become bigger and more energy-hungry, as the gut became smaller. However, meat was rare for most ancient humans, so they would still have relied heavily on plants, including wild grains.

COOKING

Our ancestors developed cooking before *Homo sapiens* evolved 200,000 years ago. Cooking made food easier to digest, meaning they could extract more calories from it, and didn't have to spend so much time and energy chewing and processing it. In addition to broadening their diets, cooking may have allowed their jaw muscles and guts to become smaller, and their brains to expand further.

15,000 YA
Invention of bread (unleavened)

800,000 YA
Archaeological evidence of controlled fire

70,000 YA
More widespread evidence of cooking hearths

| 2 million years ago (MYA) | 1 MYA | 500,000 years ago (YA) | 50,000 YA | 10,000 YA |

12,000 YA
Goat domesticated

9,500 YA
Rice cultivated

9,000 – 8,500 YA
Sheep domesticated

Our diet history

Diets have changed dramatically during human evolution, often causing our bodies to change in response. Dating these changes is challenging. Cooking may have originated 300,000 or 1.8 million years ago, depending on how experts interpret archaeological and genetic evidence. Despite this, scientists are building a picture of how our dietary history has affected us.

Dietary milestones

Our anatomy and physiology have evolved as our diet has changed over many thousands of years. Some of these pivotal events, such as meat eating or cooking, happened so long ago that our bodies have already evolved accordingly. Whether we are suited to more recent changes is still to be seen. What has become clear is that some aspects of the modern diet, with its abundance of energy-dense foods, can be very detrimental to our health. Looking back in time may even help us to eat more healthily today.

WHY ARE MANY ASIAN PEOPLE INTOLERANT TO MILK?

Intolerance to lactose in milk is more prevalent in people from Asia, because domestic cattle were introduced there much more recently than in other parts of the world.

THE GREAT COLUMBIAN EXCHANGE

When Europeans first met the native peoples of the Americas in the 15th and 16th centuries, there began an unprecedented exchange of foods that one or the other population had never seen before. Potatoes and corn rapidly became staples in the Old World, and sugarcane flourished when taken to the Americas.

EUROPE, ASIA, AND AFRICA

AMERICAS

SWEET TOOTH

For our ancestors, sweet food was a rare delicacy. Honey and ripe fruits were a great source of energy, but were scarce or seasonal. Today, we are surrounded by accessible, sweet food all the time, and our liking for it has contributed to an epidemic of obesity and its related diseases.

8,000 YA
Cattle domesticated

7,000 YA
Sugarcane cultivated

6,000 YA
Cheese invented and alcoholic drinks invented

1800 BCE
Chocolate drunk in Central America

997 CE
Word "pizza" first used in Italy

1911 CE
Home refrigerators appeared in the US

5,000 YA

1 CE

1000 CE

2000 CE

6,000 YA
Chicken domesticated

4,000 YA
Maize cultivated; leavened bread invented in Egypt

1585 CE
Chocolate introduced to Europe

8,000 YA
Potato cultivated

The cultivation of grain allowed humans to settle. This made having more children easier and they quickly out-competed hunter-gatherers in most areas. However, their limited diets and tightly packed populations meant they had poorer health than hunter-gatherers.

Humans have traded food for thousands of years, but until fairly recently, only long-life products could be transported over extended distances. The development of refrigeration and freezing, along with faster shipping, have meant that, if you can afford them, foods from all over the globe can be on your table.

REFRIGERATED GLOBAL SUPPLY CHAINS

FARMING

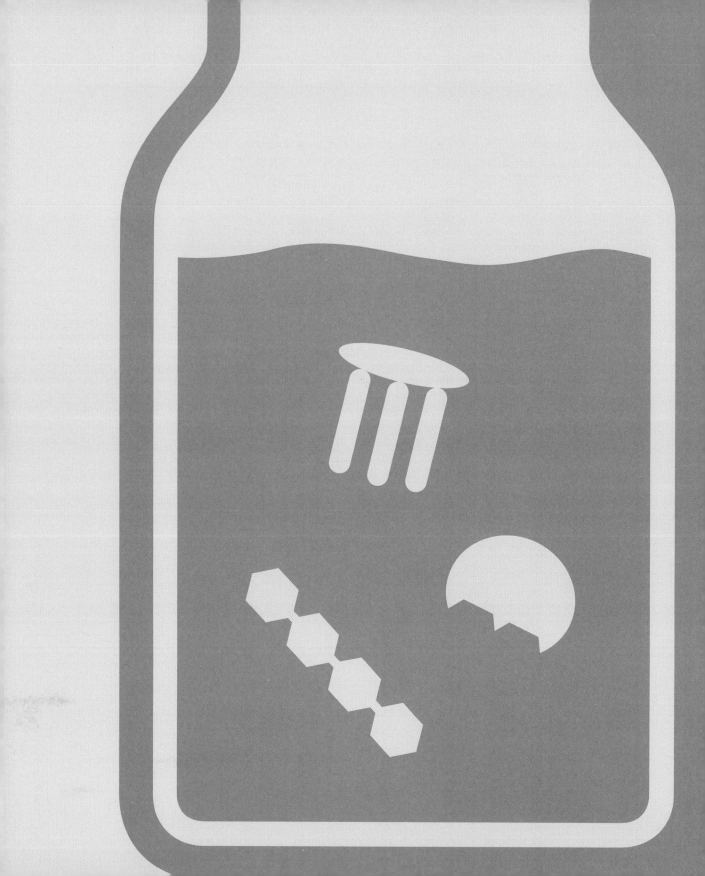

FOOD
FUNDAMENTALS

Nutrition basics

For the body to function normally it requires fuel for energy, building materials for growth and essential maintenance, plus a small but vital combination of chemical ingredients to ensure its many metabolic processes run smoothly. The body can make almost everything it needs from the nutrients in a balanced diet.

What does the body need?

An adequate combination of essential nutrients in our diet—water, carbohydrates, proteins, fats, vitamins, and minerals—should enable our bodies to work efficiently and keep us in good health. Beyond basic nutrition, there are other nutrients that, although our body doesn't necessarily need them, are certainly beneficial, such as phytochemicals in fruit and vegetables and fatty acids in some fish. Nutraceuticals, or "functional foods," including those containing probiotics (see p.87), are believed to have health benefits beyond their nutritional value, including disease prevention.

MALNUTRITION

Malnutrition results from a diet that does not contain the right amounts of nutrients. While lack of carbohydrates and protein can lead to major development and growth problems, deficiency in certain vitamins and minerals can cause specific illnesses. For example, a lack of iron may lead to anemia. Overnutrition occurs when an oversupply of nutrients causes health problems, such as obesity caused by a high-calorie diet.

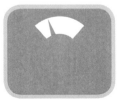

Carbohydrates

Carbohydrates are the body's primary source of energy. The body converts simple sugars and more complex starches into glucose, which fuels our body cells. Whole grains and fruits and vegetables that are high in fiber are the most healthy sources of carbohydrates.

SUGAR

Water

Around 65 percent of the body is made up of water. This is constantly being lost through digestion, breathing, sweating, and urine, and it is critical that water is replenished at regular intervals.

LARGE INTESTINE

Minerals

Present in a wide variety of foods, minerals are vital for building bones, hair, skin, and blood cells. They also enhance nerve function and help to turn food into energy. Deficiencies can cause chronic health problems.

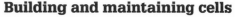

Getting what we need

When we eat food, it passes into our digestive system to be broken down and absorbed (see pp.20–21). Most nutrients are absorbed in the small intestine.

Building and maintaining cells

Cells are the basic functional units of the human body that make up its diverse tissues and organs. Every one of our trillions of cells is built and maintained by the nutrients we get through our diet. If, through poor nutrition, our cells are unable to function properly, our tissues and organs can become compromised, leading to the onset of a host of health conditions and diseases.

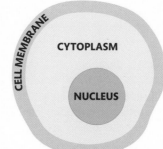

CELL MEMBRANE

CYTOPLASM

NUCLEUS

CELL STRUCTURE

Cell support

A broad range of nutrients support cell formation and growth. A cell's main structures are built from amino acids and some fatty acids, and every cell is fueled by carbohydrates and other fatty acids.

Proteins

Proteins are broken down into amino acids. Although they may be used by the body for energy, their main role is as building blocks of tissue growth and repair. Healthy protein sources include beans, lean meat, dairy, and eggs.

STOMACH

AMINO ACIDS

FATTY ACIDS

Fats

Fats are a rich source of energy and help in the absorption of fat-soluble vitamins. Essential fatty acids cannot be made by the body and must be obtained from food. The healthiest fat sources include dairy, nuts, fish, and vegetable-based oils.

SMALL INTESTINE

Vitamins

Vitamins are vital to the body's metabolic processes, especially those linked to tissue growth and maintenance. Most vitamins can't be stored in the body, so regular intake through a balanced diet is essential. As with minerals, a lack of certain vitamins can lead to deficiency diseases.

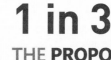

1 in 3

THE **PROPORTION OF PEOPLE** WORLDWIDE THAT SUFFER FROM **MALNUTRITION**

WHAT IS A "HEALTHY DIET"?

A healthy diet is one that provides the body with the right amounts of all the essential nutrients it needs from a variety of different food sources. This should help you achieve and maintain a healthy body weight.

Hunger and appetite

Hunger is vital to our survival, and it ensures we eat enough for our bodies to function. But a lot of the time we eat not because we are hungry but because we enjoy food—this is down to our appetite.

Hunger and satiety

Hunger is controlled by a complex interconnected system including our brain, digestive system, and fat stores. The desire to eat can be triggered by internal factors, such as low blood sugar or an empty stomach, or external triggers, such as the sight and smell of food. After we have eaten, satiety, or "fullness" signals are produced, which tell us we have had enough.

Hunger vs. appetite

Appetite is different from hunger, but the two are linked. Hunger is the physiological need for food, driven by internal cues such as low blood sugar or an empty stomach. Appetite is the desire to eat, driven by seeing or smelling food or something we link with it. Memory for how much we have eaten is also important in appetite, and people with short-term memory loss may eat again soon after eating. Stress can also increase the desire to eat. Some substances can help control appetite by specific actions on the body.

Water
Water stretches the stomach, triggering satiety. Satiety is short-lived, since water is quickly absorbed and the body responds to the lack of nutrients.

Fiber
Foods high in fiber slow the emptying of the stomach and delay the absorption of nutrients, keeping you fuller for longer.

Protein
Protein affects the release of various appetite-regulating hormones such as leptin, increasing feelings of fullness.

Grapefruit
The scent of grapefruit seems to reduce activation of the vagus nerve, reducing appetite.

Nicotine
Nicotine activates receptors in the hypothalamus, reducing hunger signals.

Exercise
High-intensity aerobic exercise affects the release of hunger hormones, temporarily suppressing hunger.

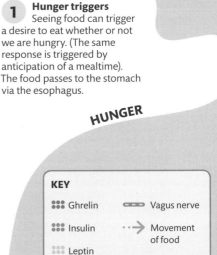

BRAIN

1 Hunger triggers
Seeing food can trigger a desire to eat whether or not we are hungry. (The same response is triggered by anticipation of a mealtime). The food passes to the stomach via the esophagus.

HUNGER

GHRELIN

KEY

::: Ghrelin

::: Insulin

::: Leptin

⊏—⊐ Vagus nerve

⋯▸ Movement of food

2 Empty stomach
When the stomach has been empty for around 2 hours, the gut muscles contract, clearing out any last debris. Low blood sugar levels exacerbate the feelings of hunger. Levels of a hunger hormone called ghrelin also rise.

PANCREAS

SMALL INTESTINE

Hypothalamus receives "full" signal from vagus nerve

6 Brain receives "full" signals
The vagus nerve sends signals straight to the hypothalamus, telling the brain that food has been consumed and reducing the hunger drive.

SATIETY

LEPTIN

INSULIN

VAGUS NERVE

5 Leptin travels to brain
Fat cells release a hunger-inhibiting hormone called leptin. After eating, more leptin is secreted and we feel full. (Conversely, leptin levels decrease with fasting, making us feel hungry.)

4 Pancreas releases insulin
The stretching stomach and the rise in glucose in the bloodstream, triggers the release of insulin. This allows the conversion of glucose to glycogen (in the liver) and then to fat. Insulin may also make the brain more sensitive to satiety signals.

STOMACH

STRETCH RECEPTORS

ADIPOSE (FAT) TISSUE

3 Stomach stretches
As the stomach fills, stretch receptors detect expansion, causing hunger-reducing chemicals to be released. (Liquids, including water, stretch the stomach temporarily, but are quickly absorbed, so hunger returns.)

Glucose released into bloodstream from digested food

APPETITE AND OBESITY

People with a tendency to obesity may respond differently to external hunger cues. They may also be less sensitive to the fullness hormone, leptin. Unfortunately, taking leptin as a drug doesn't help obesity. The body quickly adapts to be even more insensitive to leptin, even at high doses.

Hunger stimulated by external cue

Leptin released to no response

ADIPOSE TISSUE

Cravings

Cravings are a dramatic and specific desire for a certain type of food, and most of us have experienced them. Occasionally, they are caused by specific nutrient deficiencies, and may be the body's way of telling you about the problem. But mostly they are purely psychological, driven by stress or boredom. Normally, craved foods are high in fat or sugar (or high in both), which trigger a rush of pleasurable chemicals in the brain when eaten. It may be this feeling that we crave rather than the actual food.

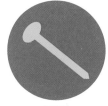

IRON

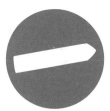

CHALK

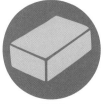

SOAP

WHY DOES MY STOMACH RUMBLE WHEN I'M HUNGRY?

After eating, your stomach muscles contract to push food through to the intestines. With an empty stomach, this still happens, but with nothing to dampen the sound, you hear the growls!

Strange tastes
Some people, especially pregnant women or very young children, experience cravings for nonfood substances, including soil, chalk, iron, and soap. Psychiatrists call this "pica."

Flavor

We eat food not only because we need to, but also because we enjoy it, and this is at least in part down to its flavor. Flavor is a combination of the taste and smell of food, which combine with input from our other senses to produce a pleasurable experience.

What gives food flavor?

You detect smell when volatile chemicals travel into your nose—either before you eat the food or when it is in your mouth. At the same time, the tongue and mouth detect five basic tastes, which combine with the smell to produce flavor. Other senses contribute too—touch and hearing tell you about the food's texture. Even the color of a food can impact how we perceive flavor—a study showed that changing the color of orange squash affected people's ability to identify its flavor correctly.

COULD THERE BE UNDISCOVERED TASTES?

It is quite likely; some argue that metallic tastes are a separate category, while calcium's chalky taste can be detected by mice and possibly humans, too.

Sour
Vietnamese dipping sauce uses a mixture of sour lime juice, salty fish sauce, and sweet palm sugar, along with garlic and chili, to activate almost all the receptors on your tongue at once. Sour tastes are produced when taste buds detect hydrogen ions. These come from acidic foods such as fruits and vinegar.

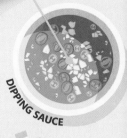

DIPPING SAUCE

Sweet
Another of the basic tastes is sweetness. Your sweet receptors respond to sugars such as fructose (in fruit) and sucrose (table sugar). Some artificial sweeteners, such as aspartame, taste much sweeter than sugar, meaning you can use less in foods.

VIETNAMESE MANGO SALAD

MANGO STRIPS

DRIED SHRIMP

"NEW" TASTES

Recently, receptors have been found on our tongues that bind to fatty acids, producing a taste of "fattiness." Whether this is a true sixth taste is still under debate. Another recent study suggested humans can also taste starch, but a receptor has not yet been found. Oil-fried chunky fries may trigger both of these proposed new classes of taste.

FRIES

Umami
Umami is the most recently discovered of the basic tastes—the name is Japanese, and it roughly translates as "savory." Glutamic acid in foods is detected as umami and it is found in high quantities in fermented and aged foods such as dried shrimp, soy sauce, and Parmesan cheese.

TOMATOES RELEASE 222 VOLATILE CHEMICALS THAT GIVE THEM THEIR **FLAVOR**

Bitter
Children often find bitter foods unpleasant, but many adults enjoy bitter tastes such as tea (including green tea), coffee, and dark chocolate. It is the most sensitive taste, probably because it evolved to prevent us from eating bitter-tasting poisonous plants.

SPRING ROLLS

VIETNAMESE TEA

VIETNAMESE TEA

SALTED PEANUTS

Salty
Table salt is sodium chloride, and we have sensors in our mouths that detect sodium ions. They are also triggered (though less strongly) by closely related atoms, including potassium.

Non-taste sensations

In addition to the five basic tastes, our tongues and mouths can detect some other sensations that are not classified as tastes. Nerves on the tongue detect temperature, touch, and pain, and foods that activate these nerves produce specific sensations. For example, the carbon dioxide in carbonated drinks doesn't only activate our sour taste receptors. Its bubbles also cause touch receptors to fire. The two combine to produce the fizzy sensation.

SENSATION	EXPLANATION
Astringent	Chemicals in tea and unripe fruit cause a puckering sensation of the mucous membrane and disrupt the saliva film, making the mouth feel dry and rough.
Cooling	Menthol in mint sensitizes the cold receptors on your tongue, giving a cool, refreshing sensation.
Spiciness	Capsaicin chemicals in chili stimulate pain and heat receptors on the tongue, causing a burning feeling.
Numbness	There is a disagreement as to the cause, but Sichuan pepper produces numbness or a tingling sensation, possibly by stimulating light touch receptors.

Smell and flavor

The smell of food can be different from its taste, despite most of a food's flavor coming from its smell. This is because when food is in our mouth, scent molecules travel up the back of the throat rather than through the nose (see p.19). This changes which molecules we detect, and in what order, creating a difference in the scent perceived. This is particularly noticeable in coffee and chocolate.

COFFEE

CHOCOLATE

Smell and taste

Molecules in food dissolve in saliva and register as tastes when they come into contact with your tongue. Airborne volatile molecules released by food are detected by your nose as smells.

Perceiving our meals

Molecules released by food in the air or by chewing dissolve when they meet moisture, such as mucus in the nose and saliva in the mouth. They can then be detected by specialized nerve cells. These cells transmit electrical signals to the brain, which identifies and categorizes each smell and taste. Our noses can pick up hundreds of different kinds of smells, but our tongues primarily detect five tastes—possibly more (see pp.16–17).

Mucus-secreting gland

Supporting cell

Olfactory receptor cell

MUCUS

How smell works
Your nasal cavity has a thin layer of mucus. When scent molecules dissolve into it, they bind to the ends of olfactory receptor cells.

Scent molecule dissolving in mucus

Scent molecule binding to receptor

WHY DOES THE SMELL OF COOKING MAKE YOU SALIVATE?

When you smell food, sensory information is passed to the brain, which sends nerve signals to the salivary glands. Saliva is produced to prepare for the first stages of digestion.

Food particle

Supporting cell

SALIVA

TASTE BUD

How taste works
The tongue's surface is full of taste receptor cells. Chemicals from food and drink dissolved in saliva come into contact with these cells.

Taste receptor cell

Sensory nerve

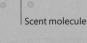

OLFACTORY RECEPTORS

ORTHONASAL OLFACTION

Scent molecule

CHEWED FOOD

TONGUE

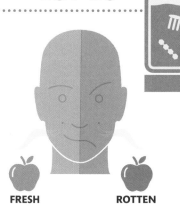

ONE PAPILLA ON THE TONGUE CAN CONTAIN **HUNDREDS OF TASTE BUDS**

To the brain
Olfactory receptor cells in the nose and taste receptor cells on the tongue send nerve signals to the brain to register smells and tastes.

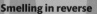

NERVE SIGNALS TO BRAIN

MUCUS

RETRONASAL OLFACTION

NERVE SIGNALS TO BRAIN

SALIVA

Smelling in reverse
Food in the mouth releases scent molecules that waft up the back of the throat (retronasal olfaction) rather than through the nose (orthonasal olfaction). Most of what you taste is actually made up of smells detected via retronasal olfaction.

Why do foods have tastes and smells?

As the first humans evolved, they made a wide range of food choices every day. This means we have evolved more taste receptors than animals who stick to one type of food. As infants, we like sweet tastes and reject bitter ones—this is thought to stem back to our evolutionary past where sweet tastes signaled high-energy foods and bitterness could be a warning for poison. Our desire for salty and umami (savory) tastes are thought to be driven by our need for salt and other minerals, and for protein.

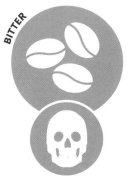

FRESH   ROTTEN

Fresh or rotten?
Distinguishing between fresh (nutritious) or rotten (potentially dangerous) fruit would have been helpful for our ancestors.

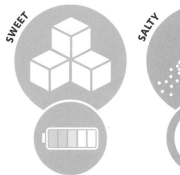

SWEET   SALTY   BITTER

High calorie
Sweet foods such as honey provide high amounts of calories.

Vital minerals
A taste for salt exists because sodium is one of the macrominerals we need to survive.

Sign of poison
Typically, bitter tastes signal poisonous foods, but with experience we can learn to like some bitter tastes.

WHY DO MEALS ON PLANES TASTE BLAND?

The dry air on a plane makes our mouths dry and our noses stuffy, interfering with the moist media in which molecules from food and drink dissolve. This means taste and smell receptors don't detect molecules properly. Our sensitivity to sweet and salty foods drops by 30 percent on planes, so in-flight meals are often salted to give them an extra kick. Oddly, umami tastes seem to be unaffected.

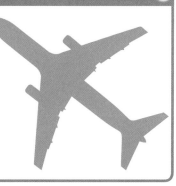

Digesting nutrients

For your body to absorb nutrients, food must first be broken down—this is the process of digestion. Most of the food you eat will reach your bowel within a few hours, but how long it stays there varies from person to person. Carbohydrates, proteins, and fats all break down at different stages of the process—fiber stays relatively intact.

What happens when we eat?

A combination of chewing, crushing, churning, and the action of digestive enzymes breaks down large food molecules into smaller ones that can be absorbed into the bloodstream. Each enzyme has a specific shape, which means it can only break down certain molecules, so we have a number of different types working in our bodies all the way from our mouth to our intestines.

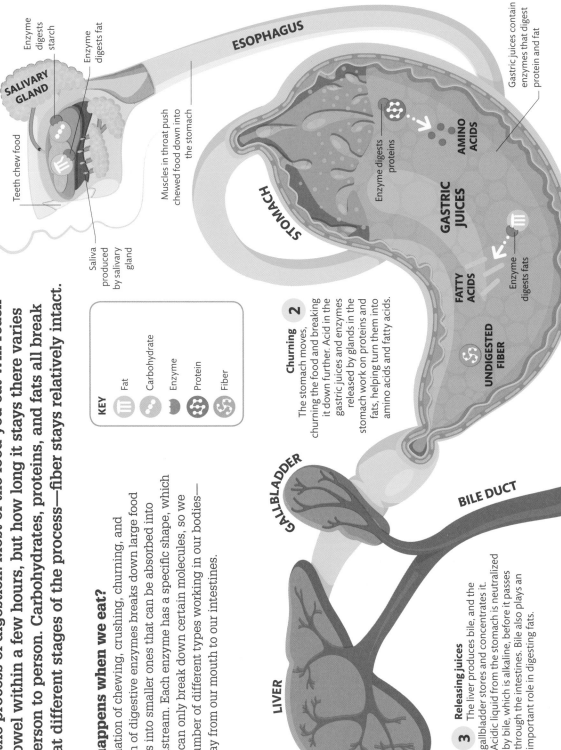

1 **Into the mouth**
Chewing breaks food down into smaller particles. This creates a larger surface area for our digestive enzymes to work on. Enzymes in the saliva begin breaking down starches (types of carbohydrate) and fats.

Enzyme digests starch

Enzyme digests fat

SALIVARY GLAND

Teeth chew food

Saliva produced by salivary gland

ESOPHAGUS

Muscles in throat push chewed food down into the stomach

STOMACH

Enzyme digests proteins

AMINO ACIDS

GASTRIC JUICES

FATTY ACIDS

Enzyme digests fats

UNDIGESTED FIBER

Gastric juices contain enzymes that digest protein and fat

2 **Churning**
The stomach moves, churning the food and breaking it down further. Acid in the gastric juices and enzymes released by glands in the stomach work on proteins and fats, helping turn them into amino acids and fatty acids.

GALLBLADDER

BILE DUCT

LIVER

3 **Releasing juices**
The liver produces bile, and the gallbladder stores and concentrates it. Acidic liquid from the stomach is neutralized by bile, which is alkaline, before it passes through the intestines. Bile also plays an important role in digesting fats.

KEY

Fat

Carbohydrate

Enzyme

Protein

Fiber

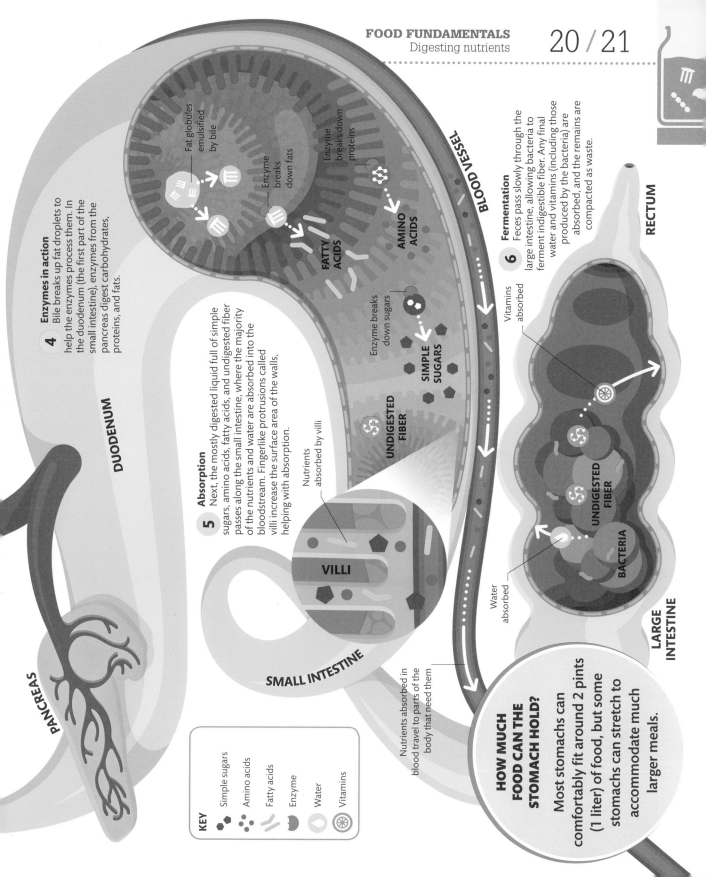

4 Enzymes in action
Bile breaks up fat droplets to help the enzymes process them. In the duodenum (the first part of the small intestine), enzymes from the pancreas digest carbohydrates, proteins, and fats.

Fat globules emulsified by bile

Enzyme breaks down fats

Enzyme breaks down proteins

FATTY ACIDS

AMINO ACIDS

Enzyme breaks down sugars

SIMPLE SUGARS

UNDIGESTED FIBER

BLOOD VESSEL

DUODENUM

PANCREAS

5 Absorption
Next, the mostly digested liquid full of simple sugars, amino acids, fatty acids, and undigested fiber passes along the small intestine, where the majority of the nutrients and water are absorbed into the bloodstream. Fingerlike protrusions called villi increase the surface area of the walls, helping with absorption.

Nutrients absorbed by villi

VILLI

SMALL INTESTINE

Nutrients absorbed in blood travel to parts of the body that need them

6 Fermentation
Feces pass slowly through the large intestine, allowing bacteria to ferment indigestible fiber. Any final water and vitamins (including those produced by the bacteria) are absorbed, and the remains are compacted as waste.

RECTUM

Vitamins absorbed

Water absorbed

UNDIGESTED FIBER

BACTERIA

LARGE INTESTINE

KEY
- Simple sugars
- Amino acids
- Fatty acids
- Enzyme
- Water
- Vitamins

HOW MUCH FOOD CAN THE STOMACH HOLD?

Most stomachs can comfortably fit around 2 pints (1 liter) of food, but some stomachs can stretch to accommodate much larger meals.

Carbohydrates

Most of the food we eat contains carbohydrates. They include sugar and starches, which provide our body with energy, and fiber, which is vital for a healthy digestive system.

What are carbohydrates?

Carbohydrate molecules are made up of carbon, hydrogen, and oxygen atoms, often in the form of hexagonal or pentagonal rings. If the rings are in ones or twos, they are sugars, but if the rings combine into unbranched or branched chains, they become starches and other complex carbohydrates. Very long, indigestible chains make up dietary fiber (see pp.24–25). In the body, sugars and starches are converted into the sugar glucose—our body's primary source of energy.

DO CARBS MAKE YOU FAT?

Carbohydrates can cause you to gain weight if you eat too many of them, but complex, high-fiber carbohydrates are a key part of a healthy diet.

STARCHES

Unrefined starches
These are found in foods including whole-grain breads, cereals, and beans. They are broken down slowly, releasing energy over a long period of time. They are also a good source of fiber, vitamins, and minerals.

WHOLE GRAINS **BEANS AND LEGUMES**

Refined starches
Only the simpler, more easily digested starches are found in refined carbohydrates such as white flour and white rice. They break down easily in the body, giving a quick energy rush, but don't keep you full for long.

WHITE RICE **CAKE** **WHITE BREAD**

SUGARS

Milk and natural sugars
Natural sugars are found in milk products, fruit, and some vegetables. The fiber in some of these foods ensures that the sugar is absorbed at a gradual rate.

APPLE **BROCCOLI** **MILK**

Free sugars
These can be added to food as refined table sugar, but are naturally present in honey, syrups, and fruit juices. These provide lots of "empty calories" and it is easy to eat too much of them.

HONEY **FRUIT JUICE** **SYRUP**

FIBER

NOT ENOUGH CARBS?

If you don't eat enough carbs, your liver converts fats into ketones and protein into glucose, which are used to generate energy. Ketogenic diets can help weight loss, but not much is known about their long-term health effects. They can also give you smelly breath!

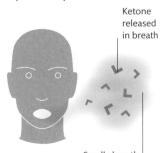

Ketone released in breath

Smelly breath caused by ketones

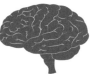

A LOW-CARB DIET MAY LEAD TO **MOOD SWINGS** AS CARBS HELP THE BRAIN MAKE **A CHEMICAL THAT STABILIZES MOODS**

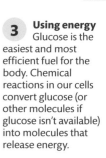

How the body uses carbohydrates

When we eat carbohydrates, our digestive tract breaks them down into sugars, which are absorbed into the blood. Glucose is used directly by our various organs and muscles as a source of energy. Fructose—a simple fruit sugar that bonds with glucose to make table sugar—can only be processed by the liver. People with high fructose diets are at higher risk of type 2 diabetes, possibly because fructose is more likely to be converted into fat.

BRAIN

The brain is the body's most energy-demanding organ

3 **Using energy**
Glucose is the easiest and most efficient fuel for the body. Chemical reactions in our cells convert glucose (or other molecules if glucose isn't available) into molecules that release energy.

SMALL INTESTINE

1 **Absorption and distribution**
Long-chain, starchy carbohydrates need to be broken down into sugars to be absorbed. Digestion begins in the mouth and continues into the small intestine, where the sugars pass into the bloodstream.

BLOOD VESSEL

MUSCLE

Muscle cells convert glucose into energy

Glucose molecules travel in the blood

Fructose molecules travel in the blood

HEART

Glucose is used or stored by the liver

The heart uses energy to pump nutrients around the body

LIVER

Glucose travels around the body

Some glucose is stored as glycogen, a complex carbohydrate like starch

Fructose is either converted to glucose or stored as fat

FAT

2 **The liver's role**
If we eat more carbohydrates than we need to use immediately, the liver stores the excess as glycogen. When blood sugar levels drop, the stored glycogen is converted back into glucose to be used by the body.

4 **Fat stores**
Once the liver's glycogen stores are full, excess glucose is converted into fat and stored around the body, to be used as fuel later if food becomes scarce.

Fiber

Fiber is the part of food that is not broken down by the body, and helps keep your digestive system functioning properly. It is found in varying amounts in plant foods.

Types of fiber

Fiber is traditionally characterized into two types. Soluble fiber dissolves in water, making a thick gel. It is found in foods such as fruit, root vegetables, and lentils, and prevents constipation by softening stools. Insoluble fiber is found in foods like cereals, nuts, and seeds. It keeps bowels healthy by increasing the weight of stools. However, studies have shown that there is crossover between the two categories and that solubility doesn't always predict how a type of fiber will behave in the body.

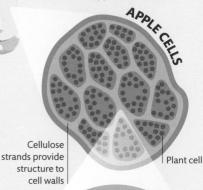

APPLE

Skin of your greens
In many plants, the most fiber-rich part is the skin. Apple skins, for example, are a great source of the insoluble fiber cellulose. This type of fiber provides structure to the apple's cell walls.

APPLE CELLS

Cellulose strands provide structure to cell walls

Plant cell

FIBER STRANDS

Chain

Sugar molecule

CELLULOSE STRANDS

CELLULOSE STRAND

Fiber strands
Fiber is a carbohydrate comprised of long chains of sugar molecules. However, unlike other carbohydrates, they resist digestion in the stomach. This means they reach the large intestine intact.

Holding it together
The long strands of cellulose in apples bond together to form a rigid framework, which provides support for the cells.

GETTING ENOUGH FIBER

Many of us don't get enough fiber in our diets. Whole grains are the most common source, but refined grains have the fiber-rich outer layer removed, so don't provide much. The UK recommends ⅝oz (18g) a day—although recommendations vary.

KEY ⅝oz (18g) of fiber   ◯ Amount required to reach ⅝oz (18g) of fiber

 WHEAT CEREAL 6¾oz (186g)

 DRIED FIGS 9½oz (260g)

 CHICKPEAS 15oz (15oz)

 BROWN BREAD 18½oz (514g)

COMPLEX FIBER FERMENTING IN COLON

Feeding your intestines bacteria

Fiber is an important source of food for your gut flora (microbes including bacteria and fungi that live in your intestines) which ferment it into fatty acids they can feed on. Keeping these bacteria healthy is vital—they produce enzymes to help digest other foods and influence your health in ways that we are only just beginning to understand.

VITAMIN K

Vitamin production
Certain strains of bacteria produce vitamins, some of which we can absorb and use. We get some of our Vitamin K this way.

Protection
Weak acids produced by fermentation make the colon less hospitable to bad bacteria, lowering the risk of stomach bugs.

FATTY ACIDS

FATTY ACIDS

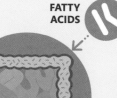

Healthy colon
More beneficial bacteria in the colon increases the mass of stools, diluting toxins and keeping the bowel healthy.

Improving immunity
Some types of bacteria in your gut improve your immune system by producing inflammation-reducing compounds.

Fiber and health

Eating plenty of fiber (see pp.198–99) reduces the risk of heart disease, certain cancers, obesity, and type 2 diabetes. A high-fiber diet counters the increased risk of colon cancer caused by eating processed meat (see p.219).

Unexpected benefit
Fiber, particularly the soluble kind, binds to bile (a bitter liquid that breaks fats down to tiny droplets), causing it to be excreted. To replace the bile, the liver must pull cholesterol out of the bloodstream, which may explain how fiber lowers the risk of heart disease.

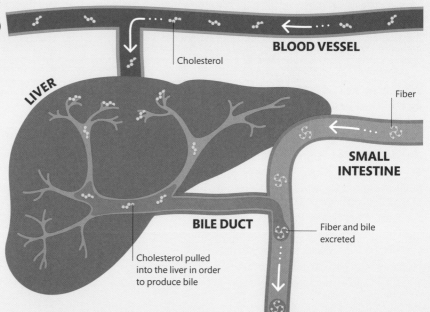

Cholesterol

BLOOD VESSEL

LIVER

Fiber

SMALL INTESTINE

BILE DUCT

Fiber and bile excreted

Cholesterol pulled into the liver in order to produce bile

Protein

Protein is a vital nutrient. The proteins we eat are broken down into their building blocks and used to make new proteins and other complex molecules needed by the body. While protein can serve as an energy source, its main function is in the creation, growth, and repair of human tissues.

What is protein?

Proteins are chains of small molecules called amino acids. While only 21 standard types of amino acid occur naturally in humans, they can join together in any combination, meaning that there are millions of different types of protein available.

When you eat foods containing protein, your body breaks them down into amino acids, then reassembles them into different sequences, producing whatever types of protein it needs.

An important property of proteins is their ability to fold and twist in on themselves, which gives each protein its distinctive shape. This is what allows proteins to have so many different uses in the body.

PROTEIN MOLECULE

SHORT PEPTIDE CHAIN

AMINO ACIDS

Bond between two amino acids

Free amino acids, with all peptide bonds digested away

Protein
Proteins are giant, complex molecules made of many amino acids connected in a chain, which often folds into a compact shape.

Protein fragment
Shorter chains of amino acids are called peptides. They form when protein is digested, but the body also makes them for many purposes.

Protein components
Amino acids are small molecules made mainly of carbon, oxygen, hydrogen, and nitrogen. There are 21 types in the human body.

Why are certain amino acids "essential"?

At some point in our evolutionary history, we lost the ability to make nine of the amino acids our body needs. This means we must consume these "essential" amino acids in our food. Proteins containing an abundance of all nine of them are called "complete." Most animal products are complete proteins, but so are quinoa, tofu, and some nuts and seeds.

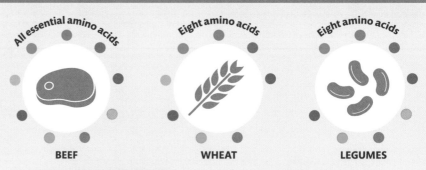

All essential amino acids

Eight amino acids

Eight amino acids

BEEF

WHEAT

LEGUMES

Complementary protein sources
Some foods such as beef have all the essential amino acids you need, but others do not. Wheat is low in the amino acid lysine but high in methionine, whereas legumes tend to have enough lysine but have lower levels of methionine. Combining these two sources of protein can provide all the essential amino acids you need.

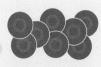

How we use protein

Dietary protein, once digested into amino acids, is involved in making a huge number of vital molecules, from DNA to hormones and neurotransmitters. Most amino acids, however, are assembled into new proteins. Some of these form the structures of our body, such as muscles. Many others act as enzymes—molecular catalysts that trigger and control the body's vital chemical processes.

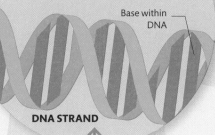

DNA

The body converts some amino acids into chemical "bases," which, once assembled in order, are the components of DNA that spell out its genetic code.

Base within DNA

DNA STRAND

PROTEIN IS PRESENT IN EVERY ONE OF OUR BODY'S TRILLIONS OF CELLS

Cell membrane proteins

A cell's membrane is its outside layer. Proteins embedded in it allow communication with the cell's surroundings—for example, by allowing molecules to pass across.

CELL   **PROTEIN**   **MEMBRANE**

Hormones

Our body uses hormones to send messages between different areas. Many hormones, including adrenaline, are proteins or peptides. They are made by glands and organs.

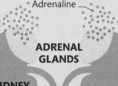

Adrenaline

ADRENAL GLANDS

KIDNEY

AMINO ACIDS

Muscle proteins

Muscles are made mainly of straight, long-chain proteins, which form muscle fibers. We need to eat proteins to build our muscles, and also to repair damage that our muscles suffer when we use them.

MUSCLE

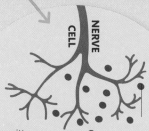

CELL   **NERVE**

Neurotransmitter

Neurotransmitters

Some amino acids are used to make neurotransmitters, which are molecules that carry messages between nerve cells throughout our brain and nervous system.

Fats

Fats are essential for our body's health. They provide energy, store excess calories for later use, and have a variety of other roles in the body, from forming cell membranes to making hormones.

What are fats?

Along with carbohydrates and proteins, fats make up one of the three main classes of macronutrients. Fats in food come as triglyceride molecules. These are made of carbon, hydrogen, and oxygen atoms arranged so the carbons form three long chains called fatty acids, joined by a short chain called glycerol. Each carbon can bond to other carbons with a single or a double bond; the number and position of these double bonds changes the type of fatty acid and its effect in the body. The fatty acids making up a fat molecule can be the same or different, giving a huge number of possible types of fat.

Fat molecule

This triglyceride, or fat molecule, has one of each type of fatty acid. The straight one is a saturated fatty acid, made only of single bonds. If a chain has one double bond, its shape is bent and it becomes a monounsaturated fatty acid. More double bonds make polyunsaturated chains with complex shapes.

Carbon atom

Glycerol holds the three fatty acids together until they are broken down in the body

GLYCEROL

Hydrogen atom

Oxygen atom

SATURATED FATTY ACID

MONOUNSATURATED FATTY ACID

POLYUNSATURATED FATTY ACID

Omega end— the carbons in the chain are counted from here

The third carbon from the omega end is the first with a double bond, making this polyunsaturated chain an omega-3 fatty acid

Bent fatty acids, such as oleic acid, found in olive oil, have one double bond

Stearic acid, found in meat, is fully saturated with hydrogen— there is no room for any more hydrogen atoms

Each carbon-carbon double bond excludes two hydrogens, which would otherwise bond with the carbons; since it is short of two hydrogens, it is not saturated with hydrogen—it is "unsaturated"

WILL FAT MAKE ME FAT?

Fat is highly calorific, so can contribute to weight gain, but compared to sweet foods, it makes you feel full for longer after eating, so a little fat may help stop you from snacking later!

Fats in the body

In addition to their use as energy stores, fats play many other crucial roles. Fats help us absorb and use some vitamins (see pp.32–33) and are involved in constructing and repairing nervous tissue. They maintain healthy skin and nails and are used to make hormones that control blood pressure, the immune system, growth, and blood clotting. Fats also form the basis of all the membranes in the body, surrounding each cell and the structures within it (see p.30).

Brain and nervous tissue are rich in fat—the brain is 60 percent fat and needs a steady supply

BRAIN

Steroid hormones, such as testosterone and estrogen, are made from fats

Fat is stored in subcutaneous (under-skin) deposits and also in deeper deposits around organs

FAT STORE

ESSENTIAL FATTY ACIDS

The human body can make most of the fats it needs from other fats or raw materials. Only two fatty acids are truly essential, because we can't make them—the omega-3 fatty acid, alpha-linolenic acid and the omega-6 fatty acid, linoleic acid. Both are found in nuts and seeds, especially linseed. Some other omega-3 oils are almost essential because the body isn't very good at making them (see fish, pp.78–79).

FLAX PLANT, SOURCE OF LINSEED

Fat or oil?

The word fat is often used to describe items that are solid at room temperature, such as butter and lard, while oils are liquid. As a rough rule, oils contain more unsaturated fatty acids. For many years, it was common to solidify vegetable oil by hydrogenating those fatty acids to make margarine—a supposedly healthy alternative to butter. The fats produced have since been found to be so unhealthy that margarine is now solidified by adding naturally solid palm oil instead.

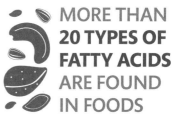

MORE THAN 20 TYPES OF FATTY ACIDS ARE FOUND IN FOODS

Oleic acid is bent

Oils
Unsaturated fats have at least some fatty acids with at least one double bond. They are found in vegetable oils, nuts, and seeds. The bends introduced by their double bonds give their molecules awkward shapes that do not pack together, so they stay liquid at room temperature.

OLIVE OIL

Stearic acid is straight

Fats
Saturated fats contain no double bonds, and their chains are straight. Their molecules pack tightly, so they solidify easily, forming solids at room temperature. They are found in animal products, such as butter and meat, and also in palm and coconut oils.

BUTTER

A trans fatty acid is often straightened, but with a kink

Hydrogenated fats
Trans fats are made by hydrogenating vegetable oils—a process that adds hydrogen to unsaturated double bonds, saturating them and straightening their chains. This forms solid fat, such as that in margarine. Trans fats have been linked to a range of health issues and are being phased out of many products.

MARGARINE

Cholesterol

A waxy, fatlike substance found in every cell of our bodies, cholesterol is made by the liver, and it is vital for normal body function. If too much builds up in the blood, however, problems such as heart disease can result. But the link between diet, cholesterol, and cardiovascular health is more complex than we thought.

CHOLESTEROL IN THE DIET

Humans can make all the cholesterol they need mainly in the liver, but they gain extra in the diet—either directly from foods such as eggs and meat, or, in some people, because saturated fats, trans fats, and some carbohydrates boost their liver's cholesterol production.

LIVER
67–75%

DIET
25–33%

Crucial chemical

Cholesterol is needed to manufacture some hormones, vitamin D, and bile acids, which form an ingredient of digestive juices (see pp.20–21). It also keeps our cell membranes—the thin layer surrounding every cell—flexible but firm. The liver regulates our cholesterol level, regardless of cholesterol in the diet, but a diet too rich in certain foods can make some people produce too much (see p.214).

Fluid inside cell is water-based

Small structures within cell are each enclosed by a membrane

Cell membrane is a thin, flexible outer envelope

CELL

Internal membranes are made the same way as the cell membrane

CELL MEMBRANE

MEMBRANE PROTEIN

Membrane made mainly of oily chemicals called phospholipids

Cholesterol stiffens the central part

Cell membrane
Each of our cells has a membrane formed of two layers of molecules. Cholesterol embedded within these layers prevents the membrane from becoming too fluid or too stiff, and gives it just the right permeability to allow the correct types and numbers of minerals and other substances to pass through. It also helps certain proteins attach to the cell—these are vital for communicating with the rest of the body.

THE HUMAN **BODY CONTAINS** AROUND **4OZ** (100G) OF **CHOLESTEROL**

Transporting fat

Fatty substances, including cholesterol, cannot mix with our water-based body fluids, so they need to be bundled into a water-friendly capsule to be transported around the body. Cholesterol is packaged into tiny capsules called lipoproteins, which come in two major types. The larger type, LDL, is referred to as "bad cholesterol," because its function is to deliver cholesterol to the blood, where excess can build up. HDL, or "good cholesterol," takes cholesterol out of the blood.

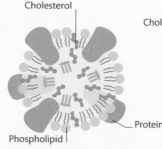

High-density lipoprotein (HDL)
HDL particles are dense, because they contain more protein and less cholesterol and other fatty parts.

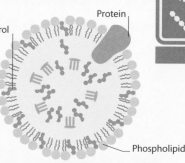

Low-density lipoprotein (LDL)
These larger particles contain more cholesterol, and a smaller proportion of their weight is protein.

The cholesterol cycle

Cholesterol cycles between the liver and the blood, performing vital functions. The process relies on a balance between the two lipoproteins—HDL and LDL. If you have more LDL than HDL circulating, plaques can build up in arteries, which can raise blood pressure and lead to heart disease (see pp.212–15). High LDL levels can be due to diet, obesity, or genes.

Bad cholesterol
Increased LDL in the blood can cause cholesterol-filled plaques (atheromas) to build up, narrowing the arteries and increasing blood pressure. If the plaque ruptures, blood clots can form, cutting off blood supply.

BLOOD VESSEL

PLAQUE

PLAQUE

HDL removes cholesterol from plaque

LDL adds cholesterol to plaque

LIVER

Liver converts excess cholesterol into bile acids and recycles or excretes them

Liver removes cholesterol from body in the form of bile salts

Good cholesterol
HDL particles transport excess cholesterol from the cells, blood, and plaques back to the liver. High HDL levels mean that more cholesterol is removed, reducing plaque formation.

HOW DO STATINS WORK?

Statin drugs lower cholesterol by slowing the liver's cholesterol production. Statins have many drawbacks, however, such as impeding the body's ability to use cholesterol to make vitamin D.

Vitamins

A group of micronutrients found in different types of food, vitamins are essential for our body's growth, vitality, and general well-being. Most of us can get the majority of the vitamins we need from a healthy, balanced diet, but in some cases, supplements can be useful.

What are vitamins?

Vitamins are organic compounds that play an essential part in controlling our body's metabolic processes. Some, such as vitamin C and E, act as antioxidants, which are thought to benefit the body by neutralizing excess free radicals (see pp.111). We need only tiny amounts, but the lack of them can impair body function and lead to deficiency diseases. Vitamins are classified according to whether they dissolve in fats or water.

Vitamin discovery
In the 1800s, doctors realized that some diseases were caused not by germs, but by nutrient deficiencies. Animal experiments using different diets and supplements led to the discovery of these micronutrients.

Fat-soluble

Some of the vitamins our body needs dissolve in fat. This means they are mainly found in fatty foods, such as oily fish, eggs, and dairy foods, rather than fruit and vegetables. Fat-soluble vitamins aren't absorbed properly by the body if they are consumed without any fat, which means that supplements of these vitamins taken without the right food may be less effective.

THE LIVER CAN STORE ENOUGH **VITAMIN A** TO LAST THE BODY **2 YEARS**

Storage of vitamins

Our body can store fat-soluble vitamins in the liver, so we don't need to eat them every day. But because of this, if we take in too much, levels can build up in the body and become toxic. Water-soluble vitamins can't be stored and any excess is excreted in urine. This means we need to consume them more frequently.

Water-soluble vitamins ingested often

Liver stockpile
Fat-soluble vitamins are stored in the same cells that store fat, mainly in the liver but also elsewhere in the body.

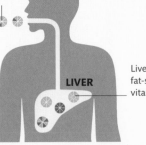

LIVER

Liver stores fat-soluble vitamins

Vitamin A
Needed for vision, growth, and development. Lack of vitamin A can lead to poor vision or blindness, especially in children.

Vitamin D
Aids uptake of some minerals. Low levels can lead to calcium deficiency and poor bone health, including rickets in children.

Vitamin E
An antioxidant. Protects cell membranes, maintaining healthy skin and eyes, and strengthens the immune system.

Vitamin K
Needed to make blood-clotting agents. Low consumption can lead to disorders in blood clotting, bleeding, and bruising.

WHERE IS VITAMIN F?

The gaps in the vitamin alphabet are left by substances once thought to be vitamins, but later reclassified. Some were found not to be vital. Vitamin F, though essential, was found to be a pair of fatty acids that were better classified as fats instead of vitamins.

KEY

Meat	Chickpeas
Poultry	Leafy greens
Liver	Broccoli
Fish	Avocado
Oily fish	Tomatoes
Tuna	Bananas
Eggs	Oranges
Egg yolk	Strawberries
Milk	Nuts
Rice	Peanuts
Whole-wheat bread	Olive oil

Water-soluble

Water-soluble vitamins are found in a wide variety of foods, including fruit, vegetables, and protein-rich foods. Because they dissolve in water, these vitamins can easily be lost in food preparation, for example, through the boiling of vegetables. The B vitamins, together called the vitamin B complex, are often grouped in supplements and are sometimes found in the same foods.

Vitamin B1
Helps generate energy and ensures muscles and nerves function well. Low levels may cause headaches and irritability.

Vitamin B2
Important for metabolism and healthy skin, eyes, and nervous system. Deficiency produces weakness and anemia.

Vitamin B3
Maintains the nervous system and brain, the cardiovascular system and blood, skin, and metabolism.

Vitamin B5
Important for metabolism and in the production of neurotransmitters, hormones, and hemoglobin.

Vitamin B6
Involved in nerve function, metabolism, and making antibodies and haemoglobin. Deficiency can affect mental health.

Vitamin B7
Biotin. Needed for healthy bones and hair, and fat metabolism. Lack of B7 can cause dermatitis, muscle pain, and tongue swelling.

Vitamin B9
Folic acid. Vital for healthy infant development. Deficiency in an expectant mother increases the risk of spina bifida in her baby.

Vitamin B12
Involved in metabolism and making red blood cells. B12 deficiency can lead to a condition called pernicious anemia.

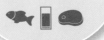

Vitamin C
An antioxidant. Helps the growth and repair of various tissues throughout the body. Deficiency can lead to poor wound healing.

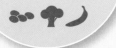

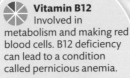

Minerals

Like vitamins, we need minerals to function properly. Our bodies require seven "macrominerals" in relatively large amounts, and only minute levels of other "trace minerals." Minerals occur naturally in certain foods, so a balanced diet should provide sufficient mineral intake but supplements may be necessary in cases of deficiency.

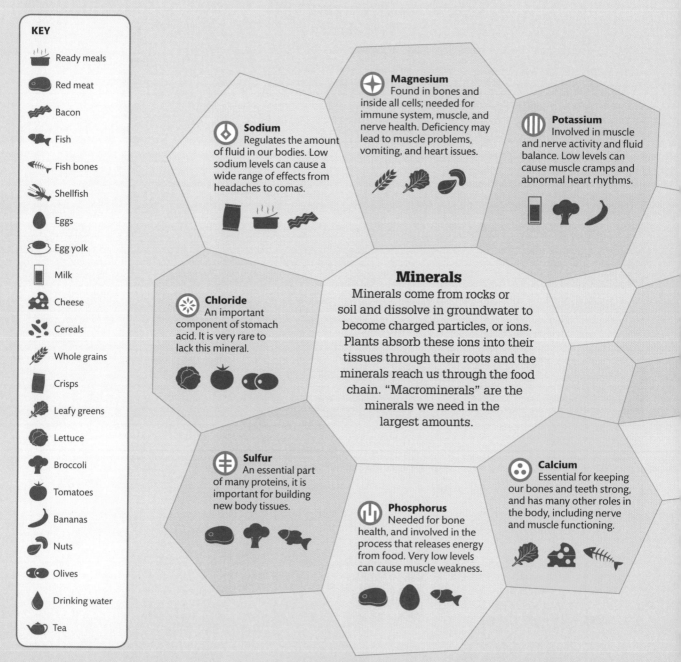

KEY

Ready meals

Red meat

Bacon

Fish

Fish bones

Shellfish

Eggs

Egg yolk

Milk

Cheese

Cereals

Whole grains

Crisps

Leafy greens

Lettuce

Broccoli

Tomatoes

Bananas

Nuts

Olives

Drinking water

Tea

Magnesium
Found in bones and inside all cells; needed for immune system, muscle, and nerve health. Deficiency may lead to muscle problems, vomiting, and heart issues.

Sodium
Regulates the amount of fluid in our bodies. Low sodium levels can cause a wide range of effects from headaches to comas.

Potassium
Involved in muscle and nerve activity and fluid balance. Low levels can cause muscle cramps and abnormal heart rhythms.

Minerals
Minerals come from rocks or soil and dissolve in groundwater to become charged particles, or ions. Plants absorb these ions into their tissues through their roots and the minerals reach us through the food chain. "Macrominerals" are the minerals we need in the largest amounts.

Chloride
An important component of stomach acid. It is very rare to lack this mineral.

Sulfur
An essential part of many proteins, it is important for building new body tissues.

Phosphorus
Needed for bone health, and involved in the process that releases energy from food. Very low levels can cause muscle weakness.

Calcium
Essential for keeping our bones and teeth strong, and has many other roles in the body, including nerve and muscle functioning.

MINERAL DEFICIENCIES

Deficiencies in mineral intake can cause various health problems. For example, long-term calcium deficiency can lead to reduced bone density and osteoporosis; lack of iron may cause anemia, with weakness and fatigue; and the early symptoms of magnesium deficiency include nausea. For each of these, dietary changes or supplement use may be recommended.

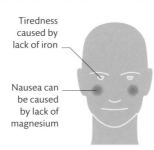

Tiredness caused by lack of iron

Nausea can be caused by lack of magnesium

YOU CAN GET ALL THE **SELENIUM** YOU NEED **EACH DAY** FROM JUST ONE OR TWO **BRAZIL NUTS**

Copper
Needed by many enzymes and for iron metabolism. Although very rare, deficiency can cause anemia.

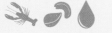

Fluoride
Helps keep our bones and teeth strong. Lack of fluoride may lead to an increase in tooth decay.

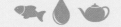

Manganese, chromium, molybdenum, nickel, silicon, vanadium, cobalt
Also needed in miniscule amounts.

Trace minerals

Minerals needed in only tiny amounts by the body are called trace minerals. Despite the fact that we need so little of them, trace minerals are no less important than macrominerals. They include iron—a mineral often deficient in our diets.

Iodine
Important for normal thyroid function. Deficiency can lead to developmental problems and physical or learning disabilities.

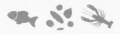

Selenium
An antioxidant that helps protect our cells from stress. People dependent on produce grown in selenium-poor soil risk deficiency.

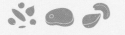

Iron
Allows red blood cells to carry oxygen, and helps with energy production. Iron deficiency anemia is quite common.

Zinc
Forms part of many enzymes without which our bodies can't function normally. Deficiency is linked to diarrhea and pneumonia.

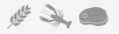

Water

Up to 60 percent of our body weight is water and it is needed to keep our organs functioning. While we can live without food for several weeks, without water, death occurs in days, showing just how important it is.

Hydration

Getting enough water keeps our skin plump and elastic, helps regulate body temperature, and ensures our kidneys filter out waste. If the water concentration in the blood is too high or too low, the body compensates by moving water into or out of our cells; both can be damaging.

A hydrated brain
Water is vital for the brain to function. The balance between water and the substances dissolved in it is important for neurons to transmit signals effectively.

Moist eyes
To keep the eyes clean and comfortable, they are continually moistened with tears, the major component of which is water.

Blood flows easily
Blood fluid (plasma) is 92 percent water. The liquid allows oxygen-carrying red blood cells, infection-fighting white blood cells, and other vital components to flow easily to where they are needed.

CAN YOU DRINK TOO MUCH WATER?

If you drink too much too quickly, cells swell as water rushes in. Swollen brain cells cause headaches, dizziness, and confusion. In severe cases, water poisoning can lead to death.

Dehydration

If more water is lost than taken in, symptoms of light-headedness and tiredness can start within hours. Thirst is the body trying to correct the problem before it becomes severe. In extreme cases, dehydration causes fits, brain damage, and death.

Decreased attention and memory
If you become dehydrated, brain tissues shrink, and it takes more effort to carry out simple tasks. Attention, mood, memory, and reaction time can be affected, and you may even become more sensitive to pain.

Dry eyes
Dehydration slows tear production which can leave the eyes feeling dry, irritated, and gritty.

Low blood pressure
If dehydration is severe, the water content of your blood falls. Blood becomes thick and viscous, making it difficult for your heart to pump it around the body. This can lead to low blood pressure, dizziness, and fainting.

DRINKING WATER

BRAIN

EYE

EYE

BLOOD VESSEL

HOW MUCH DO I NEED?

The amount of water you need varies depending on the climate and what you spend your time doing. Eight glasses per day (2–3 quarts/liters) is frequently advised for moderately active people in temperate climates, but this includes fluid from other drinks and food. For young, healthy people, the best thing to do is to listen to your body and drink when you feel thirsty! However, elderly people can become dehydrated without feeling thirsty, and so must watch their water intake.

WATER

SOUP

JUICE

THE BODY STARTS
TO ABSORB
WATER AS SOON
AS 5 MINUTES
AFTER DRINKING

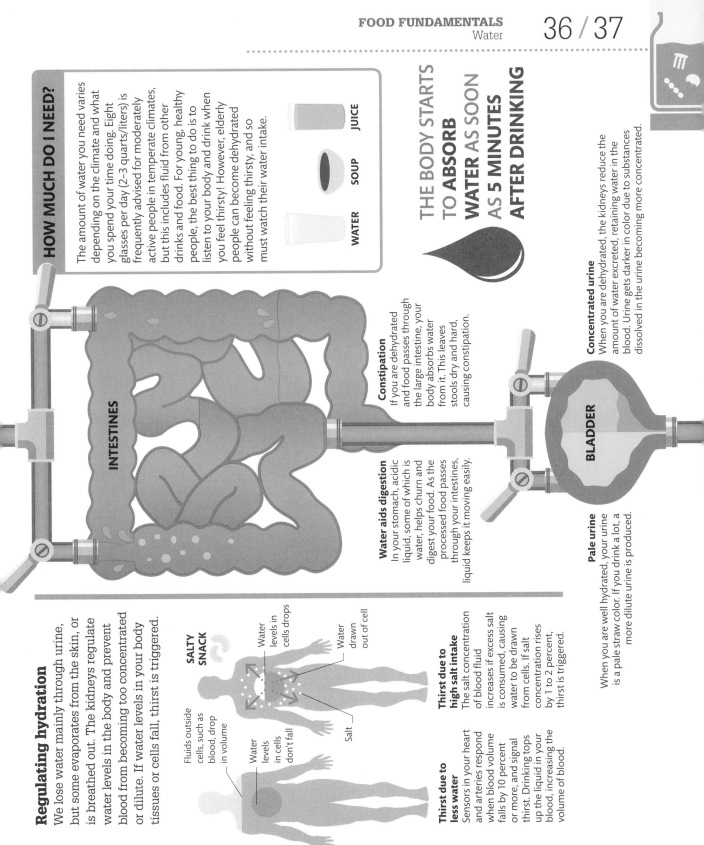

Concentrated urine
When you are dehydrated, the kidneys reduce the amount of water excreted, retaining water in the blood. Urine gets darker in color due to substances dissolved in the urine becoming more concentrated.

INTESTINES

Constipation
If you are dehydrated and food passes through the large intestine, your body absorbs water from it. This leaves stools dry and hard, causing constipation.

Water aids digestion
In your stomach, acidic liquid, some of which is water, helps churn and digest your food. As the processed food passes through your intestines, liquid keeps it moving easily.

BLADDER

Pale urine
When you are well hydrated, your urine is a pale straw color. If you drink a lot, a more dilute urine is produced.

Regulating hydration

We lose water mainly through urine, but some evaporates from the skin, or is breathed out. The kidneys regulate water levels in the body and prevent blood from becoming too concentrated or dilute. If water levels in your body tissues or cells fall, thirst is triggered.

SALTY
SNACK

Water levels in cells drops

Water drawn out of cell

Fluids outside cells, such as blood, drop in volume

Water levels in cells don't fall

Salt

Thirst due to high salt intake
The salt concentration of blood fluid increases if excess salt is consumed, causing water to be drawn from cells. If salt concentration rises by 1 to 2 percent, thirst is triggered.

Thirst due to less water
Sensors in your heart and arteries respond when blood volume falls by 10 percent or more, and signal thirst. Drinking tops up the liquid in your blood, increasing the volume of blood.

Convenience foods

With busy lives, many of us turn to ready-made convenience foods. They are quick, easy, and tasty, but not usually the healthiest option. So why are convenience foods bad for us? And are there healthier types we can choose?

What are convenience foods?

Convenience foods are preprepared or processed and include prepackaged meals, cake mixes, snack foods, preprepared fruit and vegetables, frozen ingredients, and canned food. Companies that make and sell convenience foods usually focus on taste and shelf-life rather than on nutritional value. By exploiting our evolved affinity for sweetness and our desire for quick, easy, tasty, high-calorie food, they ensure products sell in high quantities.

WHAT MAKES JUNK FOOD SO MOREISH?

Most junk food carefully balances sweetness, salt, and fat – designed to give our brains maximum pleasure and keep us coming back for more.

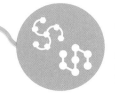

50 MILLION AMERICANS ARE SERVED AT FAST FOOD RESTAURANTS EVERY DAY

High in refined carbs
The flour used is refined and processed, removing most of the fiber and micronutrients, but leaving the high calorie count.

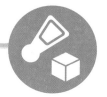

High in fat
In addition to the oil in the noodles themselves, the noodles are often fried to dry them, making them high in fat.

High in salt and sugar
Lots of salt and sugar is added to make the bland noodles tasty. This can often exceed our daily recommended amounts.

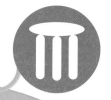

Instant noodles
Just adding water to instant noodles provides a tasty, filling snack. However, they contain few beneficial nutrients and have been linked to increased risk of obesity, diabetes, heart disease, and strokes.

Low in fiber and protein
There is little fiber or protein in instant noodles, so despite their high calorie count, they won't satisfy you for long.

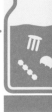

Modern eating habits

Ready-made food is all around us, from sandwich shops to takeout to fancy restaurants, and this affects the way we eat. When working hours are long and time for food preparation and cooking is short, the appeal of instant, fast food rises. However, there can be a trade-off between convenience foods and health.

Influence of takeouts

A study has shown that people who are exposed to more takeouts at home, near work, or on their route between the two, eat more takeouts and are more likely to have a higher body mass index.

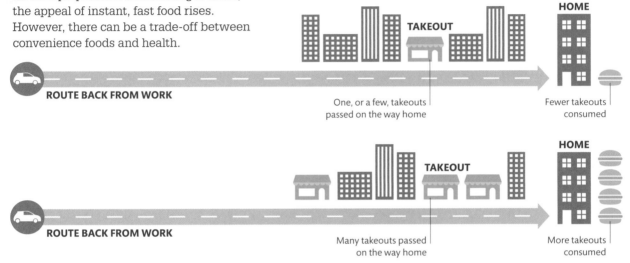

ROUTE BACK FROM WORK

TAKEOUT

HOME

One, or a few, takeouts passed on the way home

Fewer takeouts consumed

ROUTE BACK FROM WORK

TAKEOUT

HOME

Many takeouts passed on the way home

More takeouts consumed

History of convenience foods

Convenience food is not new. Food can be preserved in many ways; frozen, canned, dehydrated, or by using additives. For some, this has improved nutrition, but for others it has made it worse.

GOOD CONVENIENCE FOODS

Not all convenience foods are unhealthy. Canned and frozen fruit and vegetables, or ready-made soups, are good sources of nutrients and fiber—sometimes containing more vitamins and phytochemicals than their fresh ingredients (cooking tomatoes releases lycopene). But sugar and salt are often added to improve the taste and preserve the soup for longer.

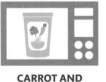

CARROT AND CILANTRO SOUP

1810 Cans first used to preserve food for sailors on long voyages.

1930s Flash-freezing invented, allowing foods to be frozen en masse and sold to the public.

Late 1960s Freezers and frozen prepared meals become mainstream.

1970s Number of women in work increases, leading to a rise in the popularity of prepared meals.

1800

2000

1894 Corn flakes invented by Dr. John Harvey Kellogg. This was one of the first ready-to-eat cereals to be mass produced.

1953–54 The first ready-to-eat meals sold, in a metal tray that could be heated in an oven.

1967 Countertop microwave ovens introduced—but it would be 20 years before they were common in the home.

1979 The first chilled ready meal, launched by a supermarket in the UK.

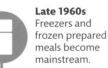

Whole foods

First introduced in the 1940s, the whole foods movement is still increasing in popularity. Its focus on eating unprocessed food is likely to increase fiber and micronutrient intake, providing health benefits, but it can be limiting if taken to the extreme.

ARE WHOLE FOODS THE SAME AS ORGANIC?

Organic foods are crops grown with natural fertilizers or pesticides or animals reared on organic feed—they are a type of whole food. But, whole foods are not always organic.

All natural
Raspberries have the highest amount of omega-3 fatty acids in any raw fruit. Also, 3½ oz (100 g) of raspberries contains more than one-quarter of your daily needs of vitamin C.

Nutrients and minerals
A whole-food diet is likely to contain a good variety of vitamins and minerals. Raspberries are particularly high in vitamins C, K, and manganese.

Antioxidants
Whole foods such as raspberries are rich in potentially beneficial antioxidants (see pp.108–09). However, sometimes these can be added artificially to foods.

What are whole foods?

Whole foods are the opposite of processed foods—they are in their natural form, or processed as little as possible. They might include fresh fruit, vegetables, meat, fish, whole grains, nuts, and seeds. Some proponents argue whole foods must also be organic, but there is little evidence for the health benefit of organic foods.

Fiber
Plant foods that are less processed tend to contain more fiber. High fiber intake benefits weight loss and protects against certain diseases (see pp.198–99).

Good fats
Whole foods don't contain the damaging trans fats common in processed products and many are high in beneficial unsaturated fats.

Fewer additives
Whole foods are "as nature intended," without added flavorings or preservatives. However, this means they often don't have as long a shelf life as processed versions.

Necessary processing

Not all foods are safe to eat without some degree of processing. Some, especially meats, need to be prepared or cooked to destroy toxins or kill dangerous bacteria. Others, such as tomatoes, become more nutritious when cooked (see p.55). Whole-food proponents advise doing this processing yourself, and keeping it to a minimum. However, even a little chopping can affect the nutrition of foods.

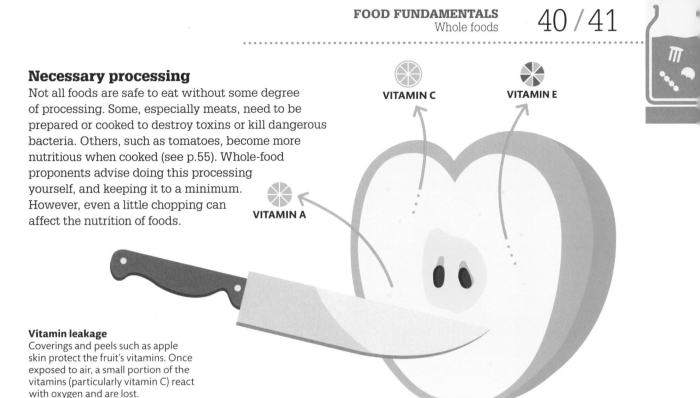

VITAMIN C

VITAMIN E

VITAMIN A

Vitamin leakage
Coverings and peels such as apple skin protect the fruit's vitamins. Once exposed to air, a small portion of the vitamins (particularly vitamin C) react with oxygen and are lost.

Whole-foods movement

Farmers and consumers in Europe in the 1920s started to seek out foods grown without insecticides. These natural foods were coined "whole foods" by Frank Newman Turner, a British organic farmer, in 1946. The "clean-eating" diet in the developed world has seen whole foods rise in popularity.

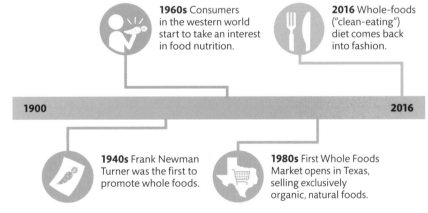

1960s Consumers in the western world start to take an interest in food nutrition.

2016 Whole-foods ("clean-eating") diet comes back into fashion.

1900

2016

1940s Frank Newman Turner was the first to promote whole foods.

1980s First Whole Foods Market opens in Texas, selling exclusively organic, natural foods.

DRAWBACKS OF WHOLE FOODS

A strict whole-food diet can be expensive and time-consuming to prepare, and difficult to stick to at social occasions or restaurants. It can also take a while to get accustomed to the taste of fresh food that contains less sugar and salt, if you are used to processed food.

PREP TIME

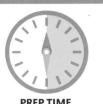

5 OZ
(150 G)
OF **STRAWBERRIES**
PROVIDES YOU WITH
ALL OF THE **VITAMIN C**
YOU NEED IN A DAY

Too much or too little?

Nutrients such as vitamins and minerals are good for us, but that does not mean that more is better. Regularly consuming too much of some vitamins, such as vitamin A, can be as dangerous as not getting enough of them.

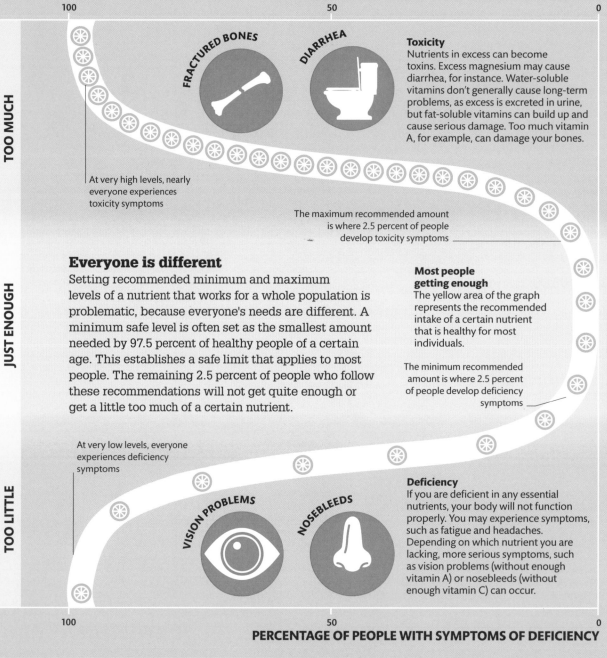

PERCENTAGE OF PEOPLE WITH SYMPTOMS OF TOXICITY

100   50   0

TOO MUCH

FRACTURED BONES

DIARRHEA

Toxicity
Nutrients in excess can become toxins. Excess magnesium may cause diarrhea, for instance. Water-soluble vitamins don't generally cause long-term problems, as excess is excreted in urine, but fat-soluble vitamins can build up and cause serious damage. Too much vitamin A, for example, can damage your bones.

At very high levels, nearly everyone experiences toxicity symptoms

The maximum recommended amount is where 2.5 percent of people develop toxicity symptoms

Everyone is different

Setting recommended minimum and maximum levels of a nutrient that works for a whole population is problematic, because everyone's needs are different. A minimum safe level is often set as the smallest amount needed by 97.5 percent of healthy people of a certain age. This establishes a safe limit that applies to most people. The remaining 2.5 percent of people who follow these recommendations will not get quite enough or get a little too much of a certain nutrient.

JUST ENOUGH

Most people getting enough
The yellow area of the graph represents the recommended intake of a certain nutrient that is healthy for most individuals.

The minimum recommended amount is where 2.5 percent of people develop deficiency symptoms

AMOUNT OF NUTRIENT IN THE DIET

At very low levels, everyone experiences deficiency symptoms

TOO LITTLE

VISION PROBLEMS

NOSEBLEEDS

Deficiency
If you are deficient in any essential nutrients, your body will not function properly. You may experience symptoms, such as fatigue and headaches. Depending on which nutrient you are lacking, more serious symptoms, such as vision problems (without enough vitamin A) or nosebleeds (without enough vitamin C) can occur.

100   50   0

PERCENTAGE OF PEOPLE WITH SYMPTOMS OF DEFICIENCY

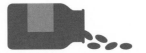

Food labeling

To make things simple, most governments turn your recommended daily need into a single guideline amount for use on packaging. Some amounts are minimum amounts of essential nutrients, such as minerals. Others are not targets, but guides to upper limits for potentially unhealthy foods, such as salt, to encourage a healthy diet. Some countries highlight where nutrients in food are likely to exceed your daily need if eaten in excess.

THE DAILY NEEDS OF **CHILDREN** AND **ELDERLY PEOPLE** ARE **NOT THE SAME** AS THOSE FOR **ADULTS**

Nutrition claims

Some foods make bold claims on the packaging about what they contain (or do not contain) and the health benefits they might have. But these claims are tightly regulated, and the food must fit certain guidelines to make a specific claim. The regulations differ slightly between countries, but some European Union (EU) examples are given below.

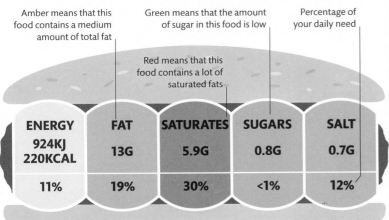

Amber means that this food contains a medium amount of total fat

Green means that the amount of sugar in this food is low

Percentage of your daily need

Red means that this food contains a lot of saturated fats

ENERGY 924KJ 220KCAL	FAT 13G	SATURATES 5.9G	SUGARS 0.8G	SALT 0.7G
11%	19%	30%	<1%	12%

EACH GRILLED BURGER (94G) CONTAINS:

Traffic light system
The UK's traffic light system was developed by the Food Standards Authority and aims to make choosing healthy food easier (in turn avoiding long-term health effects). Exactly what "high" or "low" means depends on the food or drink and portion size, but more green on a label suggests a healthier food.

NUTRITION FACTS

Serving size 1 cup (228g)
Servings per container 2

Calories 250
Calories from Fat 110

% DAILY VALUE

Total Fat *12g*	**18%**
Saturated Fat *3g*	**15%**
Trans Fat *3g*	
Cholesterol *30mg*	**10%**
Sodium *470mg*	**20%**
Total Carbohydrate *31g*	**10%**
Dietary Fiber *0g*	**0%**
Sugars *5g*	
Protein *5g*	
Vitamin A	**4%**
Vitamin C	**2%**
Calcium	**20%**
Iron	**4%**

MACARONI AND CHEESE

Labeling is not color coded

Recommended daily values for nutrients such as fat and salt are maximums, not targets

Percentages of daily need
Many countries, including the US, have food labels that show quantities of each nutrient as a percentage of your daily need. They also show the total calories per serving. Quantities of certain micronutrients (such as iron) must also be shown.

CLAIM	RULING
Sugar-free	If a food is labeled as sugar-free, it must contain less than 1 percent sugar by weight.
Low-fat	Low-fat foods must contain less than 3 percent fat by weight.
High in fiber	If they claim to be high in fiber, foods must have at least 6 percent fiber by weight.
Source of vitamin D	A food can be called a source of vitamin D if it provides 15 percent of your daily need per 3½oz (100g).
Reduced-fat	Reduced-fat products must contain 30 percent less fat than a similar product. This does not mean it is necessarily low in fat compared to other foods!

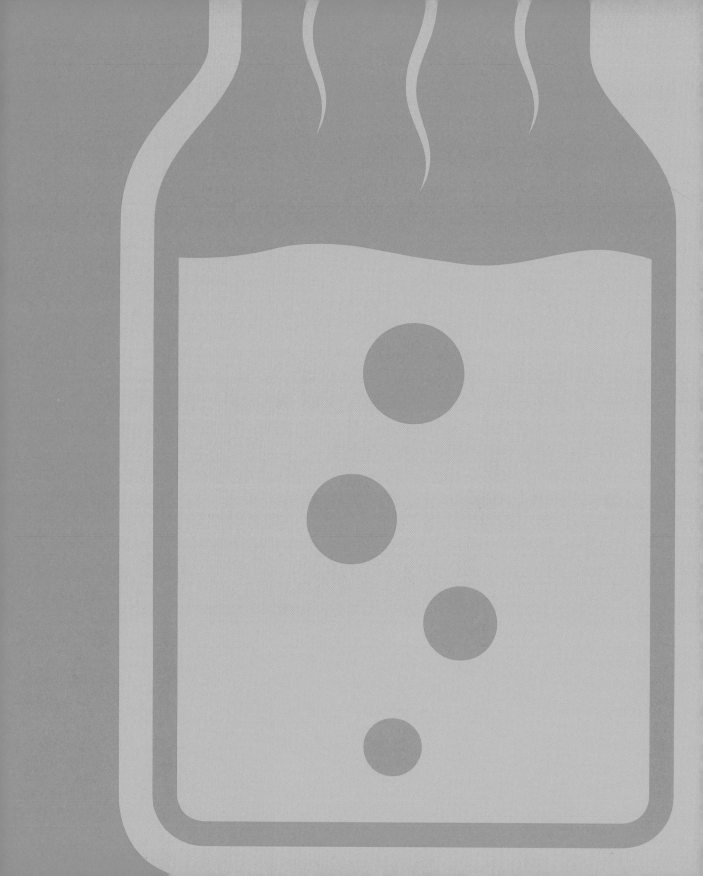

STORING AND COOKING

How fresh is fresh?

Freshness has become an important concept in evaluating the quality and desirability of food. But what does "fresh" actually mean? What are the factors influencing freshness and how do food labels help us to assess the freshness of food?

SUNLIGHT

WRINKLING

Post-harvest, a combination of a loss of water supply, sunlight, and wind can cause wrinkling

BRUISING

Decreasing freshness

While some fruit and vegetables only reach peak ripeness or desirability after harvesting, most foods will start to lose flavor and nutritional value from the moment they are harvested or butchered. This is the point at which a number of processes that make foods spoil begin. These include the release of destructive enzymes; the natural breakdown processes, such as oxidation, that degrade nutrients; and the growth of microbes as defense mechanisms in the food's cells start to stall. In some fruit and vegetables, natural metabolic and physiological processes may actually accelerate after harvesting.

From ripe to rotten
A complex combination of physical and organic processes operates on a piece of fruit to affect its freshness and determine the rate at which it declines.

SHOULD I FREEZE FOOD AS SOON AS I BUY IT?

One common myth is that food must be frozen on the day of purchase. In fact, you can freeze food at any time up to the use-by date on the label.

Time limit for freshness?

Some plant foods can remain fresh for remarkably long periods, if stored correctly. Potatoes can stay fresh for three months in a cool, dark place. Pears and apples can be stored for up to a year in special atmospherically controlled facilities.

Food's journey
Produce such as fruit and vegetables grown in the southern hemisphere will pass through many stages on its journey to markets in the US.

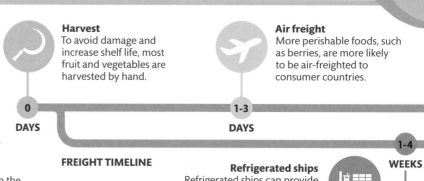

Harvest
To avoid damage and increase shelf life, most fruit and vegetables are harvested by hand.

Air freight
More perishable foods, such as berries, are more likely to be air-freighted to consumer countries.

0 DAYS

1-3 DAYS

1-4 WEEKS

FREIGHT TIMELINE

Refrigerated ships
Refrigerated ships can provide highly controlled temperatures to keep produce as fresh as possible.

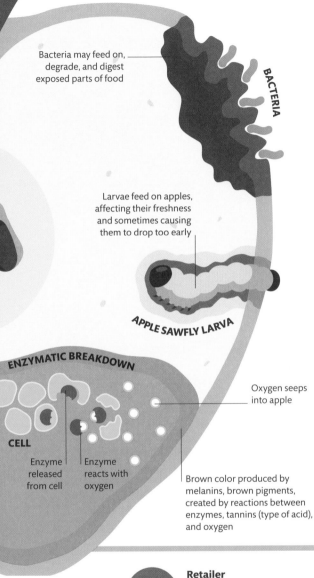

Bacteria may feed on, degrade, and digest exposed parts of food

BACTERIA

Larvae feed on apples, affecting their freshness and sometimes causing them to drop too early

APPLE SAWFLY LARVA

ENZYMATIC BREAKDOWN

CELL

Enzyme released from cell

Enzyme reacts with oxygen

Oxygen seeps into apple

Brown color produced by melanins, brown pigments, created by reactions between enzymes, tannins (type of acid), and oxygen

Loss of nutrients

Nutrients are lost at an accelerating rate as a food's freshness declines. They are particularly affected by oxidation, heat, sunlight, dehydration, and enzymes. Vitamin C can be extremely vulnerable to degradation over time, although this varies between foods. Chilling and freezing are especially helpful in delaying or preventing nutrient loss.

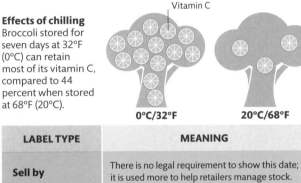

Vitamin C

Effects of chilling
Broccoli stored for seven days at 32°F (0°C) can retain most of its vitamin C, compared to 44 percent when stored at 68°F (20°C).

0°C/32°F   20°C/68°F

LABEL TYPE	MEANING
Sell by	There is no legal requirement to show this date; it is used more to help retailers manage stock.
Display until	Similar to "Sell by," this label is used by retailers to help manage their stock levels.
Best before	The "Best before" date refers to food quality, rather than safety.
Use by	In some countries, this label has legal force. Food is not safe for use after this date.

Types of date labels
Date labels on food are supposed to inform the consumer, but can be confusing.

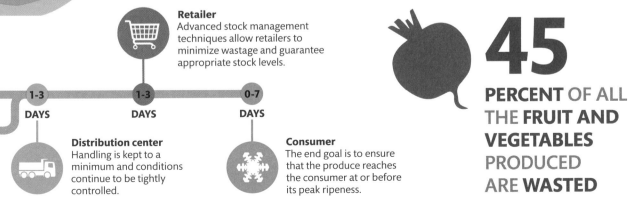

Retailer
Advanced stock management techniques allow retailers to minimize wastage and guarantee appropriate stock levels.

1-3 DAYS

1-3 DAYS

0-7 DAYS

Distribution center
Handling is kept to a minimum and conditions continue to be tightly controlled.

Consumer
The end goal is to ensure that the produce reaches the consumer at or before its peak ripeness.

45
PERCENT OF ALL THE **FRUIT AND VEGETABLES** PRODUCED ARE **WASTED**

Preservation

The very things that make food nutritious also make it vulnerable to contamination and degradation, so preserving food has always been a key concern of food science and cultures since ancient times.

SPICES AND HERBS WERE USED AS PRESERVATIVES BY **ANCIENT CIVILIZATIONS**

Types of preservation

Natural processes, including microbial growth, oxidation, heat and light, and the action of enzymes can contaminate foods or degrade them by breaking down their key components. The rate of the biochemical reactions that drive these processes depends on favorable conditions, so altering these in different ways can help to preserve foods. Some preservation methods, such as drying, have been used for tens of thousands of years. Artificial chemical preservatives are common today—but their implications for our health remain uncertain.

 Chilling and freezing
Reducing temperature decreases the rate of biochemical reactions. Freezing suspends them.

 Drying
Water is necessary for most biochemical activity, so removing moisture can prevent microbial growth.

 Salting
Increasing the concentration of salts in food kills most microbes by dehydrating them.

 Pickling
Making food more acidic can kill many microbes but will also affect the food's taste and characteristics.

 Chemical
Artificial preservative chemicals, such as nitrates, are commonly used in foods such as meats (see pp.74–75).

 Canning
In addition to sealing food, canning also involves extreme heat treatment to kill off any microbes.

 Smoking
Smoking infuses foods with a variety of antimicrobial, antioxidant, and acidifying compounds.

 Storing
Storing food in cool, dark conditions prolongs its shelf life, as will reducing exposure to oxygen and ambient microbes.

How nutrients degrade

Some categories of nutrients, such as vitamins and antioxidants, are reactive since they are composed of fragile molecules. Such vulnerable molecules will degrade naturally over time, a process that speeds up greatly with heat, physical damage, exposure to sunlight, and exposure to oxygen – the last of which generates destructive free radicals (see p.111). Different nutrients are more sensitive to certain threats than others.

NUTRIENT	LEVEL OF STABILITY	NUTRIENT	LEVEL OF STABILITY
Proteins, carbohydrates	Relatively stable	Vitamin B1 (thiamine)	Highly unstable; sensitive to air, light, and heat
Fat	Can become rancid (see p.74), particularly at higher temperatures	Vitamin B2 (riboflavin)	Sensitive to light and heat
Vitamin A	Sensitive to air, light, and heat	Vitamins B3 (niacin), B7 (biotin)	Relatively stable
Vitamin C	Highly unstable; sensitive to air, light, and heat	Vitamin B9 (folic acid)	Highly unstable; sensitive to air, light, and heat
Vitamin D	Somewhat sensitive to air, light, and heat	Carotenes	Sensitive to air, light, and heat

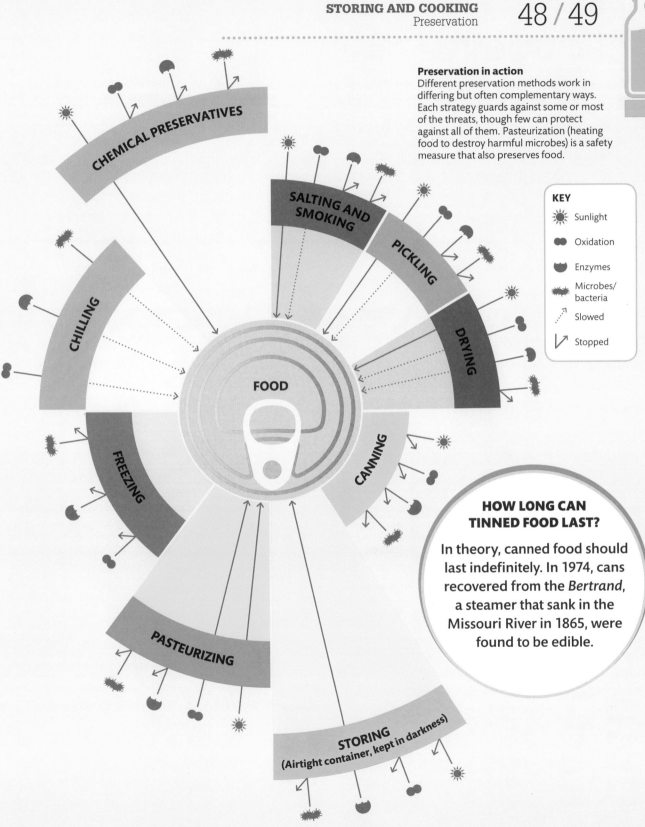

Preservation in action
Different preservation methods work in differing but often complementary ways. Each strategy guards against some or most of the threats, though few can protect against all of them. Pasteurization (heating food to destroy harmful microbes) is a safety measure that also preserves food.

KEY
- ☀ Sunlight
- ● Oxidation
- ▬ Enzymes
- ✺ Microbes/ bacteria
- ⇢ Slowed
- ↗ Stopped

CHEMICAL PRESERVATIVES

SALTING AND SMOKING

PICKLING

DRYING

CHILLING

FOOD

CANNING

FREEZING

PASTEURIZING

STORING
(Airtight container, kept in darkness)

HOW LONG CAN TINNED FOOD LAST?

In theory, canned food should last indefinitely. In 1974, cans recovered from the *Bertrand*, a steamer that sank in the Missouri River in 1865, were found to be edible.

Chilling and freezing

By extending the life of perishable foods—making it possible to store them for long periods and transport them across great distances—refrigeration and freezing have transformed the food economy and broadened our diets.

Freezing suitability

Vegetables that hold water, such as lettuce and cabbage, get mushy when thawed. When the water in their cells freezes, ice crystals puncture the cell walls, breaking the food's structure. Meat and fish can be frozen because their cells are flexible.

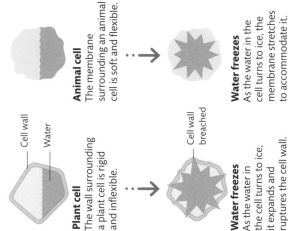

Plant cell
The wall surrounding a plant cell is rigid and inflexible.

Cell wall

Water

Water freezes
As the water in the cell turns to ice, it expands and ruptures the cell wall.

Cell wall breached

Animal cell
The membrane surrounding an animal cell is soft and flexible.

Water freezes
As the water in the cell turns to ice, the membrane stretches to accommodate it.

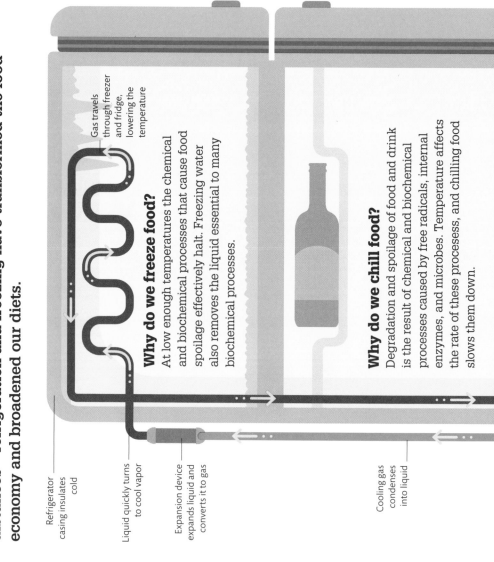

Refrigerator casing insulates cold

Liquid quickly turns to cool vapor

Expansion device expands liquid and converts it to gas

Gas travels through freezer and fridge, lowering the temperature

Cooling gas condenses into liquid

Why do we freeze food?

At low enough temperatures the chemical and biochemical processes that cause food spoilage effectively halt. Freezing water also removes the liquid essential to many biochemical processes.

Why do we chill food?

Degradation and spoilage of food and drink is the result of chemical and biochemical processes caused by free radicals, internal enzymes, and microbes. Temperature affects the rate of these processess, and chilling food slows them down.

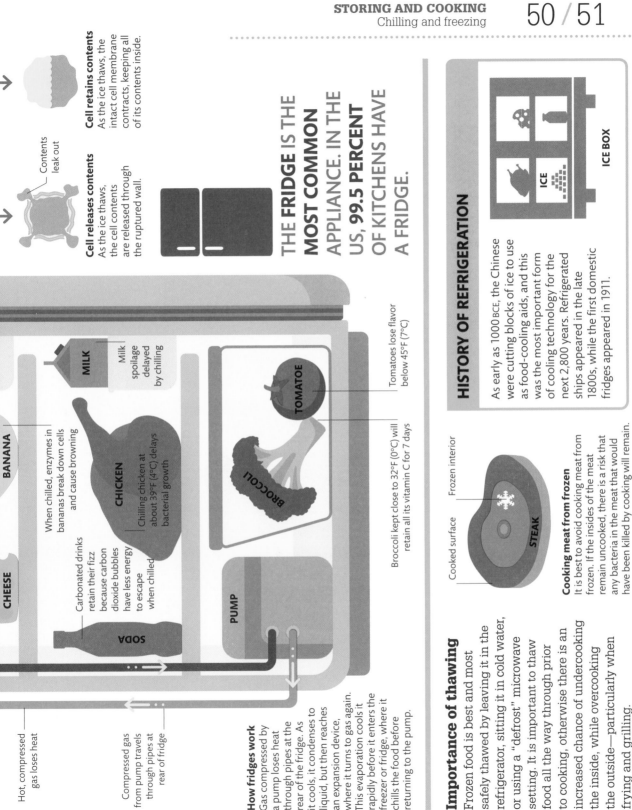

Cell retains contents
As the ice thaws, the intact cell membrane contracts, keeping all of its contents inside.

Contents leak out

Cell releases contents
As the ice thaws, the cell contents are released through the ruptured wall.

THE **FRIDGE** IS THE **MOST COMMON** APPLIANCE. IN THE US, **99.5 PERCENT** OF KITCHENS HAVE A FRIDGE.

ICE BOX

ICE

HISTORY OF REFRIGERATION

As early as 1000 BCE, the Chinese were cutting blocks of ice to use as food-cooling aids, and this was the most important form of cooling technology for the next 2,800 years. Refrigerated ships appeared in the late 1800s, while the first domestic fridges appeared in 1911.

CHEESE

BANANA

When chilled, enzymes in bananas break down cells and cause browning

Carbonated drinks retain their fizz because carbon dioxide bubbles have less energy to escape when chilled

CHICKEN
Chilling chicken at about 39°F (4°C) delays bacterial growth

MILK

Milk spoilage delayed by chilling

SODA

TOMATOE

Tomatoes lose flavor below 45°F (7°C)

BROCCOLI

Broccoli kept close to 32°F (0°C) will retain all its vitamin C for 7 days

PUMP

Cooked surface

Frozen interior

STEAK

Cooking meat from frozen
It is best to avoid cooking meat from frozen. If the insides of the meat remain uncooked, there is a risk that any bacteria in the meat that would have been killed by cooking will remain.

Hot, compressed gas loses heat

Compressed gas from pump travels through pipes at rear of fridge

How fridges work
Gas compressed by a pump loses heat through pipes at the rear of the fridge. As it cools, it condenses to liquid, but then reaches an expansion device, where it turns to gas again. This evaporation cools it rapidly before it enters the freezer or fridge, where it chills the food before returning to the pump.

Importance of thawing
Frozen food is best and most safely thawed by leaving it in the refrigerator, sitting it in cold water, or using a "defrost" microwave setting. It is important to thaw food all the way through prior to cooking, otherwise there is an increased chance of undercooking the inside, while overcooking the outside—particularly when frying and grilling.

Fermentation

Used across the globe throughout history, fermentation is a simple form of food preservation requiring no heat or artificial energy source. In the absence of oxygen, microbes can convert sugars into acids, alcohol, and gas.

Why do we ferment foods?

As microbes such as *Lactobacillus* thrive in an oxgen-free environment, their success suppresses the growth of spoilage microbes, generating preservative by-products and interesting flavors. Fermentation microbes are often the same as the ones found in our gut, so eating fermented food can be a good way to top up gut flora.

Fermented cabbage
Sauerkraut, originating from Europe, is one of the most popular preparations of fermented cabbage.

2 Teasing out the sugar
Salt helps to draw water and cell contents (including sugars) out of the plant cells, so that the fermenting microbes can get to work.

Water and sugars drawn out of cells by salt

WATER   SUGAR

1 Salted and soaked
Salt is applied as a brine, cutting off oxygen supply to competing microbes. The cabbage must be kept below the surface.

SALTY WATER

Salt

SHREDDED CABBAGE

IN THE 1700S FERMENTED CABBAGE WAS **USED BY SAILORS** TO COMBAT **VITAMIN C** DEFICIENCY AND **SCURVY**

Other foods that are fermented

In addition to helping to preserve foods, fermentation can leaven dough through generating gas, and produce browning reactions, adding color and flavor. Different methods of fermentation are used in breadmaking; alcoholic drinks and vinegar production; making yogurts and cheeses; pickling fruit and vegetables; curing meats; making soy and fish sauces; softening olives and removing their bitterness; and producing chocolate from cocoa beans.

Fermented milk
Milk has a very short shelf-life, but fermented dairy products can last for months. These range from yogurt and crème fraiche, fermented for just a few hours, to large cheeses prepared over many months.

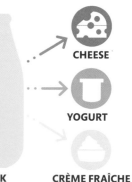

CHEESE

YOGURT

MILK

CRÈME FRAÎCHE

3 Fermentation
A succession of fermenting microbes consumes the sugars, generating a complex mixture of alcohols, acids, and flavor compounds. Fermentation also helps to retain the nutritional value of the cabbage. The layer of carbon dioxide gas protects vitamin C from oxidation, while B vitamins are produced.

ICELANDIC DELICACY

Pre-industrial societies used fermentation to prevent spoilage of fish, resulting in delicacies of strong odor and flavor. Iceland's Hákarl is Greenland shark that has been gutted and beheaded, buried in a sandy pit and left to ferment for six to 12 weeks before being wind-dried, shaved, and cut into small pieces.

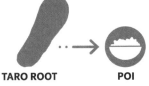

HÁKARL

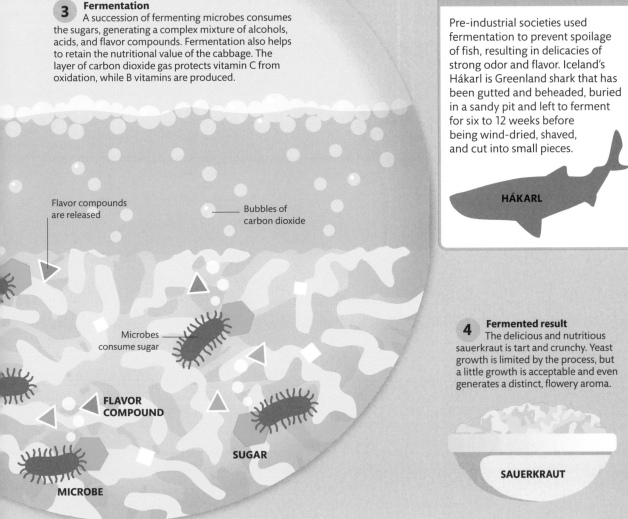

Flavor compounds are released

Bubbles of carbon dioxide

Microbes consume sugar

FLAVOR COMPOUND

SUGAR

MICROBE

4 Fermented result
The delicious and nutritious sauerkraut is tart and crunchy. Yeast growth is limited by the process, but a little growth is acceptable and even generates a distinct, flowery aroma.

SAUERKRAUT

Fermented soy
Soybeans have high levels of protein and oil, which can be extracted as a kind of milk. This is fermented in a similar fashion to milk and with outcomes as equally diverse—from the thick miso paste used for soups and seasoning to tempeh, a cultured soybean cake.

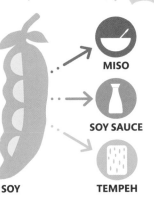

SOY

MISO

SOY SAUCE

TEMPEH

Fermented cucumber
Cucumbers are turned into pickles using lactic acid bacteria and brine with five to eight percent salt concentration.

CUCUMBER → **PICKLE**

Fermented taro root
Rich in starch but toxic when raw, taro are used in Hawaii to make poi, a fermented preparation rich in flavorful volatile acids.

TARO ROOT → **POI**

Raw foods

Raw food appeals to many because cooking can damage or lower levels of vitamins and minerals. There is a growing trend for raw food diets, but eating raw foods does not always mean maximum nutrient intake.

VITAMIN C

23% RAW

6% BOILED

3½ oz (100g) of CARROTS

Best raw foods

Vitamin C and flavonoids (see p.110) are examples of beneficial nutrients that are particularly vulnerable to heat. The best raw foods are likely to be those with high levels of these fragile nutrients. For instance, green, leafy vegetables (see pp.112–13) are rich in vitamin C and other antioxidants to help the plant deal with the damaging effect of sunlight. Raw foods do not tend to raise blood sugar levels (see p.141) since they contain fewer simple sugars.

3½ oz (100g) of KALE

Carrot
When carrots are boiled, vitamin C levels decline precipitously since this type of vitamin dissolves (is soluble) in boiling water and is then poured away.

VITAMIN C

200% RAW

89% BOILED

KEY
A percentage of your daily need of certain vitamins and minerals can be measured in raw and cooked portions of food.

● Raw

● Cooked

Kale
This leafy vegetable is rich in vitamin C. The large surface-area-to-volume ratio of kale and other leafy greens makes them particularly vulnerable to nutrient loss in boiling water.

DOES COOKING "KILL" FOOD?

There are a few plant enzymes that remain active in the stomach, but digestion changes their shape and they become inactive. They are not "alive" in the strictest sense.

RAW FOODISM

Raw foodism is a typically vegan practice of eating about 70-100 percent uncooked food. Claimed effects range from weight loss to curing diabetes and cancer. It is based on beliefs that "live foods" have natural energy, and on misconceptions about the role of plant enzymes in digestion. For instance, some plant enzymes do help digest certain kinds of protein, but most plant enzymes will be broken down by stomach acid. However, certain nutrients are missing from a purely raw food diet.

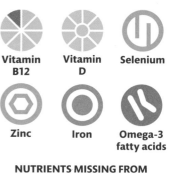

Vitamin B12

Vitamin D

Selenium

Zinc

Iron

Omega-3 fatty acids

NUTRIENTS MISSING FROM A RAW FOOD DIET

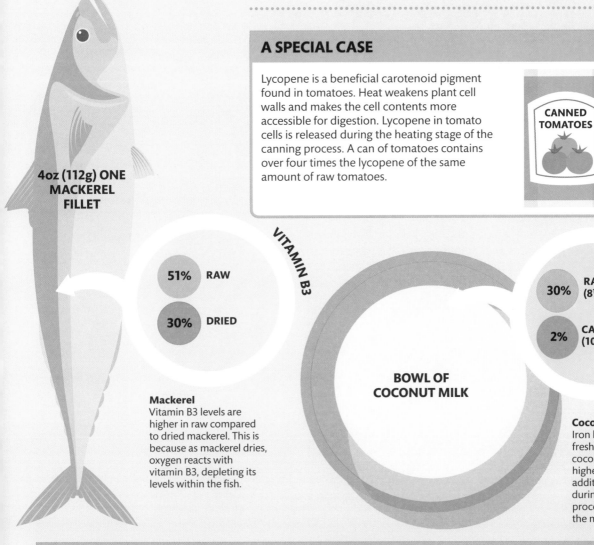

4oz (112g) ONE MACKEREL FILLET

A SPECIAL CASE

Lycopene is a beneficial carotenoid pigment found in tomatoes. Heat weakens plant cell walls and makes the cell contents more accessible for digestion. Lycopene in tomato cells is released during the heating stage of the canning process. A can of tomatoes contains over four times the lycopene of the same amount of raw tomatoes.

CANNED TOMATOES

VITAMIN B3

51% RAW

30% DRIED

Mackerel
Vitamin B3 levels are higher in raw compared to dried mackerel. This is because as mackerel dries, oxygen reacts with vitamin B3, depleting its levels within the fish.

IRON

30% RAW (8½oz, 240g)

2% CANNED (10½oz, 296g,)

BOWL OF COCONUT MILK

Coconut milk
Iron levels within freshly squeezed coconut milk are higher because the addition of water during the canning process dilutes the milk.

Limitations of raw foods

People on raw food diets can experience nutritional deficiencies and even food poisoning. Many cooking processes can actually enhance the nutritional value of foods. We cook food for safety, practical reasons, or even just to improve flavors (see pp.60–61, 64–65). Raw foods can pose risks to health—through toxins in food that do not get broken down and pathogens that are not killed.

RAW FOODS	WHAT HAPPENS
Brassicas	If eaten in excessive amounts, brassicas such as broccoli and kale contain goitrogens—substances that can interfere with hormone production in the thyroid gland.
Green potatoes	Green parts and sprouts in potatoes contain solanine, a toxic alkaloid, which if eaten can cause bouts of nausea or diarrhea.
Fava beans	Also known as broad beans, these contain alkaloids that can cause a condition, known as favism, in which your red blood cells deteriorate.
Salad bars	Many disease outbreaks *E. coli*, *Salmonella*, and *Staphylococcus* have been linked to improperly washed raw vegetables at salad bars.

Food processing

"Processed" has become a dirty word in today's food culture, but the definition of a processed food can vary greatly. Very few foods do not undergo some degree of processing, much of which is absolutely essential. Sometimes, though, we can take processing too far.

What is food processing?

Processing is generally defined as any change that is made to food or drink to alter its quality or shelf life. After harvesting crops and slaughtering livestock, methods of preservation are often put in place so food can be available at a later date. In addition to preservation, we change foods from their natural state for three main reasons: to make food edible, to improve its nutrition, and to make food safer to eat.

IS RAW MILK SAFE TO DRINK?

Bacteria in raw milk can cause food poisoning. Pasteurization is a very important process that kills harmful bacteria, which makes milk safe to drink.

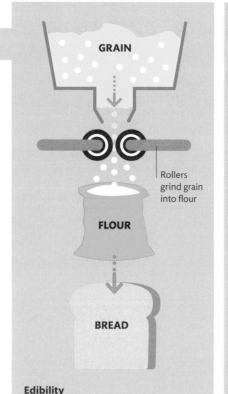

Edibility
Processing is necessary to make some foods edible. The edible parts of grain are extracted and then ground into flour, which is processed further, by forming dough and baking, into bread.

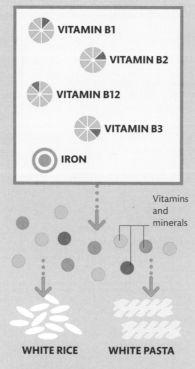

Improved nutrition
Food can be enriched in the factory with extra nutrients. In grain products, this is carried out because refining, which makes white rice from brown, removes many nutrients, which must then be replaced—sometimes by law.

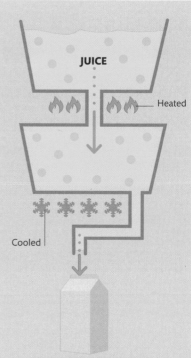

Safety
Drinks such as juice and milk are sometimes required to be processed in order to make them safe to drink. Pasteurization is a process of heating and cooling that kills harmful bacteria.

HIDDEN INGREDIENTS

Many highly processed foods are high in added sugar, salt, fat, and low in dietary fiber—with the aim of improving their taste and palatability, and to make them last longer. If levels of these ingredients are high, some authorities require food producers to highlight them on the packaging (see p.43). However, in some countries it is possible to avoid drawing attention to unhealthy or unpopular ingredients by listing complex constituents such as tomato paste or corn syrup (themselves processed from many parts) singly, without an analytical breakdown.

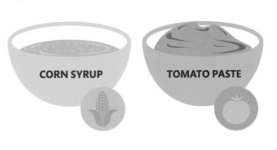

CORN SYRUP   TOMATO PASTE

How potato snacks are made
The journey from potato to reconstituted snack can be a long and convoluted one. A range of changes are made to a simple potato to make it look almost unrecognizable—and taste completely different.

1 Reconstitution
Potatoes are cooked, mashed, dehydrated, and milled into flour. Starches from corn and wheat may be added, and the resulting flour is mixed.

Processed starch added to milled flour

Mashed, half-cooked potato

Potato flour

2 Extrusion
A dough is made with the flour and squeezed through shaped nozzles at high pressure to create partially cooked, shaped snacks.

Half-cooked snack shaped by nozzle

3 Frying
The half-cooked potato snacks are dried and passed through a continuous frying machine to assure rapid, even cooking.

Potato snack deep-fried in oil

4 Flavoring
The cooked chips are shaken free of excess oil, sprayed or dusted with flavorings, salt, and other additives, and finally packaged for distribution.

Flavorings, salt, and additives sprinkled onto chips

Highly processed foods

When we think of processed foods, we are probably thinking of highly processed foods, such as chips, snacks, and chocolate – in which the main ingredients have themselves been milled, refined, cooked, or otherwise significantly altered in ways we cannot do in the kitchen. Highly processed foods are almost always high in calories, sugar, and fats, and low in nutrients and fiber.

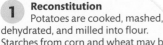

WITHOUT PROCESSING 50–60 PERCENT OF FRESH FOOD COULD BE LOST AFTER HARVEST

Main chemical additives

Additives are classed into several main groups according to their role, for example, as sweeteners, flavorings, or preservatives. In most countries, all these additives must pass strict safety regulations before they are allowed in food, although an additive approved in one country may not necessarily be approved in another.

 5 PERCENT OF THE WORLD'S POPULATION HAS A **SENSITIVITY** TO **ONE OR MORE** FOOD **ADDITIVES**

Preservatives
These prevent spoilage and prolong shelf life by slowing the growth of microbes and retarding natural chemical reactions that would otherwise make food unpleasant or inedible.

Sweeteners
These alternatives to sugars include aspartame and saccharine. They are used to reduce calories, since they are either much lower in calories than sugar, or can be used in very small amounts.

Nutrients
These replace vitamins and minerals destroyed during processing, or enrich foods with nutrients they do not contain naturally.

Stabilizers
These prevent emulsions (foods such as mayonnaise) from separating into their oily and watery constituents after they have been mixed, helping to maintain the food's texture and consistency.

Antioxidants
These are chemicals that inhibit oxidation. They are used to delay browning and decay caused by oxidation, prolonging shelf life. Ascorbic acid (vitamin C) is a commonly used example.

Additives

Additives are found in a wide variety of processed foods. They are crucial in extending the shelf life of foods, replacing lost nutrients, preserving appealing textures, and adding taste and color.

Not all bad

Additives can include natural and artificial substances, although the dividing line between them is fuzzy. Some of the additives are natural substances that have been used since ancient times for enhancing or preserving food—sodium chloride (common salt), for example. Newer additives are tested extensively before being approved for use.

WHAT IS A BATTLE BUTTIE?

The US Army developed a sandwich that will not become stale for at least two years. This is due to a packet of iron filings in each sandwich bag that absorbs the oxygen that microbes need to grow.

Emulsifiers

Emulsions are mixtures of liquids that do not normally mix, such as oil and water. Emulsifiers promote such mixing in foods—in mayonnaise, for example.

Flavorings

Artificial or natural flavorings are added to replace or enhance natural flavors lost in processing. Taste and smell are closely linked, so many flavorings also have smell components.

Colors

These are used to add or improve colors lost in processing or to add color to white or dull-looking foods in order to make them look fresher and more attractive.

Acidity regulators

These are used to control the acid–alkaline balance (pH) of food for taste (acid foods taste "sharp" or sour; alkaline ones, bitter), and to inhibit the growth of microbes so that food remains safe to eat when it has a long shelf life.

Anti-caking agents

These help to prevent powdered or granulated foods (such as flour and salt) from absorbing moisture and clumping together.

Leavening agents

These are added to doughs and batters to help them rise by promoting the production of gas (usually carbon dioxide); a common example is baking soda.

What's in a burger?

There may be more than you think. Even a 100 percent meat patty may have stabilizers to make sure the meat keeps its shape while cooking and flavorings such as salt, pepper, and onion powder. The bun and toppings may also have additives, to help prevent the growth of microbes and keep them fresh-looking.

BURGER BUN

PICKLES

CHEESE

BURGER PATTY

KETCHUP

BURGER BUN

TASTE BUD TICKLER

The savory umami flavor comes mainly from the amino acid glutamic acid, and an artificial preparation of this acid—monosodium glutamate (MSG)—is widely used as a flavor enhancer, especially in Asian dishes. In the 1960s, MSG was linked to symptoms such as migraines and palpitations, but later studies showed that MSG does not cause health problems, except in a few people who have a specific sensitivity to it.

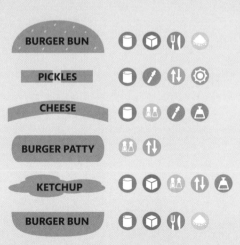

Cooking

Heat produces chemical and physical changes in food, making it softer, more digestible, and causing the food to release nutrients. However, sometimes nutrients are degraded when certain foods are cooked.

Why do we cook food?

Some scientists think that the discovery of cooking (see pp.8–9) was a key trigger in our evolution. Cooking improves and generates new flavors, aromas, and textures. One such example is a browning reaction, in which sugars in food lose water when heated, producing flavor. Raw foods are often tough, fibrous, difficult to chew, and hard for digestive processes to attack. Unless cooked, many food components cannot be broken down by our digestive system. Also, cooking helps to kill or suppress pathogens and renders many toxins inactive.

GRILLING

Grilling (applying dry heat from below) is probably the earliest method of cooking, since it can be done with an open fire. Grilling with a heat source above the food is called broiling. Grilling imparts very high temperatures to foods, enabling browning reactions, but there is a risk of charring.

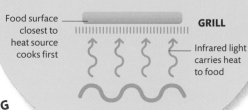

Food surface closest to heat source cooks first

GRILL

Infrared light carries heat to food

BAKING/ROASTING

An oven transfers heat, from a gas flame or electric element to the food mainly by convection, as hot air circulates in the oven. Direct infrared radiation from the oven's hot walls also heats the food.

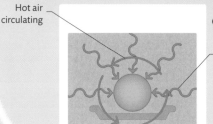

Hot air circulating

OVEN

Infrared radiation

STEAMING

Steaming transfers heat to food through air convection (as in baking), but also through condensation of vapor. Just as it takes a lot of energy to convert water into steam, so steam gives up a lot of heat energy as it condenses back into water as it reaches and moistens the food.

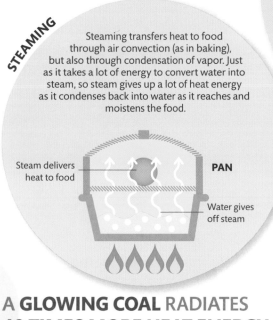

Steam delivers heat to food

PAN

Water gives off steam

BOILING

Boiling is one of the most efficient methods of cooking, since all of the food is in direct contact with the heat transfer medium (water). Browning reactions are not triggered because of the constant presence of water.

Convection currents in water carry heat from source to food

PAN

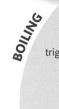

A **GLOWING COAL** RADIATES **40 TIMES MORE HEAT ENERGY** THAN THE EQUIVALENT AREA OF AN OVEN WALL

FRYING

Oil can reach higher temperatures than water, and in shallow frying it is used to conduct heat directly from the source (pan base) to food. This means browning reactions happen quicker. In this method all of the immersed food surface is in contact with the heat transfer medium (oil).

Heat from flame transferred to food through pan

Bottom surface of food cooks first

PAN

HOW MICROWAVES WORK

A microwave has a transmitter that sends out waves of around 5in (12cm) in length. They are shorter than radio waves, but longer than infrared waves from grills and ovens. A turntable rotates the food to ensure all parts are cooked.

Microwaves bounce off reflective wall

Food

Turntable

Wave guide

Transmitter, or "magnetron"

DEEP FRYING

Deep frying uses convective heat transfer, but since the medium (oil) can reach a much higher temperature than water, food can be cooked much more quickly than frying and browning reactions happen faster.

Convection currents in oil carry heat from source to food

Oil reaches temperatures above 212°F (100°C)

PAN

MICROWAVING

Microwaves agitate the water in foods, generating heat and thereby cooking the food. It may seem as though microwaves heat foods from the inside out but they tend to heat all molecules at the same time. However, microwaves will cook the wet interior of dry-cased foods (such as pie) more quickly.

Agitated water molecules generate heat

Microwave—a wave with a frequency of around 2,450MHz

MICROWAVE

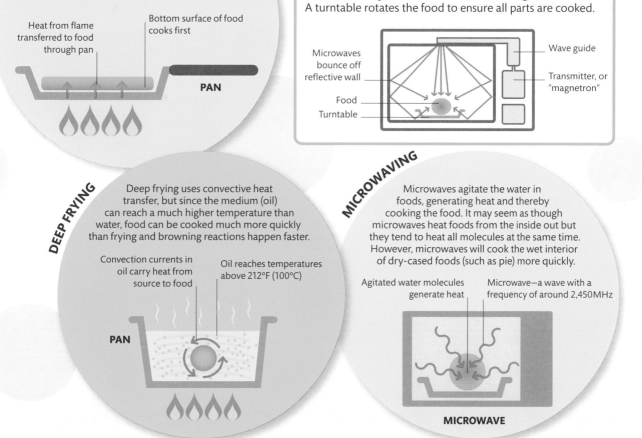

Fast and slow cooking

Cooking quickly can minimize damage to easily degraded nutrients, and can seal the outside of meat or fish to limit moisture loss, but it is harder to heat food evenly and the interior is likely to remain undercooked. Slow cooking heats through more evenly but can degrade nutrients and dry out food.

Turning up the heat

Flame grilling and barbecuing are better for thin foods with high surface area to volume ratios, since this raises the likelihood that food will be cooked through.

Oven wall during roasting
480°F/250°C

Coal in a barbeque
2,000°F/1,100°C

Gas flame in a grill
2,900°F/1,600°C

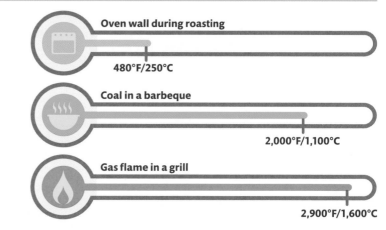

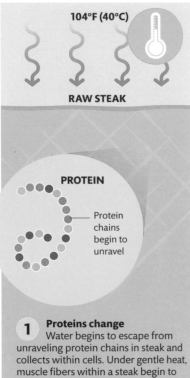

104°F (40°C)

RAW STEAK

PROTEIN

Protein chains begin to unravel

1 **Proteins change**
Water begins to escape from unraveling protein chains in steak and collects within cells. Under gentle heat, muscle fibers within a steak begin to relax and unfold, while the meat's own enzymes actively break them down.

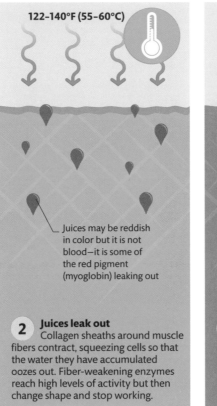

122–140°F (55–60°C)

Juices may be reddish in color but it is not blood—it is some of the red pigment (myoglobin) leaking out

2 **Juices leak out**
Collagen sheaths around muscle fibers contract, squeezing cells so that the water they have accumulated oozes out. Fiber-weakening enzymes reach high levels of activity but then change shape and stop working.

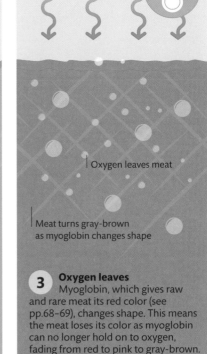

149–167°F (65–75°C)

Oxygen leaves meat

Meat turns gray-brown as myoglobin changes shape

3 **Oxygen leaves**
Myoglobin, which gives raw and rare meat its red color (see pp.68–69), changes shape. This means the meat loses its color as myoglobin can no longer hold on to oxygen, fading from red to pink to gray-brown.

How food cooks

At the molecular level, cooking involves a complex series of interactions between heat, water, and individual food components, and between the components themselves. When cooking, the perfect balance between temperature, time, and the desired change in chemistry must be achieved.

What happens when food cooks?

Food, especially meat, is composed of molecules similar to ours—proteins and fats. Plants mostly comprise of carbohydrates. Heating these molecules changes their nature, causing some to combine into new molecules, others to break down into smaller ones, and some to degrade. When heated, large molecules in food, such as enzymes, change shape and stop working. Water is a crucial factor: dry cooking causes water to evaporate; wet cooking can have the opposite effect, causing food to absorb water, as with rice or pasta.

DO FOODS LOSE NUTRIENTS WHEN COOKED?

Some foods lose a portion of vitamins when cooked. In others, the chemical reactions and release of nutrients while cooking can improve their nutritional value.

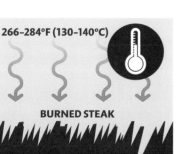

167–194°F (70–90°C)

Meat shrinks; becomes tough and fibrous from loss of juices and fluids

Water evaporates as steam

4 **Water boils off**
Collagen begins to break down and liquefy. In a pan-fried steak, water evaporates, and it becomes dense and dry. In wet-cooked meat (such as in a stew) the collagen melts, so the meat remains succulent and juicy.

230–239°F (110–115°C)

COOKED STEAK

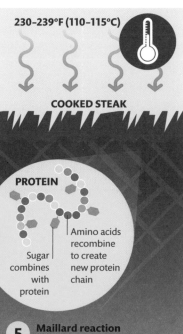

PROTEIN

Sugar combines with protein

Amino acids recombine to create new protein chain

5 **Maillard reaction**
At the meat's surface nearest the heat source, where water has boiled away, Maillard reactions take place—combining amino acids and sugars that turn the meat brown and provide it with aromas and flavor.

266–284°F (130–140°C)

BURNED STEAK

Carcinogenic compound

6 **Surface chars**
If meat is exposed to high temperatures, such as those from coals or flames on a barbeque, or left to cook for too long, combustion reactions will take place that produce carcinogenic compounds (see pp.68–69).

The story of steak
Many changes happen at the molecular level to steak meat as its temperature rises and cooking progresses from one extreme to the other.

COOKING WITH A **PRESSURE COOKER** IS EQUIVALENT TO **COOKING WITH AN OPEN PAN 3.6 MILES (5.8 KM) BELOW SEA LEVEL**

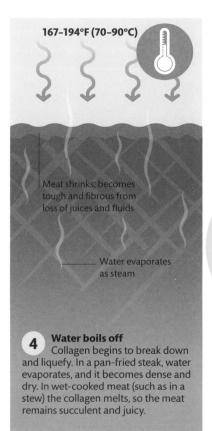

Cooking vegetables

Vegetables are composed mainly of carbohydrates, which are generally much tougher and more heat resistant than proteins. The cell walls of plants in particular are hard to break down, although heat will weaken them, allowing water from inside the cells to leak out. Vegetables turn tender when boiled because pectin (a type of carbohydrate), which sticks cells together like bricks with mortar, dissolves at boiling point. Blending cooked vegetables will eventually break down cell walls altogether—this is how vegetable puree is made.

1 **Pectin**
Long chains of linked sugars (carbohydrates) hold vegetables such as carrots together—making them tough and fibrous.

Pectin molecule

2 **Bonds broken**
When heat is applied to pectin chains, they dissolve at boiling point, making carrots tender.

Sugars break apart when heated

Safe cooking

As well as transforming food's flavours and textures, cooking makes it safe to eat by destroying toxins and killing microbes, though if not done properly, it risks making food less safe.

Contamination

Your skin and immune system protect you from harmful organisms, but if they enter your body via your food, they may cause food poisoning. Unfortunately, the scale and complexity of modern food production greatly increase the risk of contamination. From farming to processing and distribution, contamination can happen at any point in the food production chain. The most common threats are the bacteria *Salmonella*, *E. coli*, *Campylobacter*, and *Listeria*, the parasite trichinosis, and the viruses hepatitis E, hepatitis A, and norovirus.

Killing bacteria

Bacteria can be robust and persistent, but few living things survive being heated to extreme temperatures. Heat disrupts chemical bonds and drives off water, causing the bacteria's cell components to break down, their enzymes to change shape and lose their function, and their cell walls to breach. As each species of bacterium has a different composition, they have varying levels of tolerance to heating.

SALMONELLA
158°F (70°C)

LISTERIA
165°F (74°C)

LOW   HIGH

TRICHINOSIS
136°F (58°C)

E. COLI
154°F (68°C)

Safe temperatures
You can remove bacteria from your food by making sure it reaches certain temperatures. For example, to kill *E. coli* you need to make sure that the center of the food reaches at least 154°F (68°C); for *Listeria* it needs to reach 165°F (74°C).

Preventing contamination
At home, you can reduce the risk of contamination either by rinsing and washing to remove the dangerous microbes or cooking and heating to kill them with elevated temperatures.

WASHING FRUIT AND VEGETABLES

Importance of rinsing
Fruit, vegetables, and salad can be contaminated with *Listeria* and norovirus, especially if grown with certain types of fertilizer, or if prepared by someone with poor hygiene. Contaminants confined to the surface of plant foods can be washed away, which is preferable to peeling, as the outer layers are often the most nutritious.

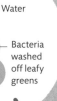
Water

Bacteria washed off leafy greens

Listeria

Norovirus

WASHING LEAFY GREENS

WASHING SILVERWARE AND SURFACES

What washing kills
A major source of food contamination is poor kitchen hygiene. Work surfaces and implements can spread germs easily. Soap or disinfectant kills bacteria, but dirty cloths can harbor germs.

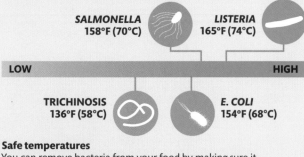

Bacteria removed by soap

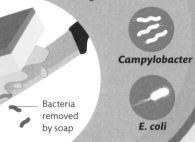
Campylobacter

E. coli

WASHING UTENSILS

YOUR **KITCHEN SINK** MAY CONTAIN 100,000 TIMES MORE **GERMS** THAN YOUR **BATHROOM**

COOKING MEAT CORRECTLY

Appropriate cooking

There is a high chance of the surface of a piece of meat being contaminated. It is hard for microbes to enter the interior of red meat, so just the outside needs cooking. Because poultry is more easily penetrated by bacteria, it needs to be cooked all the way through.

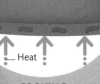

Bacteria only on outer surface of meat

Heat

COOKING BEEF STEAK

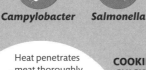

Campylobacter

Salmonella

Heat penetrates meat thoroughly

COOKING CHICKEN

SHOULD I WASH RAW CHICKEN?

Washing chicken may splash bacteria, such as *Campylobacter*, off the chicken and onto surrounding surfaces where they may proliferate.

REHEATING LEFTOVER FOOD

Sufficient heat

Leftovers can be safe to eat. First, limit microbial contamination by taking leftovers away from the heat source so it can cool quickly. Hot leftovers in the fridge can raise the temperature of surrounding chilled foods, initiating microbial growth within them. Stirring reheated foods from the microwave will help spread the heat and kill any leftover bacteria.

Bacteria live throughout leftovers

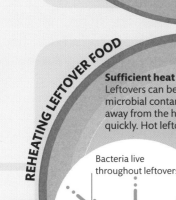

Heat

Clostridium

REHEATING MEALS

REHEATING RICE

Illness associated with reheated rice is called "fried-rice syndrome," and is caused by the bacteria *Bacillus cereus*. Spores in freshly cooked rice that sits at room temperature will grow into bacteria, which release toxins that cause vomiting and diarrhea. Reheating rice might kill the bacteria, but their spores may survive.

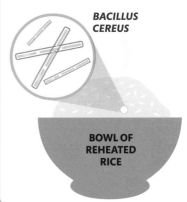

BACILLUS CEREUS

BOWL OF REHEATED RICE

TYPES OF FOOD

Red meat

Meat has played a central role in human nutrition for at least 2 million years. In the modern world, meat—especially red meat—has accounted for an increasingly high proportion of our diet, with consequences for obesity, cardiovascular health, and cancer rates.

What makes red meat red?

Meat usually refers to muscle, however, the term can also encompass organ meats. Red meat gets most of its color from iron-containing myoglobin, a richly pigmented protein that provides cells with oxygen, similar to hemoglobin in red blood cells. Energy is supplied to muscle by fats, which are broken down by cytochromes—a type of protein in muscle fibers that is also red.

Myoglobin and cytochromes

MUSCLE TISSUE

Muscle fiber

Muscle fiber
In muscles that are constantly at work—such as leg muscles—there are lots of myoglobin and cytochromes, which provide the muscle fibers with all the oxygen and energy, respectively, that they need to function.

WHY CAN MEAT SOMETIMES TASTE METALLIC?

Very lean cuts of red meat lack flavorsome fat, which contributes to the typical beef taste. This can accentuate the metallic flavor from the high quantities of iron in red meat, especially muscle meat and liver.

BOWEL CANCER RISK

Although some large-scale studies have implied that that consumption of red meat (particularly chargrilled or barbecued) correlates with a risk of colorectal (bowel) cancers, the association is weak. Furthermore, the reason for a link is unclear, and may be because fatty red meat contributes to obesity (a high BMI is associated with a risk of colorectal cancer), rather than the ingested fat itself. An analysis of 27 independent studies found no clear patterns of a direct relationship between higher red meat intake and increased risk of cancers.

Red meat and nutrition

Red meat is a complete protein source, providing all of the essential amino acids that our bodies cannot create. It is also a rich source of iron and B vitamins. Significant health concerns remain, however. The red meat we consume tends to be high in fat—the higher the fat content, the greater the flavor and tenderness of the meat. Higher fat content means a greater number of calories, more saturated fats, and the health risks associated with them.

RED BLOOD CELLS

The body needs iron to make oxygen-carrying hemoglobin in the blood, as well as myoglobin in our own muscles.

CELL CONSTITUENTS

We need the amino acids provided by meat to construct the proteins that make up our cells, including their membranes and all the cell machinery.

MUSCLES

Our own muscle fibers are built from protein that we can only make if we get the right balance and supply of amino acids in our diet.

CHOLESTEROL

The fat-burning nature of red muscle means that red meat is high in saturated fats and cholesterol, which can affect our cardiovascular health (see pp.214–15).

CARCINOGENS

Carcinogens are naturally found in many foods, but in such small quantities that they are offset by other nutrients. Smoking or charring meat can also produce carcinogens.

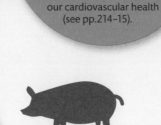

SINCE 1961, **GLOBAL PORK CONSUMPTION** HAS **INCREASED** BY **336 PERCENT**

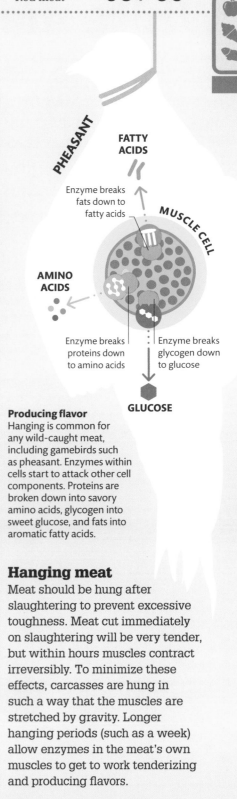

PHEASANT

FATTY ACIDS

Enzyme breaks fats down to fatty acids

MUSCLE CELL

AMINO ACIDS

Enzyme breaks proteins down to amino acids

Enzyme breaks glycogen down to glucose

GLUCOSE

Producing flavor
Hanging is common for any wild-caught meat, including gamebirds such as pheasant. Enzymes within cells start to attack other cell components. Proteins are broken down into savory amino acids, glycogen into sweet glucose, and fats into aromatic fatty acids.

Hanging meat

Meat should be hung after slaughtering to prevent excessive toughness. Meat cut immediately on slaughtering will be very tender, but within hours muscles contract irreversibly. To minimize these effects, carcasses are hung in such a way that the muscles are stretched by gravity. Longer hanging periods (such as a week) allow enzymes in the meat's own muscles to get to work tenderizing and producing flavors.

White meat

White meats include chicken, turkey, duck, and pigeon—some definitions include veal, piglet, rabbit, certain game birds, and frog. The different function and physiology of white meat gives it unique characteristics of flavor and nutritional value, which in turn have led to an explosion in global production and consumption of poultry.

What makes white meat white?

White muscles are specialized for short bursts of intense action (they are full of what are known as "fast-twitch fibers"). They burn glycogen (made of linked glucose molecules) and can work without oxygen for brief periods, although they must rest in between bursts of activity. This means they have less oxygen-carrying pigments (red pigments that deliver oxygen to muscle) than red meat. Chicken legs, which always support the body, will have slightly more red pigments, giving dark meat. Also, these redder muscle fibers have their own fat supply, making dark meat more flavorful.

Myoglobin and cytochromes (oxygen-carrying pigments)

CHICKEN BREAST

Muscle fiber

Light meat
White muscle cells do not need as rich a bloody supply as red muscle cells, so they contain less oxygen-carrying red pigments—making white meat lighter in color.

UPSIDE-DOWN ROASTING

In Western cultures, there is a chef's trick to roasting chickens and turkeys—place them breast-down in the oven. This is because most of the bird's fat is located on its back, so when placed upside down and cooked, the fat trickles into the bird's meat—providing a rich flavor and moist texture. If cooked breast upward, the flavorsome fat just pools at the bottom of the pan and is wasted!

Fat from back drips into meat

HEAT

Pasture-raised or caged chickens?

Nutritionists argue that there is a nutritional difference between hens raised inside in cages and those allowed to roam and feed outside in pastures. Pasture-raised chickens have a different diet, a more active foraging strategy, and lower stress levels than caged, barn-raised, or free-range chickens (see pp.232–33). There is evidence that this not only improves the amount of essential fatty acids and vitamins in the meat, but also reduces the levels of unhealthy fatty acids.

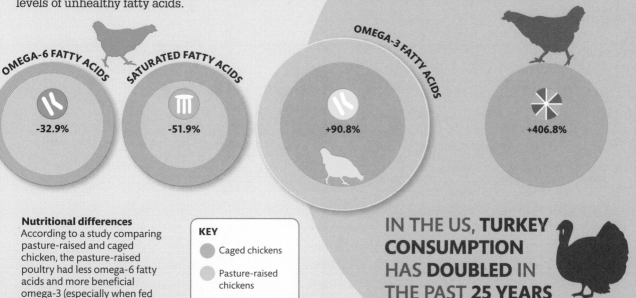

OMEGA-6 FATTY ACIDS
-32.9%

SATURATED FATTY ACIDS
-51.9%

OMEGA-3 FATTY ACIDS
+90.8%

VITAMIN E
+406.8%

Nutritional differences
According to a study comparing pasture-raised and caged chicken, the pasture-raised poultry had less omega-6 fatty acids and more beneficial omega-3 (especially when fed on soybeans), less fat overall (including saturated fat), and much more vitamin E.

KEY
- Caged chickens
- Pasture-raised chickens

IN THE US, **TURKEY CONSUMPTION HAS DOUBLED IN THE PAST 25 YEARS**

RESTORATIVE PROPERTIES OF CHICKEN SOUP

In several cultures, most notably in Ashkenazi Jews, chicken soup has long been described as particularly effective against colds. One study was conducted in which blood samples of those who ate chicken soup and had a cold were analyzed. The study found that chicken soup did have anti-inflammatory and decongestant properties that eased symptoms such as runny noses, as well as promoting good digestion, boosting fluid intake, and providing healthy nutrients.

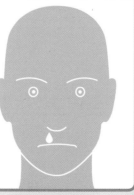

DOES TURKEY MAKE YOU DROWSY?

No, not at all—this is a myth that stems from the fact that there is an amino acid called tryptophan found in turkey that is used to create the sleep-inducing hormone melatonin.

Cuts of meat

The nutrition, taste, texture, nutrition, and even the cooking method of a piece of meat is ultimately determined by its original location on the animal's body—and how active that part was in life.

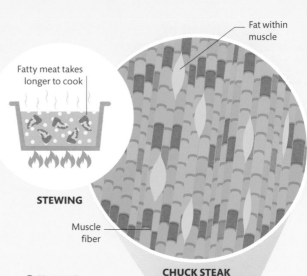

Fatty meat takes longer to cook

Fat within muscle

Muscle fiber

STEWING

CHUCK STEAK

Taste and texture

Each cut encompasses a different set of muscles on the animal. The guiding principle behind evaluating different cuts of meat is that more active muscles (such as those found on the legs) have thicker fibers and more connective tissue, and so will have tougher and chewier meat. More active muscle will also have more fat, however, and so may be more flavorsome. Butchers divide most animals into a broadly similar set of cuts, with the same terminology applying to cows, sheep, goats, and pigs—the French have the most types of cut when it comes to beef.

Fatty meat
Fattier cuts of meat can benefit from slow cooking to render down their fat. Globules of fat are scattered in-between muscle fibers that would have provided the muscle with energy (see p.68).

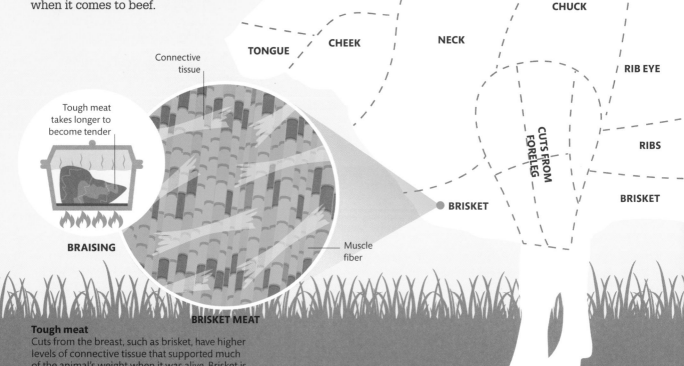

Connective tissue

Tough meat takes longer to become tender

Muscle fiber

BRAISING

BRISKET MEAT

TONGUE   CHEEK   NECK   CHUCK   RIB EYE

CUTS FROM FORELEG

RIBS

BRISKET   BRISKET

Tough meat
Cuts from the breast, such as brisket, have higher levels of connective tissue that supported much of the animal's weight when it was alive. Brisket is cooked for longer and often in liquid to dissolve the connective tissue and make the meat less tough.

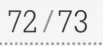

Muscle fiber

Lean tender meat can be cooked in a shorter time

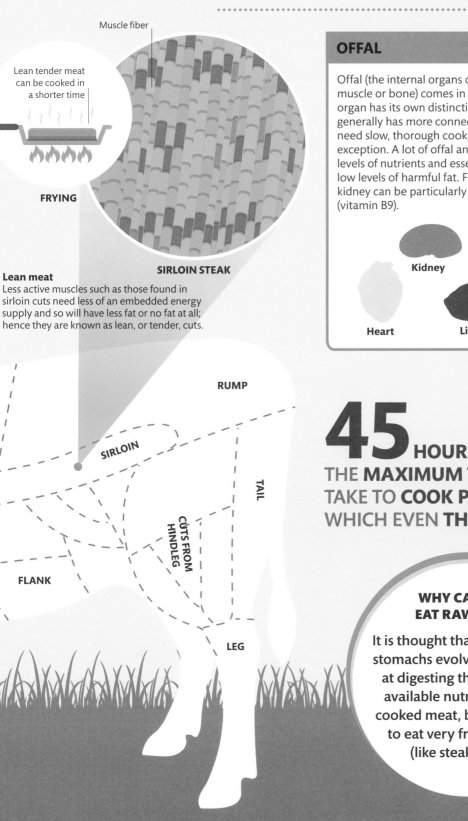

FRYING

SIRLOIN STEAK

Lean meat
Less active muscles such as those found in sirloin cuts need less of an embedded energy supply and so will have less fat or no fat at all; hence they are known as lean, or tender, cuts.

OFFAL

Offal (the internal organs of an animal, not including muscle or bone) comes in many forms, and each organ has its own distinctive flavor and texture. Offal generally has more connective tissue and tends to need slow, thorough cooking; livers are a popular exception. A lot of offal and organ meat has high levels of nutrients and essential fatty acids, and low levels of harmful fat. For instance, liver and kidney can be particularly high in iron and folate (vitamin B9).

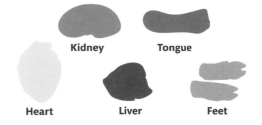

Kidney

Tongue

Heart

Liver

Feet

RUMP

SIRLOIN

TAIL

CUTS FROM HINDLEG

FLANK

LEG

45 HOURS IS

THE **MAXIMUM TIME** IT CAN TAKE TO **COOK PIGS' FEET**—AFTER WHICH EVEN **THE BONE IS EDIBLE**

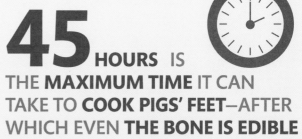

WHY CAN'T WE EAT RAW MEAT?

It is thought that our teeth and stomachs evolved to be better at digesting the more easily available nutrients in safer, cooked meat, but we are able to eat very fresh raw beef (like steak tartare).

Processed meats

Since ancient times, meat has been processed to extend its lifespan and to add flavors and aromas that can only be produced through the unique biochemical processes involved—resulting in a wide range of products.

Why do we alter meat?

Meat is metabolically active. It is fragile on the cellular level and rich in moisture and nutrients, so it is at high risk of rapid spoiling. Spoiling includes fats going rancid (oxidizing), and growth of microbes from animal hides and intestines if they contaminated the meat during butchering. Processing meat helps to delay or halt spoilage and generates complex and interesting flavors and textures. It can also mean turning whole meat into ground and reconstituted forms, sometimes known as meat mixtures. These bring their own culinary possibilities, but also their own health risks.

Meat mixtures
Meat mixtures were traditionally a way to maximize use of every part of a valuable animal carcass so that nothing went to waste. Today, meat mixtures are thought of as cheaper, lower quality products, often with negative health impacts.

Grinding
Surfaces are the risk zones for meat contamination, and grinding radically increases meat's surface area. Producers therefore ensure any bacteria are killed by blanching the meat (very briefly heating and cooling it) before grinding.

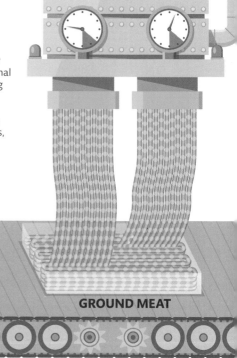

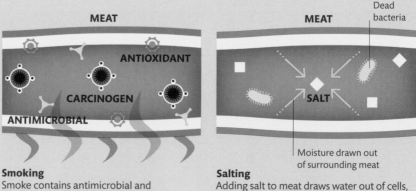

GROUND MEAT

THERE IS A **42 PER-CENT HIGHER RISK** OF DEVELOPING **HEART DISEASE** FOR EVERY **HOT DOG** YOU **EAT PER DAY**

Methods of preservation

Curing encompasses a range of preservation techniques, including the traditional methods of smoking and salting (which can often be used together). In modern times, preservative chemicals such as potassium nitrate are also used. Bacteria in the meat process it into nitrite, which reacts with oxygen in the meat to form nitric oxide. This binds with the iron in the meat to prevent oxygen from affecting fat and making it rancid. Meat gains a rosy color and a piquant flavor.

MEAT

ANTIOXIDANT

CARCINOGEN

ANTIMICROBIAL

Smoking
Smoke contains antimicrobial and antioxidant compounds and helps to prevent fat from going rancid. However, smoke also contains carcinogenic (cancer-causing) compounds.

MEAT

Dead bacteria

SALT

Moisture drawn out of surrounding meat

Salting
Adding salt to meat draws water out of cells, depriving microbes of the moisture they need to thrive. High salt levels cause protein filaments to spread out so that they no longer scatter light, making meat translucent.

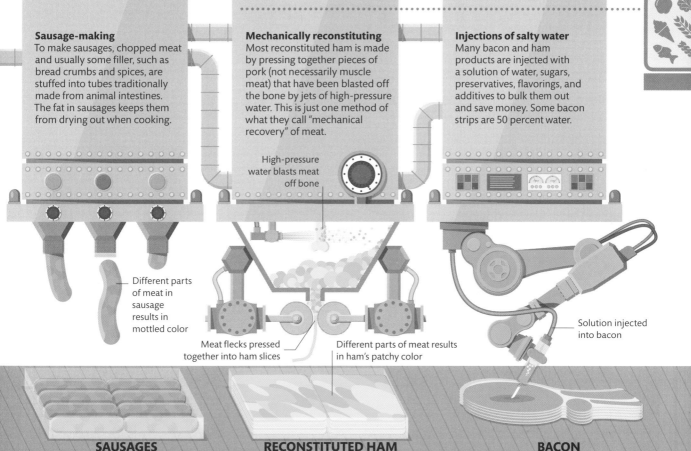

Sausage-making
To make sausages, chopped meat and usually some filler, such as bread crumbs and spices, are stuffed into tubes traditionally made from animal intestines. The fat in sausages keeps them from drying out when cooking.

Mechanically reconstituting
Most reconstituted ham is made by pressing together pieces of pork (not necessarily muscle meat) that have been blasted off the bone by jets of high-pressure water. This is just one method of what they call "mechanical recovery" of meat.

Injections of salty water
Many bacon and ham products are injected with a solution of water, sugars, preservatives, flavorings, and additives to bulk them out and save money. Some bacon strips are 50 percent water.

High-pressure water blasts meat off bone

Different parts of meat in sausage results in mottled color

Meat flecks pressed together into ham slices

Different parts of meat results in ham's patchy color

Solution injected into bacon

SAUSAGES

RECONSTITUTED HAM

BACON

WHY DOES RECONSTITUTED HAM HAVE A RIND OF FAT?

Manufacturers of re-formed ham often add a coating of fat to give an illusion of authenticity to their product, as if it has been cut directly off the carcass!

PRESERVATIVE HEALTH CONCERNS

Nitrite has been a popular preservative for the flavor and color it adds to meat, and is often used in salamis. It is especially good at delaying the growth of bacteria that produce toxins that cause botulism. However, nitrite can react with amino acids in the meat to produce carcinogenic compounds called nitrosamines. Although there is little hard evidence that nitrites in cured meats increase cancer risk, its use is now often carefully regulated.

Meat substitutes

Consumers prize meat for its flavor, texture, and nutritional value, but many are concerned by the negative health, environmental, and ethical impacts of meat consumption and production. One solution to these problems is the use of increasingly popular meat substitutes.

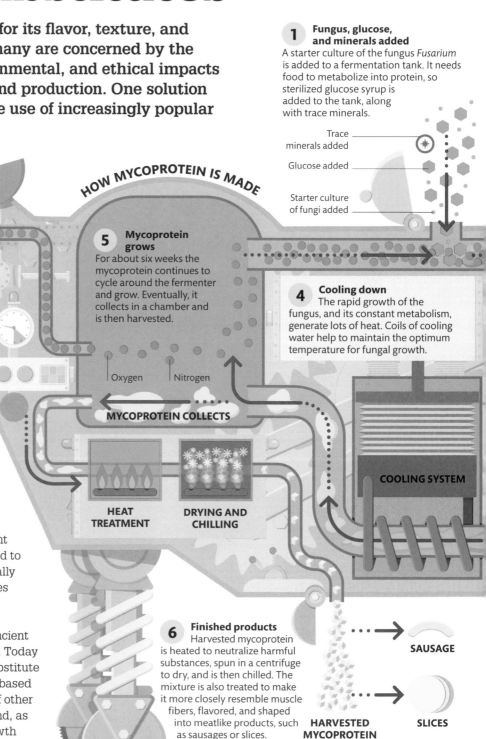

HOW MYCOPROTEIN IS MADE

1 Fungus, glucose, and minerals added
A starter culture of the fungus *Fusarium* is added to a fermentation tank. It needs food to metabolize into protein, so sterilized glucose syrup is added to the tank, along with trace minerals.

Trace minerals added

Glucose added

Starter culture of fungi added

5 Mycoprotein grows
For about six weeks the mycoprotein continues to cycle around the fermenter and grow. Eventually, it collects in a chamber and is then harvested.

4 Cooling down
The rapid growth of the fungus, and its constant metabolism, generate lots of heat. Coils of cooling water help to maintain the optimum temperature for fungal growth.

Oxygen   Nitrogen

MYCOPROTEIN COLLECTS

2 Ammonia and air added
Fungal growth is boosted by adding nitrate from ammonia and oxygen from air. These gases are bubbled through the mixture to help mix it.

COOLING SYSTEM

HEAT TREATMENT

DRYING AND CHILLING

Using meat substitutes

Although meat substitutes might seem like a modern trend related to health benefits, they have actually been popular since ancient times through cultural and religious prohibitions against meat. For example, tofu was created in ancient China by vegetarian Buddhists. Today the primary sources of meat substitute are soy-based products, gluten-based products from grains, the use of other protein sources such as nuts, and, as shown here, the controlled growth of mycoproteins from fungi.

6 Finished products
Harvested mycoprotein is heated to neutralize harmful substances, spun in a centrifuge to dry, and is then chilled. The mixture is also treated to make it more closely resemble muscle fibers, flavored, and shaped into meatlike products, such as sausages or slices.

SAUSAGE

SLICES

HARVESTED MYCOPROTEIN

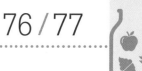

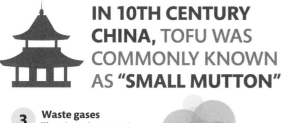

IN 10TH CENTURY CHINA, TOFU WAS COMMONLY KNOWN AS "SMALL MUTTON"

3 Waste gases
The air and ammonia bubbled through the mixture, along with waste gases produced by the metabolism of the fungus, are extracted from the fermenting vessel.

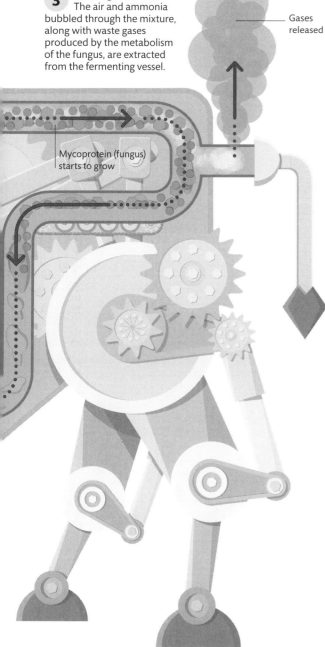

Gases released

Mycoprotein (fungus) starts to grow

Versatility of soy

Soy is rich in proteins and oils, which makes it an extremely useful base for meat substitutes. Fermenting the soy releases its rich cargo of nutrients and these can then be processed in similar fashion to milk and dairy products. Many different soya products have been developed.

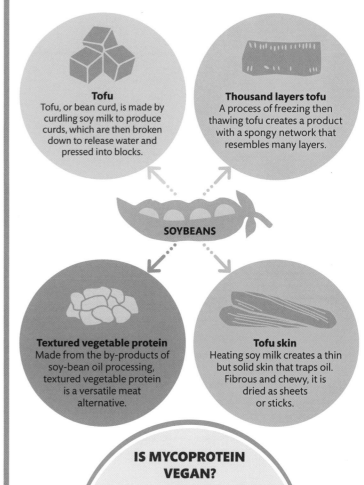

Tofu
Tofu, or bean curd, is made by curdling soy milk to produce curds, which are then broken down to release water and pressed into blocks.

Thousand layers tofu
A process of freezing then thawing tofu creates a product with a spongy network that resembles many layers.

SOYBEANS

Textured vegetable protein
Made from the by-products of soy-bean oil processing, textured vegetable protein is a versatile meat alternative.

Tofu skin
Heating soy milk creates a thin but solid skin that traps oil. Fibrous and chewy, it is dried as sheets or sticks.

IS MYCOPROTEIN VEGAN?

Although pure mycoprotein probably would be vegan, most marketed products are not because they use egg white as a binder and milk ingredients during processing.

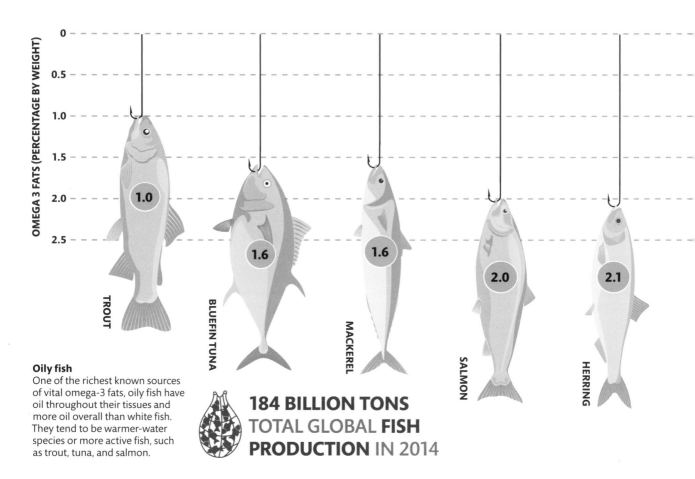

OMEGA 3 FATS (PERCENTAGE BY WEIGHT)

0 — 0.5 — 1.0 — 1.5 — 2.0 — 2.5

1.0 TROUT

1.6 BLUEFIN TUNA

1.6 MACKEREL

2.0 SALMON

2.1 HERRING

Oily fish
One of the richest known sources of vital omega-3 fats, oily fish have oil throughout their tissues and more oil overall than white fish. They tend to be warmer-water species or more active fish, such as trout, tuna, and salmon.

184 BILLION TONS
TOTAL GLOBAL FISH PRODUCTION IN 2014

Oily fish and white fish

Fish are high in protein, rich in nutrients such as iodine, calcium, and B and D vitamins, and low in cholesterol. Fish are often divided into oily (or fatty) and white fish. Oily fish have more fat than white fish and are particularly rich in omega-3 fatty acids (see pp.28–29), notably EPA and DHA. These two omega-3s can be made in the human body from another omega-3, alpha linolenic acid (ALA), but only in small amounts—so EPA and DHA are best obtained from the diet. White fish have less fat than oily fish. They also contain omega-3s, but less than oily fish.

Fish

The largest single source of wild food in the human diet as well as the product of a rapidly growing branch of farming, fish are a source of important nutrients such as protein and omega-3 fatty acids.

SASHIMI

Fish sashimi, thin slices of raw fish prepared Japanese-style, is popular worldwide. However, because the fish is raw, there is the risk that it may be contaminated with parasites or microbes, and the fish must therefore come from high-grade sources and be prepared carefully.

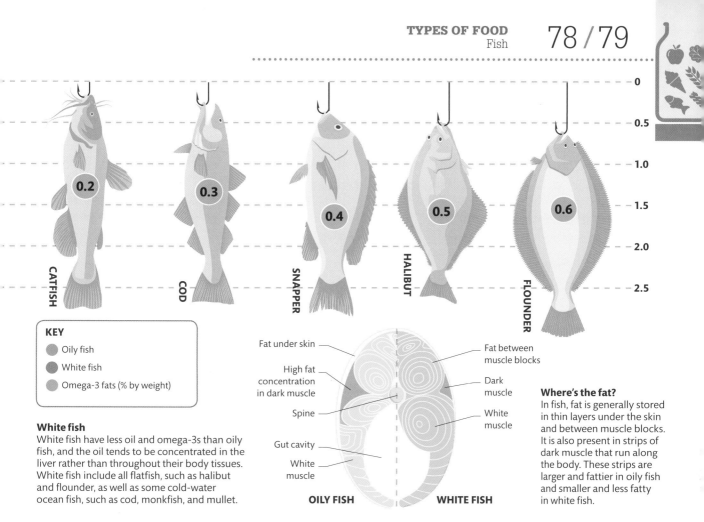

- 0
- 0.5
- 1.0
- 1.5
- 2.0
- 2.5

CATFISH — 0.2
COD — 0.3
SNAPPER — 0.4
HALIBUT — 0.5
FLOUNDER — 0.6

KEY
- Oily fish
- White fish
- Omega-3 fats (% by weight)

Fat under skin
High fat concentration in dark muscle
Spine
Gut cavity
White muscle

Fat between muscle blocks
Dark muscle
White muscle

OILY FISH | WHITE FISH

White fish
White fish have less oil and omega-3s than oily fish, and the oil tends to be concentrated in the liver rather than throughout their body tissues. White fish include all flatfish, such as halibut and flounder, as well as some cold-water ocean fish, such as cod, monkfish, and mullet.

Where's the fat?
In fish, fat is generally stored in thin layers under the skin and between muscle blocks. It is also present in strips of dark muscle that run along the body. These strips are larger and fattier in oily fish and smaller and less fatty in white fish.

Concentration of toxins
The ocean is the ultimate repository of much of the pollution generated by natural and manmade sources. Pollutants that are not readily broken down naturally, such as mercury, heavy metals, and persistent organic pollutants (POPs, see pp.202–03), may be present in low levels in small prey animals but accumulate through the food chain, becoming concentrated in top predators, such as sharks.

Toxins in the food chain
Persistent pollutants become concentrated as they move up the food chain. Sharks, swordfish, and other top predators may contain dangerous levels of these pollutants.

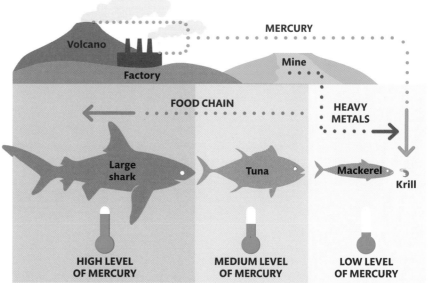

MERCURY
Volcano
Factory
Mine
FOOD CHAIN
HEAVY METALS
Large shark
Tuna
Mackerel
Krill
HIGH LEVEL OF MERCURY
MEDIUM LEVEL OF MERCURY
LOW LEVEL OF MERCURY

Shellfish

Colossal heaps of discarded shells at prehistoric sites attest to the historic importance of shellfish in the human diet, and today this diverse group of aquatic organisms is still a valuable source of nutrition.

The value of shellfish

Shellfish—crustaceans such as crabs and shrimp, and mollusks such as oysters and octopus—are a superfood category all of their own, being an excellent source of lean protein. They are also rich in B vitamins, iodine, and calcium. From a flavor point of view, seafood is rich in tasty amino acids, such as glycine, which tastes sweet, and umami (savory) glutamate.

WHY DOES COOKING CRUSTACEANS TURN THEM RED?

The shells of crustaceans contain carotenoid pigments linked to proteins. Cooking alters the proteins, releasing the reddish-colored carotenoids.

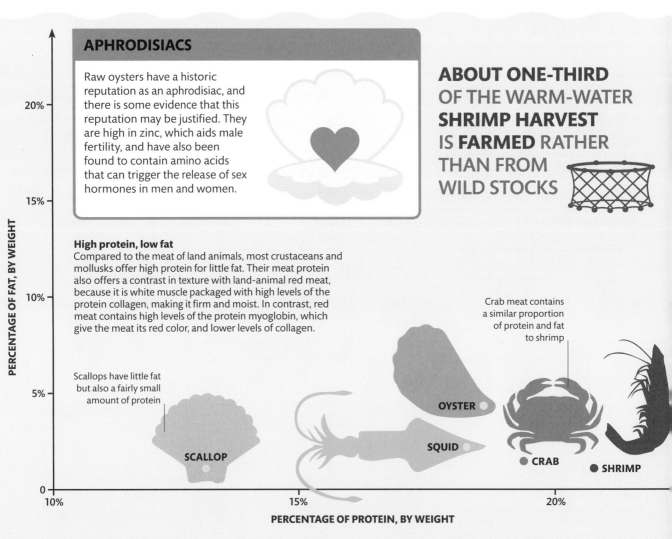

APHRODISIACS

Raw oysters have a historic reputation as an aphrodisiac, and there is some evidence that this reputation may be justified. They are high in zinc, which aids male fertility, and have also been found to contain amino acids that can trigger the release of sex hormones in men and women.

ABOUT ONE-THIRD OF THE WARM-WATER **SHRIMP HARVEST** IS **FARMED** RATHER THAN FROM WILD STOCKS

High protein, low fat

Compared to the meat of land animals, most crustaceans and mollusks offer high protein for little fat. Their meat protein also offers a contrast in texture with land-animal red meat, because it is white muscle packaged with high levels of the protein collagen, making it firm and moist. In contrast, red meat contains high levels of the protein myoglobin, which give the meat its red color, and lower levels of collagen.

Crab meat contains a similar proportion of protein and fat to shrimp

Scallops have little fat but also a fairly small amount of protein

PERCENTAGE OF FAT, BY WEIGHT

20%

15%

10%

5%

0

OYSTER

SQUID

SCALLOP

CRAB

SHRIMP

10%   15%   20%

PERCENTAGE OF PROTEIN, BY WEIGHT

When to eat shellfish

Many types of shellfish are best avoided at certain times of the year, for a number of reasons. First, many species breed in the summer and expend their energy reserves during this period, becoming meager and less tasty. Second, summer is also the period when toxin levels are highest. The best period for eating many shellfish is during the winter months, when they are fattening up in preparation for the breeding season and when toxin levels are low.

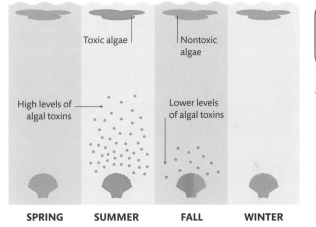

Toxic algae

Nontoxic algae

High levels of algal toxins

Lower levels of algal toxins

SPRING   **SUMMER**   **FALL**   **WINTER**

KEY
- Safe
- Dangerous

Seasonal toxicity
The summer months are often the worst for toxic blooms of algae and for harmful microorganisms, which proliferate in warmer waters and can accumulate in filter feeders, such as many mollusks and crustaceans.

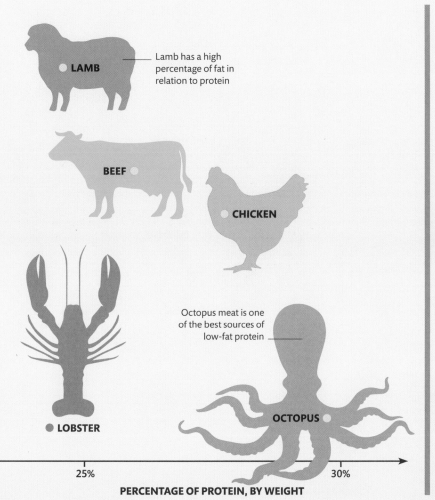

LAMB — Lamb has a high percentage of fat in relation to protein

BEEF

CHICKEN

Octopus meat is one of the best sources of low-fat protein

LOBSTER   OCTOPUS

25%   30%

PERCENTAGE OF PROTEIN, BY WEIGHT

Shellfish poisoning

Many shellfish feed by filtering out food particles from the water. However, they also trap toxins and microbes, which may build up and, if enough contaminated shellfish are eaten, may cause poisoning. The toxins are not destroyed by cooking. Symptoms of the main types of shellfish poisoning are outlined below.

Paralytic shellfish poisoning
Numbness and tingling, loss of coordination, difficulty speaking, nausea, vomiting. May be fatal.

Amnesiac shellfish poisoning
Memory problems, which may be long term, or even permanent brain damage. May be fatal.

Neurotoxic shellfish poisoning
Nausea, vomiting, slurred speech. No known fatalities.

Diarrheal shellfish poisoning
Diarrhea, nausea, vomiting, abdominal pain. No known fatalities.

Eggs

After a decade or more in the shadow of a health scare in the developed world, eggs are reemerging as what many consider to be the perfect food. Handy self-contained packages of healthy protein, eggs are rich in almost every desirable nutrient.

Nutrition powerhouse

The egg white, or albumen, contains 90 percent of an egg's water and half of its protein. The most plentiful protein in egg white is ovalbumin. Accounting for around one-third of the mass of the egg is the yolk, which contains half the egg's overall protein, three-quarters of the calories, and all the iron, thiamin (vitamin B1), fat, cholesterol, and vitamins A, D, E, and K. In fact, eggs are one of the few food sources of vitamin D. Also present in the egg yolk are essential fatty acids.

EGG INGREDIENTS
Icon sizes show total amount of each nutrient.

0.1–9 mcg

0.01–9.9 mg

10 mg–0.9 g

1–5 g

Rich in protein, but low in fat and cholesterol, egg white is extremely useful in cooking

The yolk contains the vast majority of the egg's rich load of vitamins, minerals, and other trace nutrients

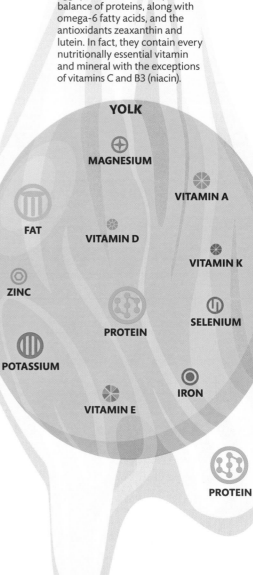

SHELL

EGG WHITE

Inside chicken eggs
Eggs provide an almost perfect balance of proteins, along with omega-6 fatty acids, and the antioxidants zeaxanthin and lutein. In fact, they contain every nutritionally essential vitamin and mineral with the exceptions of vitamins C and B3 (niacin).

YOLK

MAGNESIUM

VITAMIN A

FAT

VITAMIN D

VITAMIN K

ZINC

SELENIUM

PROTEIN

POTASSIUM

IRON

VITAMIN E

PROTEIN

EGGS AS EMULSIFIERS

Emulsifiers blend substances that are unmixable, such as oil and water. The result is an emulsion—tiny droplets of one substance suspended in the other. Egg proteins can create emulsions useful in cooking, such as mayonnaise, which is an emulsion of oil in vinegar or lemon juice.

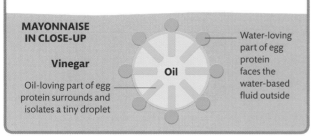

MAYONNAISE IN CLOSE-UP

Vinegar

Oil

Oil-loving part of egg protein surrounds and isolates a tiny droplet

Water-loving part of egg protein faces the water-based fluid outside

Cooking eggs

Eggs are versatile cooking ingredients, but the quality of an egg diminishes over time, partly because the shell is highly porous, allowing moisture to escape. As an egg dehydrates, it becomes more alkaline, which makes the egg white runnier and the membrane around the yolk weaker. Freshness, therefore, is essential in making the best fried and poached eggs.

Eggs have proteins that harden when heated or beaten, resulting in a range of useful cooking effects.

RAW EGG

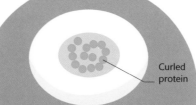

Curled protein

In a raw, unbeaten egg, the protein chains are folded and curled up, enabling them to remain separate, self-contained units suspended in water; the egg remains liquid.

179

THE **NUMBER OF EGGS** PER PERSON AVAILABLE FOR **CONSUMPTION GLOBALLY** IN 2014

COOKING EGGS

Uncurled protein with cross-links

Heating gives energy to the protein chains, which shake themselves out into long chains that can cross-link. Cross-linked protein assemblages cause the egg to harden and become opaque.

BEATING EGGS

Trapped air bubble

Uncurled protein

Whisking or beating eggs is another way to put energy into the system. As with heating, the protein chains acquire energy and unravel and interlink, trapping bubbles of air to form a foam.

BAKING EGGS

Air bubble expands

The scaffolding provided by long, interlinked egg proteins helps to give cake mixtures structural integrity, allowing the trapped air bubbles to expand without breaking or bursting open.

WHAT'S THE DIFFERENCE BETWEEN WHITE AND BROWN EGGS?

The color of a chicken egg in no way reflects differences in taste or nutritional value. It is merely determined by the breed of the hen that produced it.

A BAD REPUTATION

In recent years, eggs have experienced bad press, but most concerns are unfounded. For instance, egg yolk is high in cholesterol, but contrary to what scientists once thought, dietary cholesterol does not greatly affect blood cholesterol levels. *Salmonella* contamination, which has hit the headlines in some countries, is in fact the main risk in eating eggs, but the risk is now very low thanks to hen vaccination. Vulnerable people (such as the elderly) can further lower the risk of becoming ill by cooking or pasteurization of their eggs.

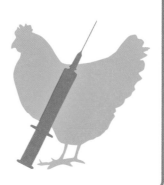

Milk and lactose

Humans are unique among mammals in continuing to consume milk after infancy, but our ability to cope—to a greater or lesser degree—with the milk-sugar (lactose) opens up for us a delicious and nutritious world of dairy products.

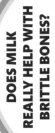

DOES MILK REALLY HELP WITH BRITTLE BONES?

Milk is rich in calcium and phosphate—two minerals that help to contribute to healthy bones. For those who can't tolerate milk, other foods can supply these important minerals.

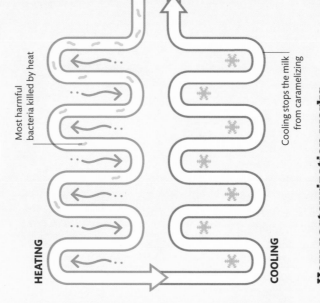

HEATING

Most harmful bacteria killed by heat

COOLING

Cooling stops the milk from caramelizing

How pasteurization works

In the 1860s the French chemist Louis Pasteur investigated microbial activity in food and developed a heat treatment that killed potentially harmful microbes without significantly affecting flavor. This process is applied to milk to make it safe to drink.

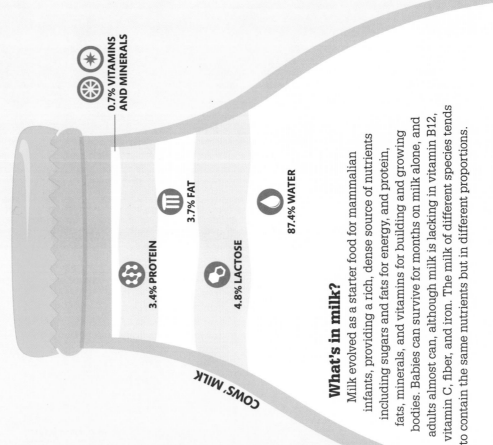

0.7% VITAMINS AND MINERALS

3.4% PROTEIN

3.7% FAT

4.8% LACTOSE

87.4% WATER

COWS' MILK

What's in milk?

Milk evolved as a starter food for mammalian infants, providing a rich, dense source of nutrients including sugars and fats for energy, and protein, fats, minerals, and vitamins for building and growing bodies. Babies can survive for months on milk alone, and adults almost can, although milk is lacking in vitamin B12, vitamin C, fiber, and iron. The milk of different species tends to contain the same nutrients but in different proportions.

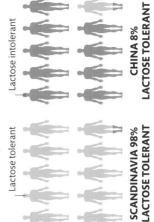

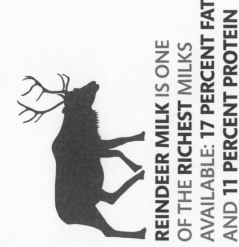

REINDEER MILK IS ONE OF THE RICHEST MILKS AVAILABLE: 17 PERCENT FAT AND 11 PERCENT PROTEIN

LACTOSE TOLERANCE

Bovine milk-drinking is a behavior that has become widespread relatively late in human evolution, and so the genes that make it possible are unevenly distributed among world populations. In most people, the level of lactase, the enzyme that allows us to digest lactose, decreases rapidly after infancy, so that adults can become lactose intolerant. However, in some parts of the world, especially in Scandinavia, populations have evolved to continue making lactase into adulthood.

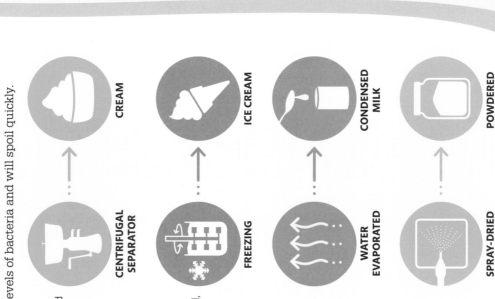

Lactose tolerant

Lactose intolerant

SCANDINAVIA 98% LACTOSE TOLERANT

CHINA 8% LACTOSE TOLERANT

Diversity of dairy products

The varied composition of milk gives it great value, both as a food source in its own right and as the base for a wonderful range of dairy products, both fermented and unfermented. Processing is important for milk products with medium-to-long shelf life, because even pasteurized milk contains high levels of bacteria and will spoil quickly.

How cream is made
Cream forms naturally in fresh, untreated milk, because it is an emulsion that will separate under gravity. In industrial production, a centrifugal separator will spin milk at high speeds in order to separate the cream.

CENTRIFUGAL SEPARATOR → **CREAM**

How ice cream is made
Milk is not simply frozen—if it were, the fat and protein would coagulate. Instead, it is frozen and spun at the same time in order to force air into the mixture. This freezes the ice crystals at a steady rate, producing a smooth, consistent texture.

FREEZING → **ICE CREAM**

How condensed milk is made
Boiling milk to evaporate half its water leaves behind condensed milk. Its shelf life is prolonged as spoilage microbes cannot survive with much of the water removed. Sugar is often added to improve taste.

WATER EVAPORATED → **CONDENSED MILK**

How powdered milk is made
Continuing to evaporate the water until about 90 percent is lost results in a highly concentrated syrup, which is then freeze-dried or spray-dried by scattering tiny droplets into hot air. Powdered milk is proof against microbial attack but can go rancid.

SPRAY-DRIED → **POWDERED MILK**

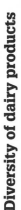

Yogurt and live cultures

Milk contains agents of extraordinary transformation—bacteria that can produce a galaxy of fermentation products that improve nutrition. The same microbes that produce yogurt may also benefit your gut, promoting a healthy balance and diversity of gut flora.

What is yogurt?

Yogurt is curdled (separated) milk. The fat droplets that are usually dispersed within milk have been captured by unraveled protein chains, creating the thicker, clumpier composition of yogurt. This change in structure is caused by bacteria (such as *Lactobacillus*) that acidify the milk. Yogurt was probably first made by accident – today, it is produced on a large scale using industrial methods.

IS THERE ANOTHER WAY TO BOOST GUT FLORA?

People with digestive problems due to too few microbes in the gut can gain those essential bacteria by undergoing a fecal transplant. Feces of someone with rich gut flora are liquidized and inserted into the colon of the patient.

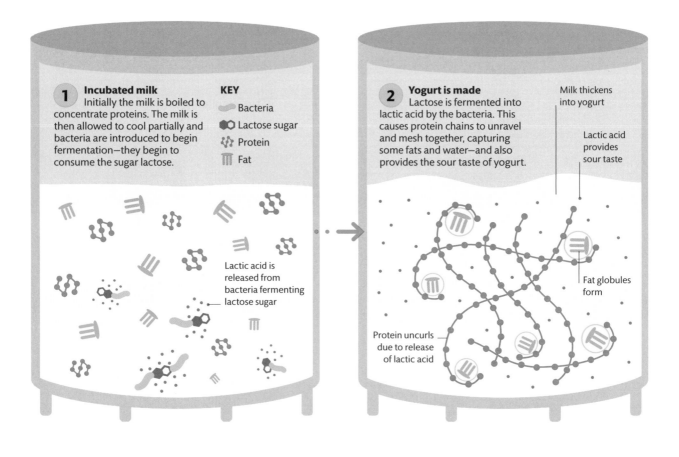

1 **Incubated milk**
Initially the milk is boiled to concentrate proteins. The milk is then allowed to cool partially and bacteria are introduced to begin fermentation—they begin to consume the sugar lactose.

KEY
- Bacteria
- Lactose sugar
- Protein
- Fat

Lactic acid is released from bacteria fermenting lactose sugar

2 **Yogurt is made**
Lactose is fermented into lactic acid by the bacteria. This causes protein chains to unravel and mesh together, capturing some fats and water—and also provides the sour taste of yogurt.

Milk thickens into yogurt

Lactic acid provides sour taste

Fat globules form

Protein uncurls due to release of lactic acid

Do live cultures survive digestion?

Live cultures in both yogurts and probiotic supplements are carefully selected and tested to ensure they do survive the acidic conditions of our stomach. Some supplements are even coated in substances that protect them until they reach the alkaline conditions of the small intestine.

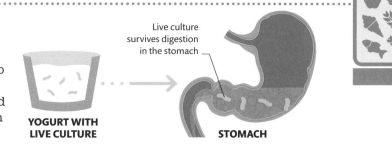

Live culture survives digestion in the stomach

YOGURT WITH LIVE CULTURE

STOMACH

Probiotic foods

Probiotic (pro meaning "for," biotic meaning "life") are bacteria that, when eaten, can live on in our gut and become part of our gut flora—a community of beneficial microbes (see p.25). Some bacteria in yogurt, such as bifidobacteria (also present in the infant gut and gained from breast milk), *Lactobacillus fermentum*, *L. casei*, and *L. acidophilus*, all colonize the human gut, helping to suppress bad bacteria by outcompeting them and making the gut environment unfavorable for them, shielding the intestinal wall, and producing antibiotics. They also suppress immunity and reduce inflammation, help to reduce cholesterol (see p.25), and even suppress carcinogens.

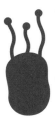

THE 100 TRILLION BACTERIA IN YOUR GUT OUTNUMBER THE CELLS OF YOUR BODY BY 10 TO 1

PROBIOTIC IN YOGURT	BENEFICIAL EFFECTS
Lactobacillus rhamnosus	Studies suggest it may reduce the risk of developing allergies, aid in weight loss in obese women, treat severe gastroenteritis in children, and reduce risk of rhinovirus infections in unborn infants.
Lactococcus lactis	Studies suggest that this species may aid in treatment of antibiotic-associated diarrhea, produce an antibacterial and potentially anti-tumor compound, and protect against an infection that causes diarrhea.
Lactobacillus plantarum	Studies suggest it may prevent endotoxin (toxins in bacteria) production, has antifungal properties, and can reduce symptoms of irritable bowel syndrome.
Lactobacillus acidophilus	This is commonly used against common causes of travelers' diarrhea. Studies suggest it may help reduce the hospital stay of children with severe diarrhea and shows antifungal properties.
Bifidobacterium bifidum	This is one of the first bacteria to colonize the infant gut after delivery. Studies suggest it may reduce the hospital stay of children with severe diarrhea; and it helps with reducing cholesterol levels.
Bifidobacterium animalis lactis	Studies suggest this strain may help treat a type of constipation in adults, reduce microbes in dental plaque, reduce the risk of upper respiratory illness, and reduce total cholesterol.

TRAVELING LIVE CULTURES

Kefir is a mildly alcoholic, yogurtlike drink made from fermented milk in eastern Europe, the Caucasus, and other regions. It is made using remarkable cultures known as "grains" (but they are not grains), which look like small cauliflower florets and combine live microbes with dairy proteins, fats, and sugars. These have been passed down through families and communities, and carried great distances by migrants. Starter cultures for many other traditional dairy fermentations have similarly been carried by migrants to new homes across the world.

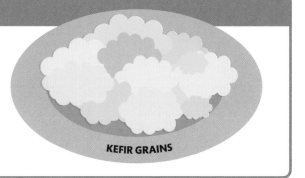

KEFIR GRAINS

Cheese

A single form of processing can lead to an astonishing profusion of products, as with the transformation of milk into cheese. Cheese can take thousands of forms, from soft and sinuous to rock hard and pungent.

How cheese is made

Milk has a short shelf life. Turning it into cheese is a way of concentrating and preserving its nutritious value, mainly by removing water that supports spoilage microbes. Curdling the milk makes it possible to remove much of its water, while salting and acidifying the pressed curds helps preserve them further. The result is a solid mix of protein and fat, with milk and microbe enzymes roped in to break down the contents into flavor-filled fragments.

THERE ARE AT LEAST 400 COMPOUNDS THAT CAN AFFECT THE FLAVOUR OF CHEESE

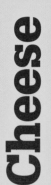

Variety of cheese

The type of cheese produced from milk depends on how it is processed; the use and degree of pressing, drying, washing, or cooking; whether mold is added, and length of aging. The protein and fat content of the milk itself (and the animal it came from) also determine the kinds of cheese that it can become.

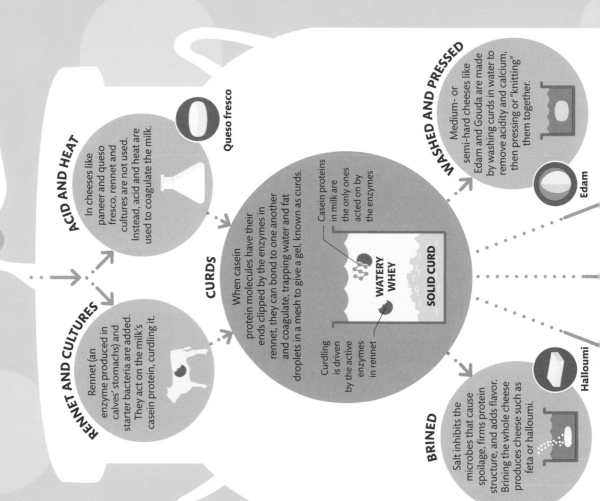

MILK

ACID AND HEAT

In cheeses like paneer and queso fresco, rennet and cultures are not used. Instead, acid and heat are used to coagulate the milk.

Queso fresco

RENNET AND CULTURES

Rennet (an enzyme produced in calves' stomachs) and starter bacteria are added. They act on the milk's casein protein, curdling it.

CURDS

When casein protein molecules have their ends clipped by the enzymes in rennet, they can bond to one another and coagulate, trapping water and fat droplets in a mesh to give a gel, known as curds.

Casein proteins in milk are the only ones acted on by the enzymes

Curdling is driven by the active enzymes in rennet

WATERY WHEY

SOLID CURD

WASHED AND PRESSED

Medium- or semi-hard cheeses like Edam and Gouda are made by washing curds in water to remove acidity and calcium, then pressing or "knitting" them together.

Edam

BRINED

Salt inhibits the microbes that cause spoilage, firms protein structure, and adds flavor. Brining the whole cheese produces cheese such as feta or halloumi.

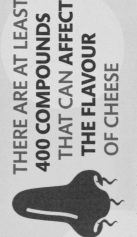

Halloumi

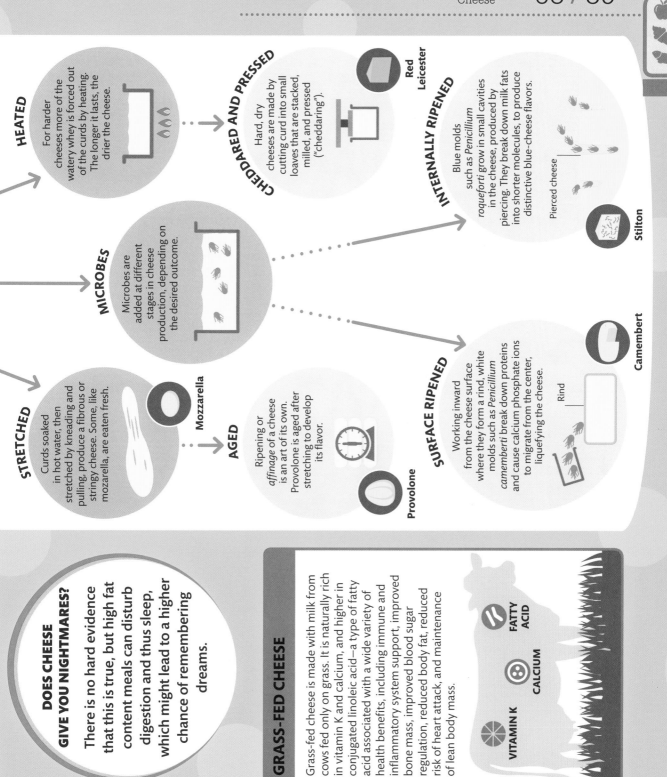

HEATED

For harder cheeses more of the watery whey is forced out of the curds by heating. The longer it lasts, the drier the cheese.

CHEDDARED AND PRESSED

Hard, dry cheeses are made by cutting curd into small loaves that are stacked, milled, and pressed ("cheddaring").

Red Leicester

MICROBES

Microbes are added at different stages in cheese production, depending on the desired outcome.

INTERNALLY RIPENED

Blue molds such as *Penicillium roqueforti* grow in small cavities in the cheese, produced by piercing. They break down milk fats into shorter molecules, to produce distinctive blue-cheese flavors.

Pierced cheese

Stilton

STRETCHED

Curds soaked in hot water, then stretched by kneading and pulling, produce a fibrous or stringy cheese. Some, like mozarella, are eaten fresh.

Mozzarella

AGED

Ripening or *affinage* of a cheese is an art of its own. Provolone is aged after stretching to develop its flavor.

Provolone

SURFACE RIPENED

Working inward from the cheese surface where they form a rind, white molds such as *Penicillium camemberti* break down proteins and cause calcium phosphate ions to migrate from the center, liquefying the cheese.

Rind

Camembert

DOES CHEESE GIVE YOU NIGHTMARES?

There is no hard evidence that this is true, but high fat content meals can disturb digestion and thus sleep, which might lead to a higher chance of remembering dreams.

GRASS-FED CHEESE

Grass-fed cheese is made with milk from cows fed only on grass. It is naturally rich in vitamin K and calcium, and higher in conjugated linoleic acid—a type of fatty acid associated with a wide variety of health benefits, including immune and inflammatory system support, improved bone mass, improved blood sugar regulation, reduced body fat, reduced risk of heart attack, and maintenance of lean body mass.

FATTY ACID

CALCIUM

VITAMIN K

Starchy foods

Although they can be rather tasteless and bland, starchy foods, such as potatoes, yams, rice, wheat, and pulses, are a primary staple of most people's diets, providing a large proportion of energy requirements as well as other nutrients, such as protein and fiber.

Types of starchy foods

Starch is used by plants to store energy, either in the plant cells themselves for short-term storage, or in roots, tubers, fruits, or seeds for long-term storage. It is these long-term stores that are the starchy foods we are familiar with—potatoes and rice, for example. However, starchy foods also include processed foods, such as flour, bread, noodles, and pasta. Most authorities recommend that starchy foods make up the main source of carbohydrate in our diets.

What is starch?

Starch is a carbohydrate formed from long chains of identical glucose units linked together. There are two types of starch: amylose, made of straight chains of glucose molecules, and amylopectin, made of branching chains. The relative proportions of amylose and amylopectin in a starchy food affects how quickly it is digested and, therefore, its glycemic index.

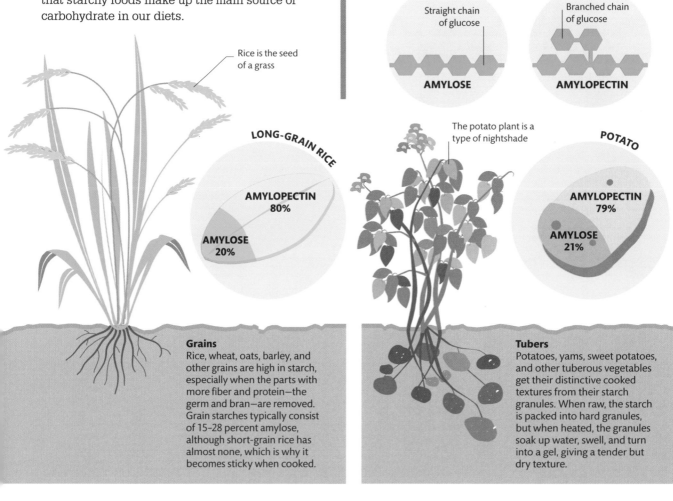

Straight chain of glucose

AMYLOSE

Branched chain of glucose

AMYLOPECTIN

Rice is the seed of a grass

LONG-GRAIN RICE

AMYLOPECTIN 80%

AMYLOSE 20%

The potato plant is a type of nightshade

POTATO

AMYLOPECTIN 79%

AMYLOSE 21%

Grains
Rice, wheat, oats, barley, and other grains are high in starch, especially when the parts with more fiber and protein—the germ and bran—are removed. Grain starches typically consist of 15–28 percent amylose, although short-grain rice has almost none, which is why it becomes sticky when cooked.

Tubers
Potatoes, yams, sweet potatoes, and other tuberous vegetables get their distinctive cooked textures from their starch granules. When raw, the starch is packed into hard granules, but when heated, the granules soak up water, swell, and turn into a gel, giving a tender but dry texture.

Blood glucose levels

Foods with a high glycemic index (GI) produce a large, rapid rise in blood sugar followed by a similarly rapid fall, leaving us feeling hungry. Low GI foods do not cause this "sugar spike," but produce a slower, smaller increase, followed by a gradual decrease.

Blood glucose rises and falls dramatically

Blood glucose rises steadily but remains low

HIGH GI

LOW GI

BLOOD GLUCOSE LEVEL

HOURS   1   2

Glycemic index

Glycemic index (GI) is a measure of how quickly a carbohydrate-containing food raises your blood sugar level when that food is eaten by itself. Carbohydrates that are digested quickly and cause a rapid increase have a high GI; examples include sugar and starchy foods with a lot of amylopectin, such as potatoes and white rice. Amylopectin is more easily digested than amylose, as it has more chain ends for enzymes to work on. But a food's GI by itself is not a good indicator of whether that food is healthy; for example, chips have a lower GI than boiled potatoes but are very high in fat.

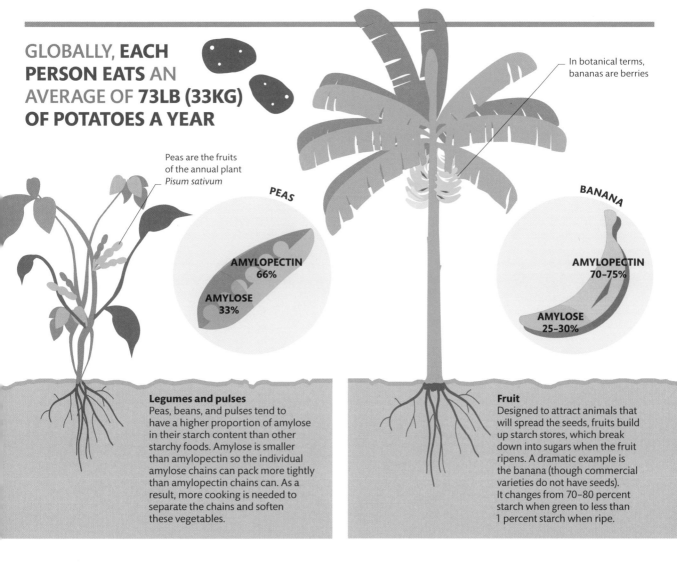

GLOBALLY, **EACH PERSON EATS** AN AVERAGE OF **73LB (33KG)** OF POTATOES A YEAR

Peas are the fruits of the annual plant *Pisum sativum*

PEAS

AMYLOPECTIN 66%

AMYLOSE 33%

In botanical terms, bananas are berries

BANANA

AMYLOPECTIN 70–75%

AMYLOSE 25–30%

Legumes and pulses

Peas, beans, and pulses tend to have a higher proportion of amylose in their starch content than other starchy foods. Amylose is smaller than amylopectin so the individual amylose chains can pack more tightly than amylopectin chains can. As a result, more cooking is needed to separate the chains and soften these vegetables.

Fruit

Designed to attract animals that will spread the seeds, fruits build up starch stores, which break down into sugars when the fruit ripens. A dramatic example is the banana (though commercial varieties do not have seeds). It changes from 70–80 percent starch when green to less than 1 percent starch when ripe.

Grains

Grains are the most important food group globally in terms of supplying calories and nutrients for the majority of the world's population.

Types of grain

Also known as cereals, grains are the edible seeds of plants of the grass family. The grains we eat most commonly, either by themselves or as ingredients in other foods, are rice, wheat, corn, oats, barley, rye, and millet. Amaranth, buckwheat, and quinoa are also commonly thought of as grains, although botanically they are not related to true grains. Nutritionally, all of them are high in carbohydrate, much of it as complex, slow-release starches.

Anatomy of a grain

Grains are seeds, designed to protect and nurture embryonic plants. They consist of three main elements: the germ (the plant embryo), the endosperm (the energy store), and the bran (the protective outer layer). Many of the most valuable nutrients are in the germ and bran, which are removed during refining.

ENDOSPERM

BRAN

GERM

MINERALS · PHYTOCHEMICALS · FIBER · B VITAMINS

Bran
An outer coating of tough, fibrous material, the bran is rich in fiber, minerals, B vitamins, and phenolic phytochemicals (which form part of the seed's defense system).

PROTEIN · CARBOHYDRATE · FATS · B VITAMINS

Endosperm
The endosperm, or kernel, of a grain is rich in starch, and significant amounts of proteins, fats, and B vitamins, although the amounts vary according to the type of grain.

MINERALS · PHYTOCHEMICALS · PROTEINS · VITAMIN A · FATS · B VITAMINS

Germ
The germ is the most nutritionally rich and flavorful part of a grain, containing large amounts of fats, proteins, vitamins, minerals, and phytochemicals.

WHOLE GRAIN VS. REFINED GRAIN

Whole grains contain all parts of the grain. Refined grains, such as white rice and white flour, have had the bran and germ removed. Refining may also involve bleaching to make the grain whiter. After refining, grains may be enriched to add back nutrients previously removed.

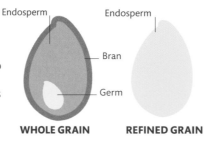

Endosperm

Endosperm

Bran

Germ

WHOLE GRAIN

REFINED GRAIN

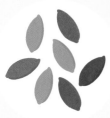

100,000
THE NUMBER OF DISTINCT
VARIETIES OF RICE

Types of rice

Rice is the largest source of calories for humans worldwide. On average, it contributes about 21 percent of the total calorie intake of every person on the planet, although there are large regional variations. For example, in southeast Asian countries such as Vietnam and Cambodia, rice provides up to 80 percent of the calories eaten by each person. There are two main subspecies: japonica and indica, with javanica being a subtype of japonica.

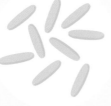

Japonica
Originating in China but now grown in many temperate and subtropical regions, japonica rice is short-grain and has a low amylose content (see p.90).

Indica
Long-grain indica rice is grown in lowland tropical and subtropical regions. It has a high amylose content so takes longer to cook.

Javanica
Grown mainly in highland tropical zones in Indonesia and the Philippines, javanica rice, like japonica, has a low amylose content.

ENERGY SOURCE

Globally, we get far more of our calories from grains than from any other type of food: overall, they provide more than half of the total calories we humans eat. Around 60 percent of the calories eaten by people in developing countries come directly from grains. In the developed world, the figure is about 30 percent, although many more of the total calories consumed come indirectly from grains via the feed eaten by animals we then eat.

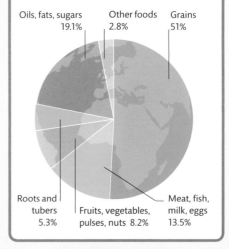

Oils, fats, sugars 19.1%

Other foods 2.8%

Grains 51%

Roots and tubers 5.3%

Fruits, vegetables, pulses, nuts 8.2%

Meat, fish, milk, eggs 13.5%

Nutrient content of grains

Overall, whole grains are a good source of calories, carbohydrates, fiber, proteins, B vitamins, and phytochemicals. Most grains contain about 70–75 percent carbohydrate, 4–18 percent fiber, 10–15 percent protein, and 1–5 percent fat. However, there is a lot of variation between the different grains in their specific nutrient content, as shown by white rice and amaranth.

Amaranth vs white rice
Compared with most other grains, amaranth contains relatively little carbohydrate but lots of fat, whereas white rice is high in carbohydrate and low in fat.

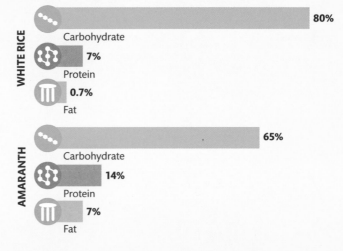

WHITE RICE
Carbohydrate — 80%
Protein — 7%
Fat — 0.7%

AMARANTH
Carbohydrate — 65%
Protein — 14%
Fat — 7%

Bread

Consisting at its most basic of a cooked mixture of flour and water—often with salt added, and sometimes with yeast or a raising agent, such as baking soda—bread is one of the oldest types of prepared food and remains an important staple even today.

Making leavened bread

Leavened bread is made with a raising agent—most commonly yeast—that causes the dough to develop bubbles of gas, expand, and rise. Mixing flour and water causes proteins in the flour to form a network of gluten (see pp.98–99) in the dough. The yeast ferments the starch and sugars in the dough into alcohol and carbon dioxide gas, which gets trapped in the gluten network. When the fermented dough is baked, the heat drives off the alcohol and carbon dioxide, leaving the familar spongelike structure of bread.

Unleavened bread

Developed before leavening, and still popular in many forms today, unleavened breads were a natural development of the use of cereals to make porridge or grain mash. They were made simply by baking the porridge or mash without using any raising agents, producing a flat bread.

UNLEAVENED BREAD	ORIGIN
Tortilla	Latin America
Johnnycake	North America
Souri	North Africa
Pita	Greece
Baladi	Egypt
Bouri	Saudi Arabia
Matzoh	Middle East
Lavash	Middle East
Chapati	India
Roti	India

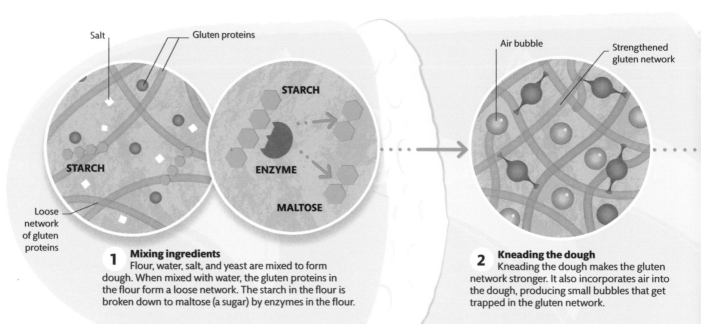

Salt Gluten proteins

STARCH

STARCH

ENZYME

MALTOSE

Loose network of gluten proteins

1 Mixing ingredients
Flour, water, salt, and yeast are mixed to form dough. When mixed with water, the gluten proteins in the flour form a loose network. The starch in the flour is broken down to maltose (a sugar) by enzymes in the flour.

Air bubble Strengthened gluten network

2 Kneading the dough
Kneading the dough makes the gluten network stronger. It also incorporates air into the dough, producing small bubbles that get trapped in the gluten network.

Sourdough bread

The first leavened breads were probably sourdoughs—breads made with a starter culture consisting of wild yeasts and specific bacteria. The wild yeasts cannot process the maltose sugar in the dough; this is done instead by the bacteria, which produce lactic acid as a byproduct. As a result, the bread has a slightly acidic, sour flavor, but it is generally more flavorful, denser, and longer lasting than other types of leavened bread.

Wild yeast

Bacteria process maltose

SOURDOUGH CULTURE

Commercially cultured yeast can process maltose

YEAST CULTURE

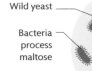

THE **FIRST PRESLICED**, WRAPPED **BREAD** WAS **PRODUCED IN 1928,** BY US INVENTOR OTTO ROHWEDDER

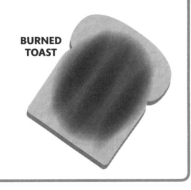

DON'T BURN IT!

Acrylamide is a cancer-causing chemical produced when bread and other starchy foods, such as potatoes, are cooked at high temperature and start to brown. The amount of acrylamide can be minimized by cooking food to the lightest acceptable color.

BURNED TOAST

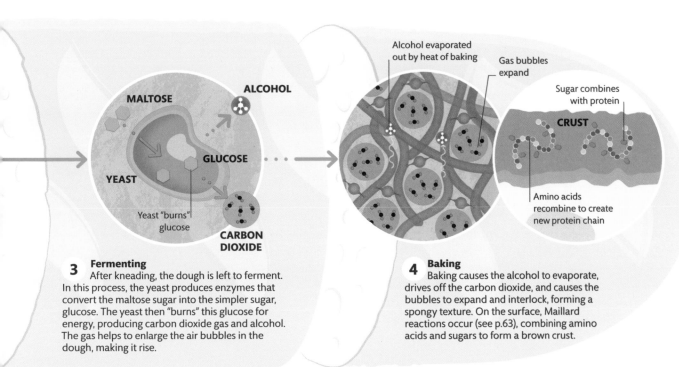

Alcohol evaporated out by heat of baking

Gas bubbles expand

Sugar combines with protein

CRUST

Amino acids recombine to create new protein chain

MALTOSE

ALCOHOL

GLUCOSE

YEAST

Yeast "burns" glucose

CARBON DIOXIDE

3 **Fermenting**
After kneading, the dough is left to ferment. In this process, the yeast produces enzymes that convert the maltose sugar into the simpler sugar, glucose. The yeast then "burns" this glucose for energy, producing carbon dioxide gas and alcohol. The gas helps to enlarge the air bubbles in the dough, making it rise.

4 **Baking**
Baking causes the alcohol to evaporate, drives off the carbon dioxide, and causes the bubbles to expand and interlock, forming a spongy texture. On the surface, Maillard reactions occur (see p.63), combining amino acids and sugars to form a brown crust.

Noodles and pasta

Noodles have a long history in east Asia, where they are a staple food in many countries. Pasta, a specific type of noodle, is a traditional Italian staple but has become popular worldwide.

What is the difference?

Noodles—sheets, ribbons, and other shapes of cooked dough—may be made from various flours. The flour is mixed with water, eggs, or both to create the dough, which is then shaped and cooked. Pasta is a type of wheat noodle made specifically from durum wheat flour, which can be made into complex shapes because of its high gluten content (see p.98).

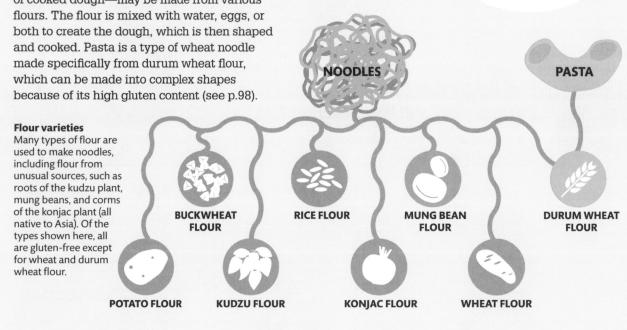

NOODLES

PASTA

Flour varieties

Many types of flour are used to make noodles, including flour from unusual sources, such as roots of the kudzu plant, mung beans, and corms of the konjac plant (all native to Asia). Of the types shown here, all are gluten-free except for wheat and durum wheat flour.

BUCKWHEAT FLOUR

RICE FLOUR

MUNG BEAN FLOUR

DURUM WHEAT FLOUR

POTATO FLOUR

KUDZU FLOUR

KONJAC FLOUR

WHEAT FLOUR

SHOULD I COOK MY PASTA *AL DENTE*?

Pasta cooked *al dente*—firm to the bite—is broken down in the body more slowly than pasta cooked until it is soft. As a result, it releases sugar more slowly and so has a lower glycemic index, which may reduce spikes in blood sugar.

How instant noodles are made

The key stage in making instant noodles is the middle one. Cooking then cooling raw noodles makes them more absorbent than normal noodles. This means that they retain more water and so have a shorter cooking time when being prepared for eating.

1 Preparing dough
Flour, water, salt, and kansui (an alkaline liquid) are kneaded to make dough, which is rolled then cut into thin noodles.

Sheet of dough

Raw noodles

2 Cooking and cooling
The raw noodles are cooked by steaming for a few minutes, then cooled to harden them.

Noodles being steamed

3 Dehydrating
Water is removed by air drying or frying and the resulting instant noodles are then packaged.

Instant noodles

DECORATIVE

FARFALLE

CONCHIGLIE

RUOTE

RADIATORI

LONG

SPAGHETTI

VERMICELLI

ANGEL HAIR

FUSILLI

RIBBON

FETTUCCINI

TAGLIATELLE

LINGUINI

LASAGNE

Pasta shapes

Pasta shapes and patterns combine aesthetics, function, and culture. Some shapes and types are associated with specific regions, such as penne with Campania in southern Italy, and farfalle with Lombardy in northwest Italy. Some shapes are particularly suitable for holding sauces: shell-shaped conchiglie, for instance, are good for thick meat or cream sauces and can even be stuffed.

CANELLONI

MACARONI

RIGATONI

PENNE

SHORT CUT

BRONZE-DIE PASTA

Pasta shapes are made by pressing the dough through perforated plates called dies. Dies made of bronze are prized because they have a rough surface that imparts a coarseness to the pasta that is good for holding sauces; bronze-die pasta also cooks more quickly.

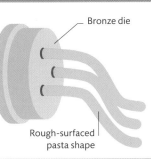

Bronze die

Rough-surfaced pasta shape

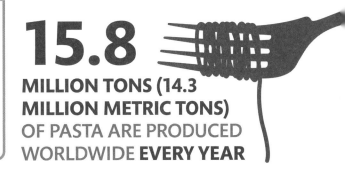

15.8
MILLION TONS (14.3 MILLION METRIC TONS) OF PASTA ARE PRODUCED WORLDWIDE **EVERY YEAR**

Gluten

Found in many grains, including wheat, gluten is a vital ingredient in a huge range of breads, pasta, and other dough products. However, some people are sensitive to gluten and suffer health problems when they eat it.

What is gluten?

Gluten is an enormous composite protein—the largest known—that consists of a strong, stretchy mesh of smaller proteins linked by molecular bonds. These smaller proteins are glutenin, which has a long, chainlike shape, and gliadins, which are shorter and round. The glutenin is what gives gluten its elasticity, whereas the gliadins give it strength. It is this combination of stretchiness and strength, together with its meshlike structure that can trap bubbles of gas, that makes gluten important in bread-making (see pp.94–95).

IS THERE GLUTEN-FREE WHEAT?

No, all wheat contains gluten. However, there is a type of wheat starch that is gluten-free. It is made by thoroughly washing wheat flour with water to remove the gluten.

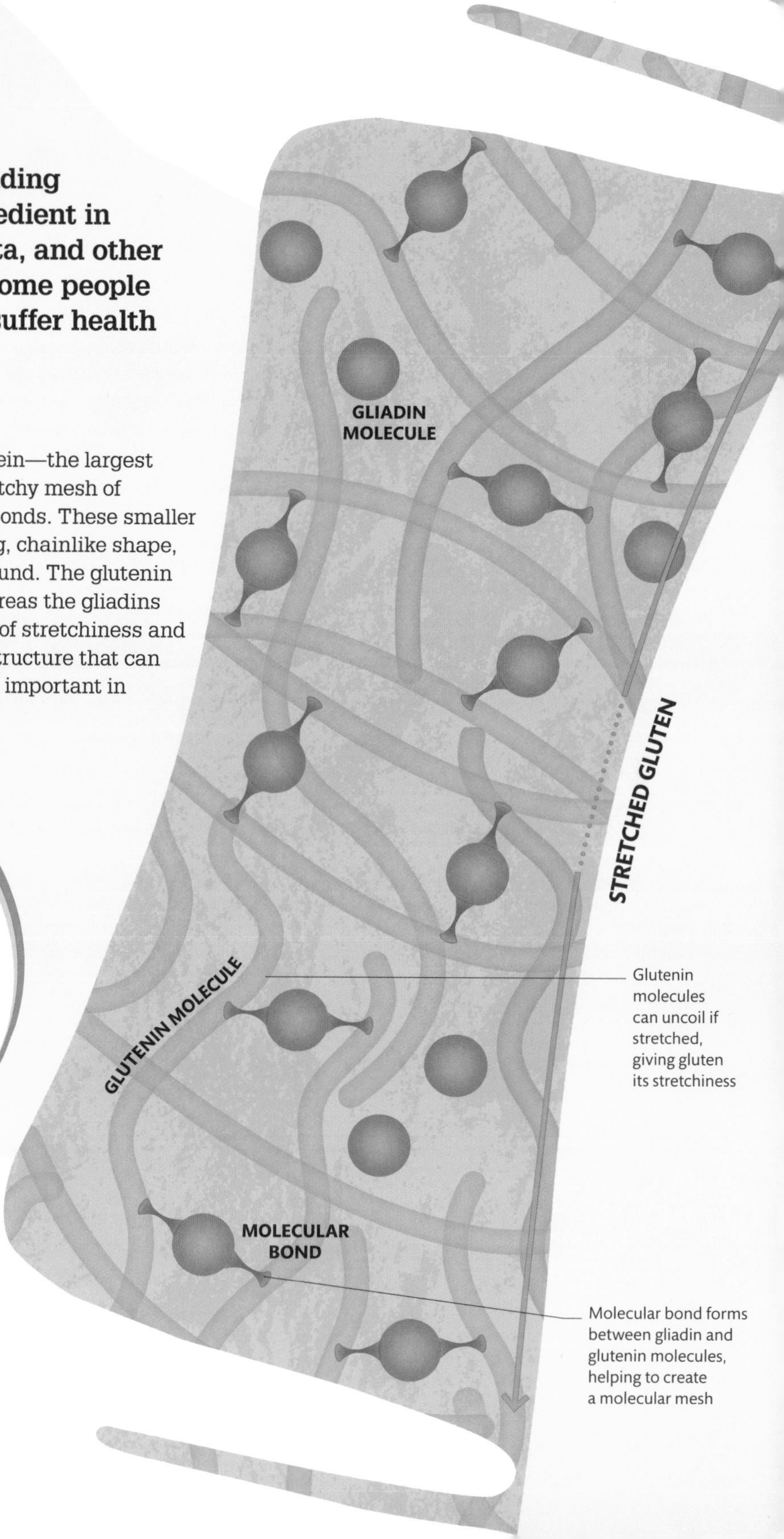

Structure of gluten
Gluten is a resilient, rubbery substance that forms when glutenin and gliadin molecules in flour are mixed with water; this happens when making dough, for example. The molecules bond together to form a mesh that can trap bubbles of gas—as occurs when dough is kneaded. Because the mesh is stretchy, the gas bubbles can expand without breaking it.

GLIADIN MOLECULE

STRETCHED GLUTEN

GLUTENIN MOLECULE

MOLECULAR BOND

Glutenin molecules can uncoil if stretched, giving gluten its stretchiness

Molecular bond forms between gliadin and glutenin molecules, helping to create a molecular mesh

Gluten sensitivity

A significant number of people cannot tolerate gluten in the diet and experience health problems from eating it (see pp.208–09). One of these problems is celiac disease, which is due to the body's immune system reacting abnormally to gluten. The other main problem is non-celiac gluten sensitivity (NCGS), the cause of which is not known. Both conditions produce similar symptoms, including stomach pain, diarrhea or constipation, headaches, and tiredness, but celiac disease is more serious and causes permanent damage to the intestines.

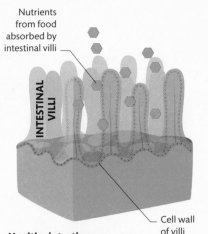

Nutrients from food absorbed by intestinal villi

INTESTINAL VILLI

Cell wall of villi

Healthy intestines
In healthy people, the inner wall of the intestine has thousands of tiny, fingerlike projections called villi, which greatly increase the intestine's surface area and so enhance its capacity for absorbing nutrients.

Antibodies mistakenly attack intestinal villi

Nutrients unable to be absorbed by body due to no intestinal villi

Intestinal villi reduced

Celiac disease
In people with celiac disease, gluten stimulates the immune system to mistakenly attack the intestinal villi, damaging and reducing them. As a result, the intestine's ability to absorb nutrients is impaired.

Gluten-free foods

There are many foods that are naturally gluten free, including fresh fruit and vegetables, potatoes, rice, legumes, and fresh meat and fish (see pp.210–11). There are also many gluten-free processed foods available. These may be made with gluten-free alternatives, such as rice flour instead of wheat flour, or use substances that mimic the properties of gluten; for example, xanthan gum can be used to make dough stretchy.

UNLESS PEOPLE ARE VERY CAREFUL, A **GLUTEN-FREE DIET** CAN LACK **VITAMINS**, **MINERALS**, AND **FIBER**

TYPES OF FOOD		NOT GLUTEN-FREE
	Grains	Wheat, rye, barley, spelt, kamut, einkorn wheat, emmer
	Vegetables	Canned vegetables or vegetables in ready meals if they contain certain emulsifiers, preservatives, thickening agents, stabilizers, or starch
	Fruits	Fruit fillings that contain thickening agents, starch, or both
	Dairy products	Types of processed cheese that contain certain additives, such as thickening agents
	Meat	Sausage products and processed meats that include additives containing gluten
	Fish and shellfish	Fish in batter and fish in bread crumbs
	Fats and oils	Margarine and vegetable oils containing additives with gluten
	Beverages	Coffee or cocoa containing additives with gluten (from drinks machines, for example), beer, malt drinks
	Other foods	Seitan (wheat gluten, also known as "wheat meat")

Beans, peas, and pulses

Beans, peas, and pulses are all legumes—a group of plants whose fruits are contained inside pods. In addition to being a good source of nutrients for us, legumes are also valuable for animal feed and help to fertilize soil.

What are pulses?

The term "pulse" refers only to the dried fruits of legumes, including dried peas and beans, lentils, and chickpeas. Fresh legumes, such as green beans and green peas, are not classed as pulses. Technically, soybeans (see pp.102–03) and peanuts (see pp.126–27) are legumes and are related to pulses, but in food science, they are not usually included with them because of their much higher fat content.

Making protein

Legumes are special because they host bacteria in their roots that can use the nitrogen in air to make ammonia, which can then be converted into protein. The ammonia also helps to fertilize the plant.

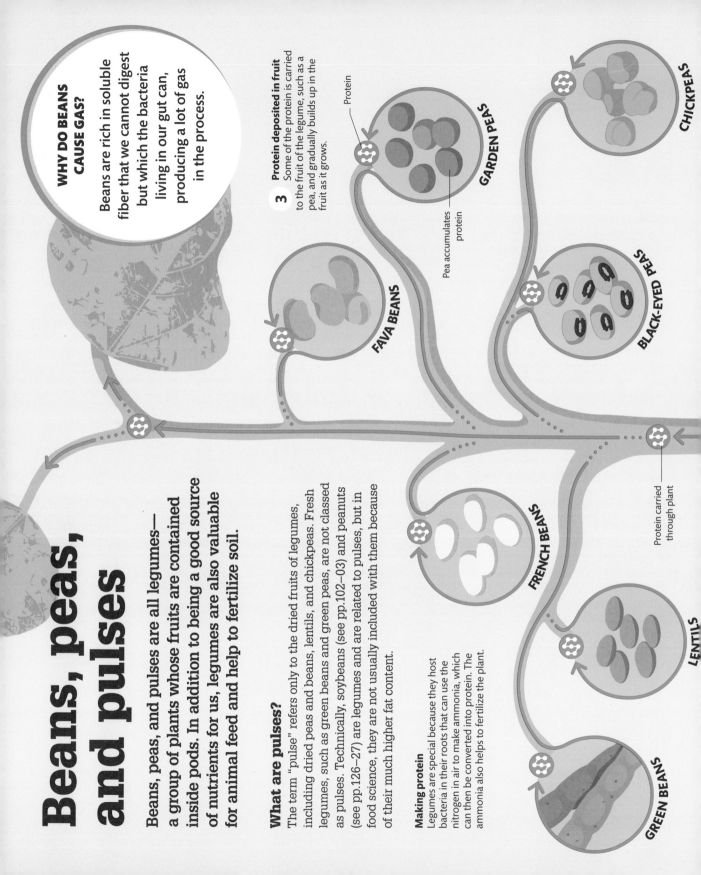

WHY DO BEANS CAUSE GAS?

Beans are rich in soluble fiber that we cannot digest but which the bacteria living in our gut can, producing a lot of gas in the process.

3 **Protein deposited in fruit**
Some of the protein is carried to the fruit of the legume, such as a pea, and gradually builds up in the fruit as it grows.

Protein

Pea accumulates protein

GARDEN PEAS

CHICKPEAS

FAVA BEANS

BLACK-EYED PEAS

Protein carried through plant

FRENCH BEANS

LENTILS

GREEN BEANS

Nutritional benefits of pulses

Pulses are a good source of protein, and compared with animal protein sources such as beef, are low in fat and high in fiber. Although pulses are high in carbohydrate, much of it is in the form of starch that is digested slowly, so they do not cause spikes in blood sugar levels. They are also rich in phytochemicals (see pp.110–11), and have high levels of minerals and B vitamins.

FAVA BEAN

Other 0.7%
Fat 0.7%
Protein 8%
Carbohydrate 17.6%
Water 73%

BEEF

Other 1%
Fat 5%
Protein 21%
Water 73%

REMOVING TOXINS

Some beans contain toxins that can cause serious poisoning if they are eaten raw. The best known example is probably red kidney beans, but lima beans and fava beans also contain toxins. The raw beans can be detoxified by soaking or cooking them thoroughly. This also softens them, which helps to make them easier to digest.

Beans soaking in water

2 Protein produced
Ammonia is converted into protein in the leaves and other parts of the plant. This protein is then distributed to cells throughout the plant.

PROTEIN

AMMONIA

Ammonia transported through plant

1 Nitrogen converted to ammonia
Rhizobium bacteria in root nodules convert nitrogen from the air into ammonia, which is then transported throughout the plant.

Nitrogen in the air

Ammonia

ROOT NODULE

Nitrogen taken up by bacteria in root nodules

Soy

Among beans, and among plant foods in general, soybeans are unusual in the completeness of the protein they provide. An important food for thousands of years in the East, soybean products have also been embraced by some in the West.

DO PLANT HORMONES IN SOY GIVE MEN MOOBS?

Some bodybuilders take soy protein to help muscles grow. Male bodybuilders may avoid it due to rumors that phytoestrogens—the plant hormones in soy—will make them feminine in physique! The levels are far too low to have such an effect.

Edamame beans

Soybeans have become familiar worldwide due to the popularity of immature beans, known as edamame in Japan. Soy milk, tofu, and soy sauce, however, are all made with mature beans.

Mature bean is yellow-brown

YOUNG SOYBEAN (EDAMAME)

MATURE SOYBEAN

Soy milk and tofu

Although they are full of nutritious protein and oil, mature soybeans are unpalatable until they are processed. In east Asia, people developed ways to extract the protein and oil and make them palatable. One method is to make soy milk by grinding and heating the beans. Soy milk is a useful product in itself, but a further step is to curdle it, making a kind of soy cheese—tofu.

5 Pressing
The curds are drained and may be broken up to release water. While still hot, the curds are pressed and cut into blocks.

CLOTH PRESS

4 Curdling
Soy milk is curdled with salts that encourage dissolved proteins to bond with protein-coated oil drops.

TOFU CURDLER

Coagulant salts mixed into soy milk to curdle it

3 Filtering
The pulp, consisting of the bean hull and fiber, is filtered out to leave soy milk.

SOY MILK PRESS

Soy milk is run off through filter

2 Cooking
The mash is cooked to inactivate enzymes that will otherwise split the oils into pungent aroma molecules.

HEATER

1 Soaking and mixing
The beans are soaked until soft and mashed into a slurry, releasing proteins and droplets of oil.

MIXER

Cooking is carried out before filtering in Japan; in China, the soy milk is filtered before cooking

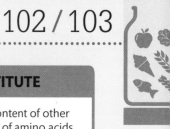

MEAT AND DAIRY SUBSTITUTE

Soybeans have twice the protein content of other beans and a nearly perfect balance of amino acids. Fortified with calcium, soy milk makes a good substitute for cow's milk. Other soy products can be used as meat substitutes, including tofu and textured vegetable protein (see pp.76–77).

36%

High-quality protein, with adequate quantities of essential amino acids

64%

Carbohydrates, fiber, minerals, oil, and water

1 Cooking
As with soy milk, the beans are soaked and cooked to prevent the plant's enzymes from producing "beany" flavors.

STEAM COOKER

2 Inoculating
The beans, along with cooked grains in Japanese-style soy sauce, are inoculated with spores of *Aspergillus* mold for a first fermentation.

GROWING FUNGUS

Temperature and humidity are controlled

Nugget of soybeans covered with mold

3 Fermenting
Immersion in brine kills the mold, but leaves its enzymes active. These aid a second fermentation carried out by bacteria and yeast.

Brine (salt and water) covers the mixture of beans, mold, yeast, and bacteria

FERMENTATION TANK

PROTEIN IN SOY MILK IS COMPLETE—IT PROVIDES ALL NINE ESSENTIAL AMINO ACIDS

4 Pressing
After around 6 months, the mix is pressed through a cloth and the raw soy sauce runs off.

CLOTH PRESS

5 Bottling
The sauce is pasteurized and filtered or clarified before bottling.

BOTTLES

Soy sauce

Soybeans are fermented to make a sauce containing much of the beans' goodness, including 10 times the antioxidants of red wine (see pp.170–71). Many modern soy sauces are produced chemically, skipping most fermentation steps, so they lack the friendly bacteria of traditional soy sauces. A necessary part of even traditional production is the addition of salt, since this prevents the growth of unwanted bacteria. Some soy sauces contain 14–18 percent salt, so they must be limited in a low-sodium diet (see pp.212–13).

Potatoes

First grown as a food crop in South America more than 7,000 years ago, potatoes were brought to Europe in the 16th century and have since become the most popular vegetable worldwide and an important source of food calories.

What's in a potato?

Potatoes are well known for having a high starch content, and a large proportion of this is in the form of amylopectin (see p.90). Amylopectin is easy to digest, so potatoes have a high glycemic index (see p.91). Potatoes are also rich in vitamin C, antioxidants, vitamin B6, and potassium; most of these nutrients, and the fiber, are in the skin.

OTHER 1.3%
FAT 0.1%
STARCH 15.4%
FIBER 2.1%
PROTEIN 2.1%
WATER 79%

Main nutrients in raw potatoes
Apart from water, potatoes consist mainly of starch. They also contain some fiber, protein, and phytochemicals (see pp.110–11), but almost no fat.

Effects of cooking

Different methods of cooking affect the relative amounts of nutrients, by driving off more or less water and also by adding components, such as extra fat during frying. Boiling can cause the starch granules in a potato's cells to soak up water. In floury potatoes, this makes the cells separate, giving a fine, dry texture, while in waxy potatoes the cells stick together, giving a denser, moister end product.

Main nutrients in cooked potatoes
The relative amounts of the main nutrients are very similar in boiled and baked potatoes but significantly different in chips and fries. This is because frying makes the potatoes absorb fat and also significantly reduces their water content.

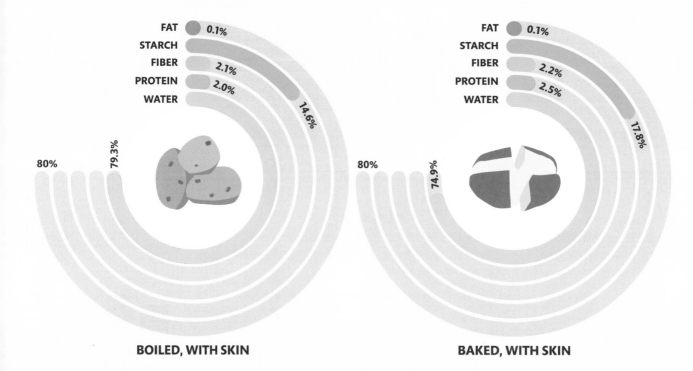

	BOILED, WITH SKIN	BAKED, WITH SKIN
FAT	0.1%	0.1%
STARCH	14.6%	17.8%
FIBER	2.1%	2.2%
PROTEIN	2.0%	2.5%
WATER	79.3% (80%)	74.9% (80%)

BOILED, WITH SKIN

BAKED, WITH SKIN

Uses of potatoes

Potatoes are extremely versatile vegetables. In cooking, floury varieties (including Yukon golds and russets) are suitable for roasting, frying, baking, and mashing, while waxy ones (such as fingerlings) are better for stews and hotpots, salads, and gratins. Because of its low cost, potato starch is also used in a wide variety of processed foods, for example, to help bind the ingredients in some cake mixtures, cookies, and even ice cream.

| STEWS AND SAUCES | COOKIES | ICE CREAM | CAKE MIXTURE | POTATO SNACKS |

Versatile starch
Potato starch is found in a surprising variety of foods, and so it is fortunate that potato seems to be one of the least allergenic foods tested.

POTATOES WERE THE **FIRST VEGETABLES** TO BE **GROWN IN SPACE**, IN A 1995 SPACE SHUTTLE EXPERIMENT

SWEET POTATOES

Sweet potatoes (which are often confused with yams but are different vegetables) originated in South America but are now popular in many countries. They owe their distinctive sweetness to an enzyme that breaks down their starch into maltose, a sugar that is sweeter than table sugar. Sweet potatoes also contain large amounts of beta carotene (which can be converted into vitamin A in the body), minerals, and plant estrogens.

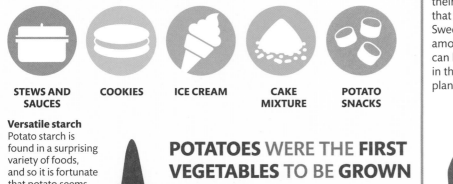

Higher percentage of fiber than baked or boiled potatoes due to lower water content

Water content reduced, resulting in increased proportions of other constituents

FAT
STARCH
FIBER
PROTEIN
WATER

3.8%
3.4%
14.7%
80%
38.6%
37.3%

FRIES, WITHOUT SKIN

Higher percentage of fat than fries due to much lower water content and greater fat absorption

Water content greatly reduced, resulting in much increased proportions of other constituents

FAT
STARCH
FIBER
PROTEIN
WATER

4.8%
7%
1.9%
80%
34.6%
47.9%

CHIPS, PLAIN, WITHOUT SKIN

Fruit and vegetables

Full of vitamins, minerals, fiber, and phytochemicals but low in fat and calories, fruit and vegetables are a vital part of a healthy, balanced diet.

Five a day

In many developed countries, the average person eats relatively little fruit and vegetables, but studies have shown that a diet high in these foods can lower the risk of some serious health problems, such as colorectal cancer, heart disease, and stroke. Because of this, the World Health Organization (WHO) has recommended that at least 14oz (400g) of fruit and vegetables should be eaten every day. Based on this recommendation, many health authorities have given guideline intakes, commonly "five a day," meaning that at least five 3oz (80g) portions of fruit and vegetables should be eaten every day.

What foods count?

Your five a day can include almost any fruit or vegetable, except for starchy ones, such as potatoes, yams, and cassavas. Beans and legumes also count, but only as one portion, no matter how much you eat. Fruit juice and smoothies can be included too, although some authorities say that they should be limited due to their high sugar content.

Reds
Red fruit and vegetables contain the carotenoid lycopene. This may lower the risk of certain cancers, although trials in humans have shown mixed results.

REDS

Purple lettuce

Five-a-day foods
To count in your five a day, fruit and vegetables do not have to be fresh. Beans and legumes also count, as do single servings of juice and smoothies.

PURPLES

Purples
The purple color is due to anthocyanin antioxidants. Some purple fruit and vegetables, such as purple lettuce and beets, are also high in nitrates, which may help to reduce blood pressure.

FRESH FRUIT AND VEGETABLES

CANNED FRUIT AND VEGETABLES

COOKED FRUIT AND VEGETABLES

FROZEN FRUIT AND VEGETABLES

BEANS AND LEGUMES

DRIED FRUIT

UNSWEETENED PURE FRUIT JUICE

UNSWEETENED SMOOTHIES

Carrot

ORANGES

Eating a rainbow

The different colors of fruit and vegetables indicate that they contain different phytochemicals (see pp.110–111). Many of these are natural antioxidants, some of which are believed to protect against disease. Although there is no strong scientific evidence to support the specific idea that "eating a rainbow" is especially beneficial, by doing so you will naturally eat a variety of fruit and vegetables, which can help to ensure you get essential nutrients, such as vitamins and minerals, and can also help toward your five a day.

Yellow and orange
Fruit and vegetables that are yellow or orange contain high levels of beta-carotene. which is converted in the body into vitamin A. Beta-carotene itself is not an essential nutrient, but vitamin A is. Carrots, grapefruit, corn, squash, sweet potatoes, and bell peppers are all high in beta-carotene.

YELLOWS

Corn

Banana

CAN I JUST EAT MY FAVOURITE FRUIT OR VEGETABLE?

No. Eating a varied selection is important because different fruit and vegetables contain different types of beneficial nutrients.

Greens
The green color is due to the pigment chlorophyll but many green-colored fruit and vegetables contain nutrients as well. For example, broccoli and kale contain lutein and zeaxanthin, phytochemicals that may aid eye health.

GREENS

PHYTOESTROGENS

These are hormones that are produced by plants and which may act as hormones in us—in particular, as oestrogens (female sex hormones). Phytoestrogens in fruit and vegetables may play a key role in maintaining health in women during and after the menopause. In studies, women who ate most fruit or who followed a Mediterranean diet were less likely to have hot flashes and night sweats.

Superfoods

The term "superfood" has no clear definition but is usually taken to mean a food that is high in beneficial substances and low in unhealthy ones, and that can help improve health, combat disease, or both.

Variety of superfoods

Superfoods are a type of functional food, said to possess unusually high levels of health-boosting nutrients with few, if any, dietary drawbacks. However, the term owes more to marketing hype and food faddism than to hard science. In practice, an enormous variety of fresh foods could qualify as superfoods, although there are some that stand out as being particularly rich in nutrients, such as kale, shellfish, and avocados.

Popular foods
The most high-profile foods often claimed to be superfoods include some genuine contenders, such as avocado and almonds, but also some unproven ones, such as goji berries and chia seeds.

POMEGRANATE

BROCCOLI

AVOCADO

ACAI BERRY

ALMOND

KALE

BLUEBERRY

Blueberries

One of the first foods to be called a superfood, blueberries are small blue fruits native to North America and are rich in vitamins C and K, fiber, the mineral manganese, and anthocyanin antioxidants (see pp.110–11). Several small-scale studies have suggested that blueberries may reduce the risk of cardiovascular disease and improve mental functioning but there is no conclusive evidence from large-scale studies to back up these, or other, more extreme health claims.

Blueberry consumption
The "superfood" label has led to a steep rise in blueberry consumption in the US, increasing five-fold in 20 years.

50 (45)
1995

100 (90)
2005

250 (225)
2015

x 1,000 TONS (METRIC TONS)

WHAT ARE FUNCTIONAL FOODS?

Foods that are said to produce health benefits beyond their basic nutritional value. The term may also be used to refer to foods that have been given extra benefits by adding more ingredients.

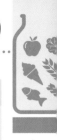

SUPERFOOD	HEALTH CLAIMS
Quinoa	High in protein, and a "complete" protein source containing all the essential amino acids; gluten-free
Broccoli	High in vitamins (especially vitamin C) and antioxidants; lowers cholesterol (limited supporting evidence); protects against some cancers (unproven)
Kale	High in iron and calcium; high in vitamins C and K; high in folate; helps to prevent or slow some age-related vision problems
Beets	Lowers blood pressure (some evidence that it may have a small effect); prevents dementia (unproven)
Garlic	Lowers blood pressure (limited supporting evidence); reduces cholesterol (true, but only a small reduction); protects against some cancers (limited supporting evidence)
Avocado	Contains monounsaturated fats that are good for the heart, fiber to help regulate blood sugar, plus vitamins K, E, and C, B vitamins, and potassium
Acai berry	High in antioxidants; may have anticancer and anti-inflammatory properties (unproven)
Blueberry	High in antioxidants and vitamin C
Goji berry	High in antioxidants; more vitamin C than an orange (untrue); increases longevity, enhances vision and fertility, slows aging (all unproven)
Pomegranate	Said to lower blood pressure and strengthen bones (both unproven, though blood pressure effect partly supported by some trials)
Almonds	Contain unsaturated fats that are good for the heart; high in fiber; high in antioxidants; high in B vitamins and vitamin E; high in minerals
Amaranth	High in protein; gluten-free; higher mineral content than many vegetables
Chia	Helps with weight loss (unproven); high in soluble fiber and protein; high in omega-3 fats
Linseed	High in omega-3 fats; high in soluble fiber
Green tea	Boosts metabolic rate (untrue); lowers cholesterol (limited supporting evidence); lowers blood pressure (some evidence that it may have a small effect); reduces risk of certain cancers (unproven)
Wheatgrass	Reduces bowel inflammation (unproven); boosts red blood cell numbers (unproven)

BEETS

GOJI BERRY

SOYBEAN

GARLIC

Manuka honey

All honey has antimicrobial properties but honey made by bees fed on manuka flower nectar has been shown to have unique antibacterial powers, proven against a wide range of pathogens. Sterile medicinal honeys are even used medically in wound gels.

Phytochemicals

More than just a passing fashion, naturally occurring phytochemicals have opened a new window into the health benefits and nutritional power of fruit, vegetables, and other plant foods.

What are phytochemicals?

Technically, phytochemicals are any chemicals produced by plants, and phytonutrients are specific types of phytochemicals that have nutritional value. However, in food science the two terms are often used to refer to the same thing—plant chemicals present in tiny amounts that are not immediately essential but which have (or are believed to have) long-term effects on health. Some foods contain large amounts of beneficial phytochemicals, offering the possibility of using them to improve health.

DO TOMATOES HELP PROTECT AGAINST CANCER?

Tomatoes are rich in lycopene, which has been linked to beneficial health effects on prostate cancer, although the scientific evidence for this effect is inconclusive.

The main phytochemicals
Phytochemicals can be categorized according to their chemical type. Some preliminary studies have reported promising health benefits but so far there is little supporting scientific evidence.

	Terpenes	Organosulfides	Saponins	Carotenoids	Polyphenols
EXAMPLES	Limonene, carnosol, pinene, myrcene, menthol	Allicin, sulforaphane, glutathione, isothiocyanate	Beta sitosterol, diosgenin, ginsenosides	Alpha and beta carotenes, beta cryptoxanthin, lycopene, lutein, zeaxanthin	Phenolic acids, stilbenes (e.g., resveratrol), lignans, flavonoids (e.g., catechins, anthocyanins, quercetin, genistein, daidzein, glycitein), tannins
HEALTH CLAIMS	May have antiseptic, antibacterial, antioxidant, anti-inflammatory, and anticancer properties	May have antioxidant, anticarcinogenic, and antimicrobial properties; the sulfur in these compounds plays a key part in protein synthesis and enzyme reactions	Mimic human steroids and hormones; may lower levels of cholesterol; may boost immune function; may have antimicrobial and antifungal properties	May inhibit growth of cancer cells; may enhance immune system response; may have antioxidant properties; some carotenoids can help to protect eye health (see p.115)	May inhibit inflammation and tumor growth; may reduce risk of asthma and coronary heart disease; some have antioxidant properties; some act as phytoestrogens (see p.107) and may reduce menopausal symptoms, such as hot flashes; some are associated with a lower risk of certain cancers in postmenopausal women
FOOD SOURCES	Citrus peel, cherries, hops, green herbs (e.g., mint, rosemary, bay, oregano, sage)	Green leafy vegetables, garlic, onions, horseradish, bok choy	Yams, quinoa, fenugreek, ginseng, soybeans, peas	Red, orange, yellow, and green fruit and vegetables	Apples, citrus fruits, berries, grapes, beets, onions, whole grains, walnuts, soy products, green beans, mung beans, kudzu root, chickpeas, coffee, tea

The antioxidant effect

Natural body processes and external factors produce free radicals (atoms or molecules missing an electron) inside cells. These are highly reactive and can cause cell damage. Normally, the body produces antioxidants that donate spare electrons and so neutralize the free radicals. But sometimes there are too many free radicals for the body to cope, in which case dietary antioxidants may help.

THERE ARE ABOUT **4,000 DIFFERENT** PHYTOCHEMICALS

3 Antioxidant action
Antioxidants have lots of spare electrons, which they can use to neutralize free radicals in the cell.

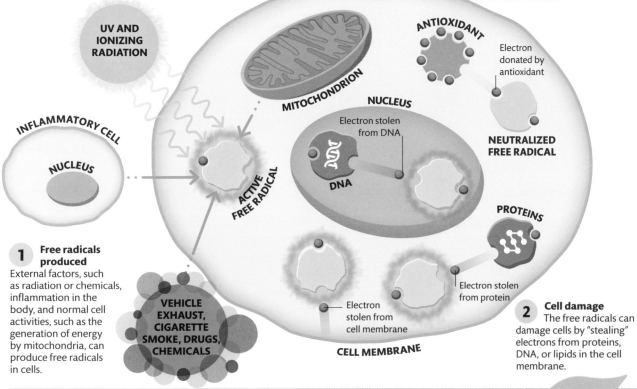

UV AND IONIZING RADIATION

ANTIOXIDANT

Electron donated by antioxidant

MITOCHONDRION

NUCLEUS

Electron stolen from DNA

NEUTRALIZED FREE RADICAL

INFLAMMATORY CELL

NUCLEUS

DNA

ACTIVE FREE RADICAL

PROTEINS

Electron stolen from protein

1 Free radicals produced
External factors, such as radiation or chemicals, inflammation in the body, and normal cell activities, such as the generation of energy by mitochondria, can produce free radicals in cells.

VEHICLE EXHAUST, CIGARETTE SMOKE, DRUGS, CHEMICALS

Electron stolen from cell membrane

CELL MEMBRANE

2 Cell damage
The free radicals can damage cells by "stealing" electrons from proteins, DNA, or lipids in the cell membrane.

Alkaloids

A diverse group of phytochemicals, alkaloids are produced by a wide range of plants to protect against disease and pests. They are the active ingredients in some plant foods, such as coffee beans (in which they are responsible for the bitter taste), and some are used medicinally, morphine, for example. Certain alkaloids, such as strychnine, are toxic.

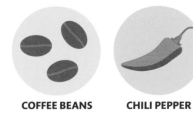

COFFEE BEANS   CHILI PEPPER

Sources of alkaloids
Many plant foods contain alkaloids, including coffee beans and chili peppers. The former contain the alkaloid caffeine; the latter contain capsaicin, responsible for the peppers' hotness.

Eat the skin

Plants typically produce most antioxidants in their outer parts, such as the skin of fruit and the outer part of leafy green vegetables, and these are therefore the best parts to eat for a good dose of antioxidants.

Fueling photosynthesis
The photons in sunlight power photosynthesis, but this same energy can damage DNA and other biological molecules. Plants produce protective antioxidants to help them overcome this stress.

Photons from sunlight hit the leaf surface

PHYTOCHEMICAL

Phytochemicals such as alkaloids and carotenoids, form a protective "shield," absorbing UV radiation

DNA

Energized free radical "steals" electron from DNA

2 Free radical production
Activated free radicals trigger chemical reactions and damage delicate molecules such as DNA by "stealing" electrons. Damage to DNA and other parts of the cell machinery can cause malfunctions and cell death.

ACTIVATED FREE RADICAL

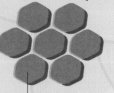

CHLOROPHYLL

1 Photosynthesis
UV radiation from the sun is absorbed by chlorophyll during photosynthesis, producing energy for the plant. Oxygen is produced as a byproduct along with activated free radicals.

Chlorophyll is abundant in green plants and gives leaves their color

DOES SPINACH MAKE YOU STRONG?

Spinach is rich in nitrate, which, when metabolized in the body, can make muscle cells more efficient. Indirectly then, spinach could help make you stronger (but you need to exercise, too!)

Leafy vegetables

The darker the leaf, the more packed it is likely to be with phytochemicals, not to mention many vitamins and minerals, all supplied in a virtually calorie-free, high-fiber package. This makes leafy greens—from spinach to curly kale—an undeniable superfood. But their strong and distinctive flavors are not for everyone.

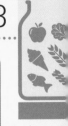

LEAFY AROMA

When a leaf is cut or crushed, enzymes are released from inside cells. These enzymes break up the long-chain fatty acids in the membranes of chloroplasts (small bodies that contain chlorophyll) to release hexanol and hexanal (leaf alcohol). These small molecules are responsible for the grassy aroma that is produced.

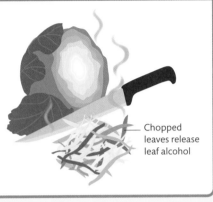

Chopped leaves release leaf alcohol

NEUTRALIZED FREE RADICAL

Antioxidant locks onto a free radical and inactivates it

ANTIOXIDANT

3 Antioxidant protection
Leaf cells are equipped with high levels of antioxidants to neutralize free radicals.

The goodness in greens

Leafy vegetables are low in calories as the plant does not use its leaves to store starch or sugars, only to make them. Leafy vegetables are also rich in fiber to support the spread and weight of the leaf, and they are packed with micronutrients to combat the biological "stress" caused by exposure to sunlight and oxygen production. The parts of the plant exposed to the most sun contain the most beneficial phytochemicals, including carotenoids and organosulfides (see pp.110–111).

A STEAK WITH A **CALORIE VALUE OF 1,700** HAS THE SAME IRON CONTENT AS **SPINACH PROVIDING JUST 100 CALORIES**

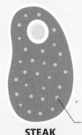

Iron from plants

Leafy greens are rich in iron (they may have higher levels than beef) but all their iron is the non-heme form, which is much less well-absorbed than the heme form found in animal meat. Because of this, vegetarians and vegans are recommended to consume up to 1.8 times more iron than meat eaters. However, adding a vitamin C source to a meal increases non-heme iron absorption up to six-fold; avoiding calcium and tannins (found in tea and coffee) also helps.

Non-heme iron

Just 10% of non-heme iron absorbed

Non-heme iron
The majority of iron in all diets is non-heme. However, only a small proportion of non-heme iron can be used by the body, so larger quantities are needed (for example, by vegetarians).

SPINACH

More heme iron absorbed

Heme iron
Heme is the iron-containing part of proteins found in blood and muscle; it is more readily used by the body than non-heme iron, with 25 percent of heme iron absorbed.

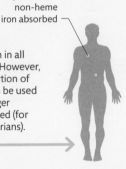

Heme iron

STEAK

Brassicas

The diverse members of the cabbage family are united by their nutritional prowess. They offer an amazing combination of healthy vitamins, minerals, and phytonutrients, but some can provoke strong reactions in consumers.

What's in them?

Brassicas are low in starch and sugars, but rich in other nutrients, particularly vitamins. They are packed with phytochemicals—plant substances thought to benefit health. Their distinctive taste and—to some—off-putting odors are mostly linked to their high levels of sulfur-containing compounds, which form part of a chemical defence system. Enzymes act on these compounds if the leaves are eaten or damaged, leading to a bitter taste.

WHY DO SPROUTS TASTE BETTER AFTER A FROST?

A cold snap stresses the plants and they respond by converting some of their stored starch into sugar for an energy boost, making them sweeter.

Brussels sprouts are the edible buds of the plant

BRUSSELS SPROUTS

CABBAGE

The whole plant is edible, not just the bulb

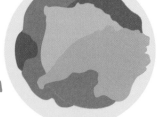

KOHLRABI

THE BRASSICA FAMILY TREE

Also called cruciferous vegetables (after their small cross-shaped flowers), the diverse brassica group sprang from two species of wild mustard, one Mediterranean and one from central Asia.

WILD MUSTARD

CAULIFLOWER

The flowering head of the plant is edible

BROCCOLI

SPRING GREENS

Kale leaves and stems are edible

KALE

Cancer fighters

Alongside health-boosting nutrients such as iron, calcium, potassium, and vitamins C, K, and A, brassicas are also rich in phytochemicals such as carotenoids, polyphenols, and particularly isothiocyanates and indoles. In addition to being anti-inflammatories, isothiocyanates and indoles are thought to fight cancer by triggering apoptosis, a process akin to cellular suicide, in which cells kill themselves. Cancer cells normally take no notice of signals for cell death, so setting off apoptosis can destroy tumors.

Anticancer activity
Scientists are interested in the phytochemicals in brassicas, and suspect they might fight cancers of the lung, prostate, breast, colon, and rectum.

BREAST

LUNG

Varying results, but evidence of a lowered lung cancer risk from brassicas, especially in women

A review of several studies concluded there was little evidence of a link between brassicas and breast cancer risk

COLORECTAL

Some evidence from small studies suggests lowered risk of cancer

PROSTATE

One Dutch study found brassicas to be a benefit to women in reducing risk of colon cancer

BIOAVAILABILITY

A food may be rich in nutrients, but how many of them will actually make it into the bloodstream? The degree to which nutrients can be accessed is known as bioavailability, and it can be boosted by other substances. For instance, uptake of iron from brassicas is increased in the presence of vitamin C, while adding a little fat or oil to green vegetables helps the body absorb more of the fat-soluble vitamins A, D, E, and K.

Oil in dressings can improve bioavailability

Eye health

The eye is vulnerable to infection and dryness, but also particularly to the damaging effects of light, especially high-energy ultraviolet light, which knocks electrons off atoms to create harmful free radicals (see p.111). These in turn can cause cell and DNA damage, boosting the risk of age-related macular degeneration and cataracts. Certain carotenoids, which are antioxidants found in brassicas, may slow the progress of macular degeneration and help to reduce the incidence of cataracts.

 ABOUT 30 PERCENT OF PEOPLE CANNOT TASTE THE BITTERNESS OF BRASSICAS

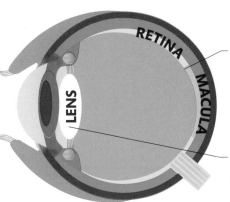

RETINA

MACULA

LENS

Carotenoids, such as lutein and zeaxanthin, concentrate in the macula and can protect eye health

The antioxidants found in brassicas may help to prevent cataracts by protecting the lens

Preserving vision
The macula is the part of the retina with the keenest vision. This is where carotenoids concentrate, giving it a distinct yellow color.

Root vegetables

Nature's storehouses, root vegetables have long been among the most accessible sources of calories for much of the world's population. Although they can be bland—and some are even toxic—root vegetables also provide minerals and other valuable nutrients.

Types of root vegetables

What we call root vegetables are the edible underground parts of plants. Not all of them are actually roots, as they include modified stems. These vegetables have evolved or been bred to be energy storage organs, a way for plants to store sugars, starch, other carbohydrates, and nutrients. They fall into three broad categories: tubers, taproot vegetables, and bulb vegetables. Taproot vegetables are true roots; they include carrots, beets, celeriac, daikon, parsnips, turnips, rutabagas, and radishes. Bulb vegetables are modified stems; they include garlic, onions, leeks, and shallots. Tubers are also modified stems; they include potatoes, sweet potatoes, yams, cassavas, and Jerusalem artichokes.

Taproot vegetables
These vegetables are true roots, helping to absorb moisture and nutrients from the ground. The taproot is the first root that the seed grows when it germinates. Carrots and parsnips are related taproots notable for their relatively low starch and high sugar content.

CARROT

CORTEX

LATERAL ROOT

EPIDERMIS

STORAGE ROOT

TAP ROOT

TOXIC TUBERS

Cassavas (also called manioc) are a staple food in many developing countries but they contain toxic cyanides, mainly in the peel and cortex layer immediately under the peel, which is why cassavas are peeled before being processed or eaten. Sweet varieties generally contain lower levels of cyanides; bitter-tasting ones contain higher levels and must be processed to remove them, often by soaking in water.

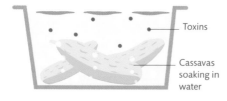

Toxins

Cassavas soaking in water

DO CARROTS HELP YOU SEE IN THE DARK?

Carrots are high in beta-carotene, which the body converts into vitamin A, vital for eye health. If your diet contains enough of these nutrients, eating more will not improve your vision.

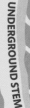

ONION

SCALE LEAF

TUNIC

ROOT

UNDERGROUND STEM

STOLON

ROOT

MOTHER TUBER

POTATO

SKIN

CORTEX

TUBER

Bulb vegetables
Onions and other bulb vegetables are underground, modified stems with specially adapted scale leaves or buds. The plant pumps these full of storage nutrients to use as an energy store during winter until it sprouts again the following spring.

Tubers
Like bulb vegetables, tubers are underground plant stems modified to store nutrients. With their high starch content, tubers have been an important calorie source since prehistoric times and remain a global food staple today.

High fiber, high starch

Root vegetables are often unfairly overlooked as "superfoods". In fact most of them are high in fiber, minerals, and vitamins. Even when they are high in carbohydrates, these tend to be "slow-burning" types with a relatively low glycemic index (see p.91) and calories. Yams are a good example. Not to be confused with sweet potatoes, true yams are native to Africa and are used widely in Asian cuisine. They are chiefly composed of complex carbohydrates and soluble dietary fiber.

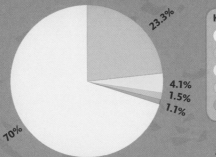

23.3%

4.1%
1.5%
1.1%

70%

KEY
- Water
- Starch
- Fiber
- Protein
- Other

Nutrients in yams
Yams are 70 percent water, but the vast majority of the rest is carbohydrate, including 23 percent starch and 4 percent fiber. They are also rich in B vitamins and vitamin C, and high in minerals such as copper, calcium, potassium, iron, manganese, and phosphorus.

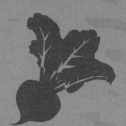

THE **RED** PIGMENT **BETALAIN IN BEETS** IS OFTEN USED AS A **FOOD COLORING**

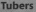

The onion family

The fearsome chemical defenses of the members of the onion family make them treasured kitchen companions for cooks seeking pungency, flavor, and a powerful punch of health-boosting phytochemicals.

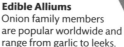

Edible Alliums
Onion family members are popular worldwide and range from garlic to leeks.

Scallions are harvested before they grow a large bulb

Meet the relatives

Onions and their relatives are edible members of the *Allium* genus, which store their energy in swollen leaf bases or scales. Crucially, their energy stores are not of starch, but of chains of fructose sugars, such as inulin, which break down with long, slow cooking to produce sweet flavors.

The bulb of an onion is not a root, but a mass of enlarged leaf bases

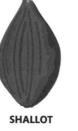

GARLIC SHALLOT ONION CHIVE SCALLION LEEK

Garlicky goodness

Like all of the onion family, garlic produces sulfur compounds designed to irritate and ward off herbivores, but which can also boost human health. Garlic's sulfur defenses consist of the antioxidant allicin, among others. As with onions, the defensive chemicals are produced by enzymes released when cells are damaged. So to get the full nutritional benefits of garlic, it is best to crush the garlic and leave the enzymes to work for a while before destroying them in the cooking pan.

30 SECONDS
THE TIME BETWEEN
CUTTING AN ONION
AND IT **MAKING YOU CRY**

Widens blood vessels
Garlic has been shown to relax peripheral blood vessels, producing a "warming" effect that boosts circulation and improves nail health.

Combats "bad" cholesterol
Allicin protects bad cholesterol from oxidation (which increases the risk it will clog up arteries). It also helps the body to expel the bad cholesterol faster.

Lowers blood pressure
Since garlic relaxes small blood vessels, it should also reduce blood pressure, and indeed there is evidence of a small but significant effect.

Fights colds
Traditionally used as a cold treatment, garlic does have antiviral properties, but more study is needed to confirm that garlic works.

Reduces blood stickiness
Sulfur compounds in garlic help to reduce the stickiness of platelets in the blood, reducing the risk that they create unwanted blood clots and subsequent blockages.

Why do onions make us tearful?

Onions release chemical weapons when they are damaged. Their chemical cascade begins with alliin, like garlic, but the important product is not allicin, but lachrymatory ("tear-jerking") factor, intended to sting the eyes of would be onion-munchers. Chefs wishing to avoid tears can try cooling the onion before cutting or using an extremely sharp knife to minimize cell damage.

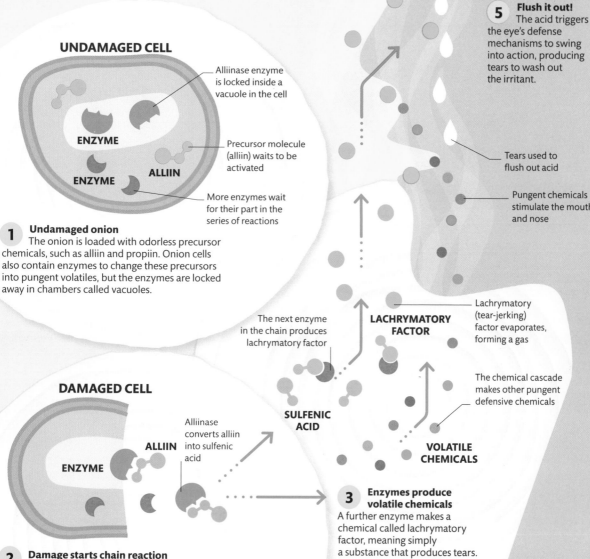

UNDAMAGED CELL

Alliinase enzyme is locked inside a vacuole in the cell

ENZYME

Precursor molecule (alliin) waits to be activated

ENZYME

ALLIIN

More enzymes wait for their part in the series of reactions

1 **Undamaged onion**
The onion is loaded with odorless precursor chemicals, such as alliin and propiin. Onion cells also contain enzymes to change these precursors into pungent volatiles, but the enzymes are locked away in chambers called vacuoles.

DAMAGED CELL

Alliinase converts alliin into sulfenic acid

ALLIIN

ENZYME

2 **Damage starts chain reaction**
Damage to the cell breaks open the vacuole and mixes the alliinase enzymes with the alliin, and the damage response sequence is set in motion.

The next enzyme in the chain produces lachrymatory factor

SULFENIC ACID

LACHRYMATORY FACTOR

Lachrymatory (tear-jerking) factor evaporates, forming a gas

The chemical cascade makes other pungent defensive chemicals

VOLATILE CHEMICALS

3 **Enzymes produce volatile chemicals**
A further enzyme makes a chemical called lachrymatory factor, meaning simply a substance that produces tears. It evaporates, along with some other volatile chemicals produced.

4 **Onion chemical forms acid in eye**
The lachrymatory factor diffuses quickly through the air to reach the eyes. It dissolves in the layer of fluid that coats the eye and some of it forms sulfuric acid, stinging the eye.

PAIN SIGNAL TO BRAIN

BRAIN

"CRY" SIGNAL FROM BRAIN

5 **Flush it out!**
The acid triggers the eye's defense mechanisms to swing into action, producing tears to wash out the irritant.

Tears used to flush out acid

Pungent chemicals stimulate the mouth and nose

Vegetable fruits

Although they are fruits in the botanical sense of the word, in a culinary sense, these plant products are definitely vegetables, lending themselves to a huge range of culinary applications and loaded with macro- and micronutrients.

Fruit or vegetable?

Botanically speaking, a fruit is the seed-bearing structure that develops from the ovary at the base of a flower. Many are sweet and fit the culinary definition of fruit (see pp.122–23), but a few are comparatively low in sugar, richer in non-sweet flavors, and generally require cooking. These fall under the culinary heading of "vegetable." They include vegetables with high levels of phytochemicals, such as pumpkin and squash, whose orange color comes from beta-carotene, capsaicin-filled chilies and peppers (see pp.128–29), and lycopene-rich tomatoes.

Types of vegetable fruits

Vegetable fruits belong mainly to three families: the nightshade family (including tomatoes, eggplants, and peppers) which tends to grow upward on a vine, the squash and cucumber family (including marrow, zucchini, and melons) which grows along vines on the ground, and the legume, or bean, family (see pp.100–01).

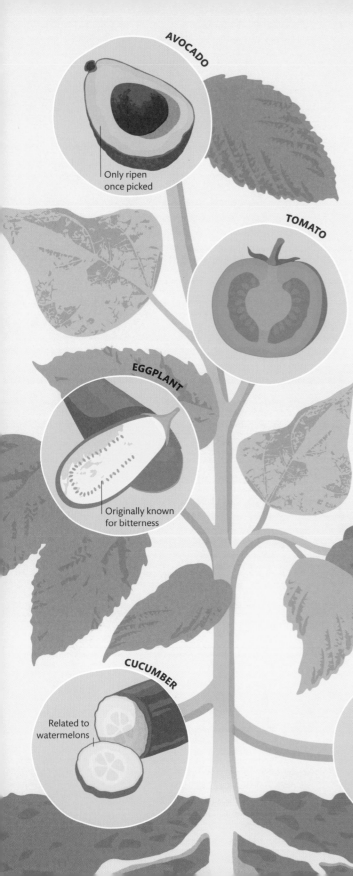

AVOCADO
Only ripen once picked

TOMATO

EGGPLANT
Originally known for bitterness

CUCUMBER
Related to watermelons

PUMPKIN
Largest fruit in the world

SQUASH
High in dietary fiber

How ketchup is made

Based on Chinese fish brine sauces brought back to the West by seamen and merchants, and combined with tomatoes native to America by New Englanders, ketchup is made by cooking and pureeing tomatoes and blending the puree with vinegar, herbs, spices, and sweeteners. Though often very high in salt, sugar, and calories, it can also contain higher levels of the powerful antioxidant lycopene than raw tomatoes.

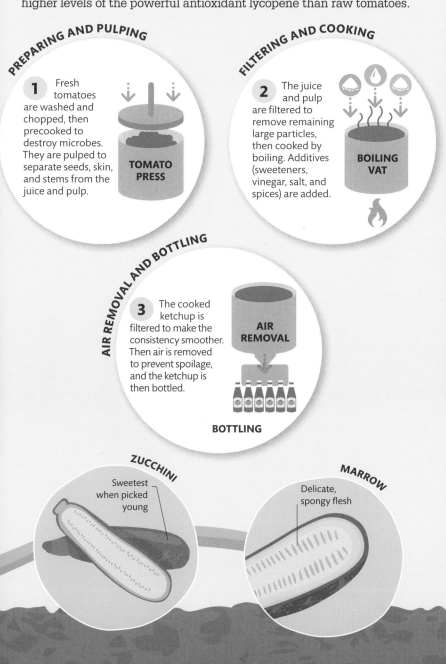

PREPARING AND PULPING

1 Fresh tomatoes are washed and chopped, then precooked to destroy microbes. They are pulped to separate seeds, skin, and stems from the juice and pulp.

TOMATO PRESS

FILTERING AND COOKING

2 The juice and pulp are filtered to remove remaining large particles, then cooked by boiling. Additives (sweeteners, vinegar, salt, and spices) are added.

BOILING VAT

AIR REMOVAL AND BOTTLING

3 The cooked ketchup is filtered to make the consistency smoother. Then air is removed to prevent spoilage, and the ketchup is then bottled.

AIR REMOVAL

BOTTLING

ZUCCHINI

Sweetest when picked young

MARROW

Delicate, spongy flesh

Unusual avocado

Avocados are extraordinarily oily, containing 15–30 percent oil and with very low levels of sugar and starch. The name comes from the Nahuatl (Aztec) word *ahuacatl*, meaning "testicle." Avocados can easily be pureed to make guacamole and other dishes.

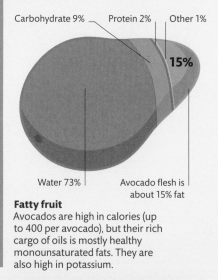

Carbohydrate 9%   Protein 2%   Other 1%

15%

Water 73%   Avocado flesh is about 15% fat

Fatty fruit
Avocados are high in calories (up to 400 per avocado), but their rich cargo of oils is mostly healthy monounsaturated fats. They are also high in potassium.

KILLER FRUITS

Zucchini can contain toxins called cucurbitacins. Cultivated varieties are bred to have low toxin levels, but ornamental varieties can have high levels. The toxin is not destroyed by cooking, and poisoning can sometimes be fatal.

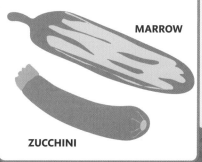

MARROW

ZUCCHINI

Sweet fruits

Evolved to appeal to animals and enhanced by humans to combine flavor, aroma, sweetness, and visual appeal, fruits are rich in vital antioxidants. There are several different categories, and many thousands of varieties found and grown worldwide.

Types of fruit

Several foods we call vegetables are technically fruits (see pp.120–21), but in culinary terms, fruits are generally distinguished by their high sugar content and the fact that they can be eaten raw. Their sweetness can give them a high glycemic load and calorie count, but this is counterbalanced by their rich loads of fiber, vitamins, and phytochemicals, particularly pigments and antioxidants, often concentrated in the skins. The simple fruits shown below grow from the ovaries of a single flower, but in aggregate fruits such as raspberries, many fruits develop from one flower, while a multiple fruit, such as pineapple, grows from many flowers.

ARE APPLE SEEDS POISONOUS?

They do contain a compound that degrades into cyanide, but you would need to eat more than 100 crushed, ground apple seeds for a lethal dose.

BANANAS NATURALLY CONTAIN A **TINY, HARMLESS AMOUNT** OF **RADIOACTIVE POTASSIUM**

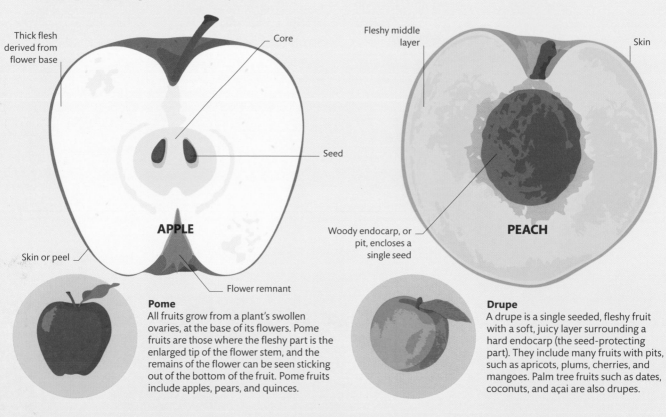

Thick flesh derived from flower base

Core

Seed

Skin or peel

APPLE

Flower remnant

Fleshy middle layer

Skin

Woody endocarp, or pit, encloses a single seed

PEACH

Pome
All fruits grow from a plant's swollen ovaries, at the base of its flowers. Pome fruits are those where the fleshy part is the enlarged tip of the flower stem, and the remains of the flower can be seen sticking out of the bottom of the fruit. Pome fruits include apples, pears, and quinces.

Drupe
A drupe is a single seeded, fleshy fruit with a soft, juicy layer surrounding a hard endocarp (the seed-protecting part). They include many fruits with pits, such as apricots, plums, cherries, and mangoes. Palm tree fruits such as dates, coconuts, and açai are also drupes.

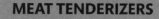
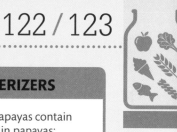

How fruit ripens

Ripening is a complex process that involves several substances. It starts when the fruit releases a burst of ethylene gas. This, in turn, triggers the release of enzymes. These enzymes act on various natural chemicals in the fruit, turning it from hard, green, and acidic into a softer, sweeter, more appealing food.

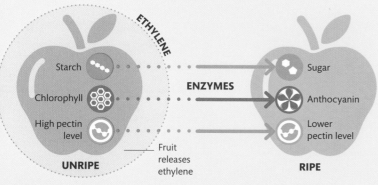

ETHYLENE

Starch

Chlorophyll

High pectin level

UNRIPE

Fruit releases ethylene

ENZYMES

Sugar

Anthocyanin

Lower pectin level

RIPE

The ripening process

During ripening, enzymes produced by the fruit convert starch into sugars, and green chlorophyll is replaced by anthocyanin pigments. They also reduce the amount of hard pectin, making the fruit softer, and reduce the amount of acid, making the fruit less sour. Ripe fruit gets its aroma from large organic molecules being broken down into smaller, volatile ones.

MEAT TENDERIZERS

Pineapples and papayas contain enzymes (papain in papayas; bromelain in pineapples) that break down proteins in meat into smaller peptide molecules; the effect of this is to make the meat tender.

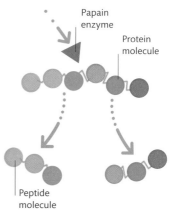

Papain enzyme

Protein molecule

Peptide molecule

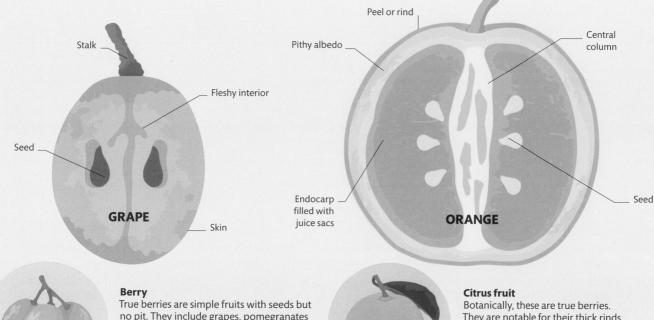

Peel or rind

Pithy albedo

Central column

Stalk

Fleshy interior

Seed

Endocarp filled with juice sacs

Seed

GRAPE

Skin

ORANGE

Berry

True berries are simple fruits with seeds but no pit. They include grapes, pomegranates (whose flesh-covered seeds are eaten), and many vegetable fruits. A number of fruits we call berries are not (such as raspberries and strawberries) while, in botanical terms, bananas and kiwis are berries.

Citrus fruit

Botanically, these are true berries. They are notable for their thick rinds and high acidity. Citrus peel is higher in vitamin C than the flesh, and is packed with antioxidants. The bitter-tasting pithy albedo is high in pectin, known to help lower cholesterol.

Mushrooms and fungi

Mushrooms are probably the most familiar examples of a unique group of organisms—fungi—that also includes molds and yeasts. Fungi are not only foods themselves but are also vital for making other items in the diet, such as bread, cheese, and alcohol.

Versatile food

Fungi are neither plants nor animals but make up their own separate group of living things. Some fungi, notably mushrooms, feed on dead and decaying matter, yet they can be healthy components of the diet and a sustainable source of protein and micronutrients; some species, however, can be highly toxic. Their relatives—yeasts and mold—are used to transform foods and are essential for processes such as fermentation (see pp.52–53).

Uses of fungi

Fungal protein (mycoprotein) may be used by itself as a food or it may be processed into other meat substitutes. Fungi are used to produce the veins in blue cheese and the rind of some soft cheeses (see pp.88–89), and the Japanese seasoning miso relies on fermentation by fungi for its unique taste. Mushrooms are also one of the few plant sources of vitamin D for vegetarians.

Use of fungi and yeasts

We use both fungi and yeasts to make soy sauce. First, a fungus ferments the soybeans and wheat, breaking down the proteins. Then yeasts carry out a second fermentation to break down the protein components to amino acids, which help to add more flavor.

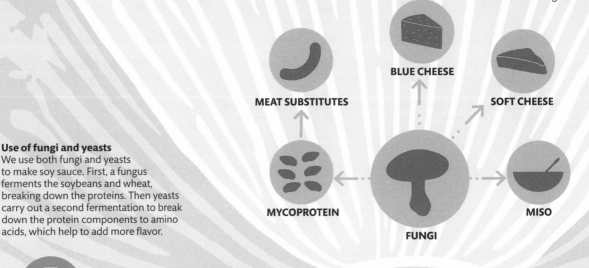

MEAT SUBSTITUTES

BLUE CHEESE

SOFT CHEESE

MYCOPROTEIN

FUNGI

MISO

SOY SAUCE

FUNGI AND YEASTS

YEASTS

THERE ARE ABOUT **100** SPECIES OF **POISONOUS MUSHROOMS** IN NORTH AMERICA ALONE

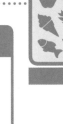
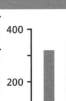

Poisonous mushrooms

Poisonous and nonpoisonous species of fungus can look very similar and live side-by-side. The various poisonous fungi produce a wide range of toxins (collectively called mycotoxins), including aflatoxins produced by molds and amatoxins produced by mushrooms. Some mushrooms, known generically as psilocybin mushrooms, also produce hallucinogens.

Fatal fungi
The difficulty in identifying mushrooms that are safe to eat means that field mushrooms should be picked only under expert supervision.

POTASSIUM SOURCE

Mushrooms are a good source of potassium. Raw white mushrooms, for example, contain almost as much potassium, weight for weight, as bananas and have the added advantage of containing much less sugar—about one-quarter of the amount in bananas.

POTASSIUM MG/100G (3.5 OZ)

Fly agaric
This red-topped mushroom contains several toxins, plus the hallucinogen muscimol

Autumn skullcap
The autumn skullcap contains the same amatoxins as the death cap

Death cap
Containing amatoxins, the death cap is a common cause of fatal mushroom poisoning

LOW TOXICITY   HIGH TOXICITY

Deadly dapperling
Resembling an edible variety, this mushroom contains amatoxins that can cause liver damage

Destroying angel
Actually several related species, destroying angels have the same amatoxins as the death cap

Aflatoxins

The mold *Aspergillus flavus* grows on peanuts and grains in humid conditions. It produces aflatoxins, which threaten the health of any animals eating contaminated nuts or grain. They are also extremely dangerous to humans, causing liver damage and, potentially, liver cancer.

BREAD

ALCOHOLIC DRINKS

Uses of yeasts
We use yeasts to produce the alcohol we use in drinks and the carbon dioxide gas that makes bread rise. The alcohol and carbon dioxide happen to be by-products of the yeast eating starch and sugar.

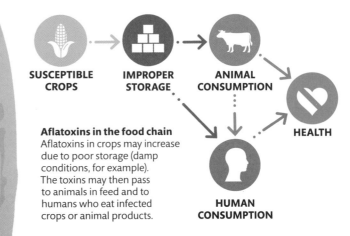

SUSCEPTIBLE CROPS → **IMPROPER STORAGE** → **ANIMAL CONSUMPTION**

HEALTH

HUMAN CONSUMPTION

Aflatoxins in the food chain
Aflatoxins in crops may increase due to poor storage (damp conditions, for example). The toxins may then pass to animals in feed and to humans who eat infected crops or animal products.

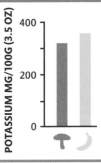

Nuts and seeds

Most nuts are seeds, so it is not surprising that nuts and seeds have a lot in common nutritionally. Both are rich sources of healthy fats and important phytochemicals.

What's the difference between nuts and seeds?

A seed is an embryo plant inside a protective outer covering. Seeds can be grains (see pp.92–93), legumes, such as peas, beans, and peanuts (see pp.100–01), or nuts. A nut is generally an edible seed with a hard shell. Botanically, a true nut is a hard-shelled pod that contains fruit with a single seed; hazelnuts are an example. Nuts can also be the seeds of drupes, which have soft flesh on the outside of the fruit. Drupe nuts include walnuts, and also almonds, which are closely related to peaches and plums (see pp.122–23).

Fruits, nuts, and seeds

Only a few nuts, including chestnuts and macadamias, represent the entire fruit of a plant. The rest are just the seeds of a larger whole. Pine nuts are exceptional in that they are produced by a cone-bearing, not a fruiting, plant. Millet can be classified as a grain rather than a seed.

NUTS

NUTS THAT ARE FRUITS

Sweet chestnuts

Hazelnuts

NUTS THAT ARE SEEDS

Peanuts

Pecan nuts

Macadamia nuts

Almonds

Walnuts

Cashews

Brazil nuts

Pistachios

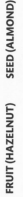
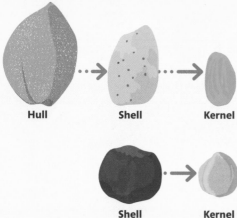

SEED (ALMOND)

Hull → Shell → Kernel

FRUIT (HAZELNUT)

Shell → Kernel

Two types of nuts

In some nuts that are seeds, a fleshy hull surrounds a shell that encloses the kernel—the edible nut. In almonds, the flesh is equivalent to the flesh of its close relatives peaches and cherries, but it is not edible. In nuts that are fruits, there is no outer fleshy hull.

HOW CAN I TELL IF NUTS HAVE GONE BAD?

With a high fat content, nuts are liable to go rancid. Their insides should be opaque or off-white; darkening or translucency is a sign they are past their best.

SEEDS

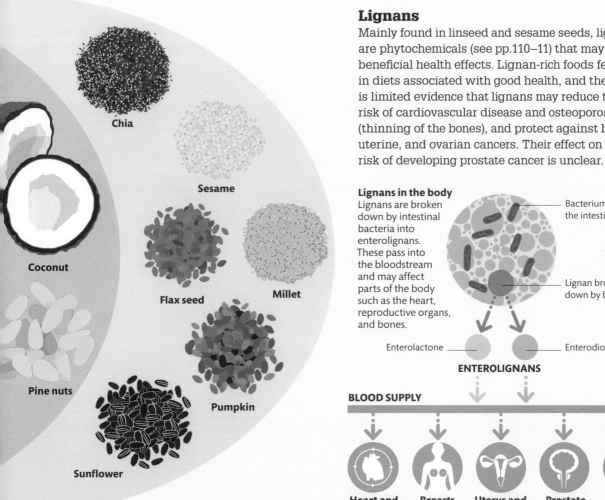

Chia

Sesame

Coconut

Flax seed

Millet

Pine nuts

Pumpkin

Sunflower

Lignans

Mainly found in linseed and sesame seeds, lignans are phytochemicals (see pp.110–11) that may have beneficial health effects. Lignan-rich foods feature in diets associated with good health, and there is limited evidence that lignans may reduce the risk of cardiovascular disease and osteoporosis (thinning of the bones), and protect against breast, uterine, and ovarian cancers. Their effect on the risk of developing prostate cancer is unclear.

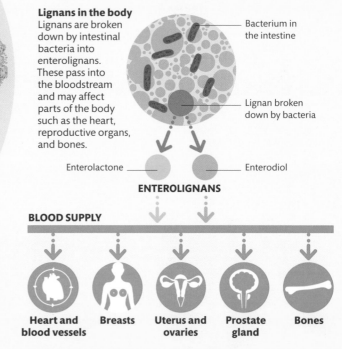

Lignans in the body
Lignans are broken down by intestinal bacteria into enterolignans. These pass into the bloodstream and may affect parts of the body such as the heart, reproductive organs, and bones.

Bacterium in the intestine

Lignan broken down by bacteria

Enterolactone

Enterodiol

ENTEROLIGNANS

BLOOD SUPPLY

Heart and blood vessels

Breasts

Uterus and ovaries

Prostate gland

Bones

Oils in nuts and seeds

Nuts and seeds are among the most calorific foods available, mainly due to their high fat content. They are particularly high in omega-6 fatty acids, which are vital for brain function and cell growth and development. However, aside from walnuts and linseeds, they are relatively low in omega-3 fatty acids (oily fish are rich sources, see pp.78–79), which may help to protect against heart disease.

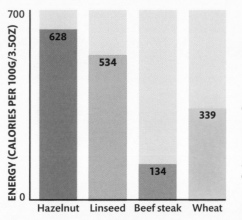

ENERGY (CALORIES PER 100G/3.5OZ)

700

0

628 — Hazelnut
534 — Linseed
134 — Beef steak
339 — Wheat

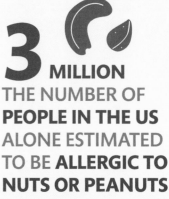

3 MILLION
THE NUMBER OF **PEOPLE IN THE US** ALONE ESTIMATED TO BE **ALLERGIC TO NUTS OR PEANUTS**

Chilies and other hot foods

Prized for adding kick to dishes, chili peppers and other hot or pungent foods, such as mustard and horseradish, come armed with powerful chemical defenses that we can use for flavor but that may also prove to have health benefits.

How hot is hot?

Chilies get their spicy heat from the chemical compound capsaicin. We measure the capsaicin concentration of chilies and chili-derived products by using the Scoville scale, devised by Walter Scoville in 1912. The scale originally indicated how many times a chili extract had to be diluted before its heat became imperceptible to a panel of five tasters. Today the Scoville scale has been updated to provide a direct measurement of capsaicin levels, using scientific analysis instead of subjectivity. In addition to creating this heat sensation, capsaicin also disrupts the mitochondria (the cell's power-stations). Cancer cells are particularly vulnerable to this, so much so that capsaicin is being tested as an anticancer drug. Other hot foods, such as horseradish and mustard, get their heat from pungent, volatile compounds, and can be judged on a pungency scale.

16 MILLION
THE SCOVILLE HEAT UNITS IN PURE CAPSAICIN

CAN CHILIES AID WEIGHT LOSS?

Research in mice found that capsaicin helped convert white fat to healthier brown fat; other research suggests that chili reduces cravings for fat and sugar.

The Scoville scale
The traditional chart topper was the habanero, but in recent years, new breeds of superhot chili peppers have been created with Scoville ratings of over 2 million. Precise levels vary from plant to plant and even between individual chilies.

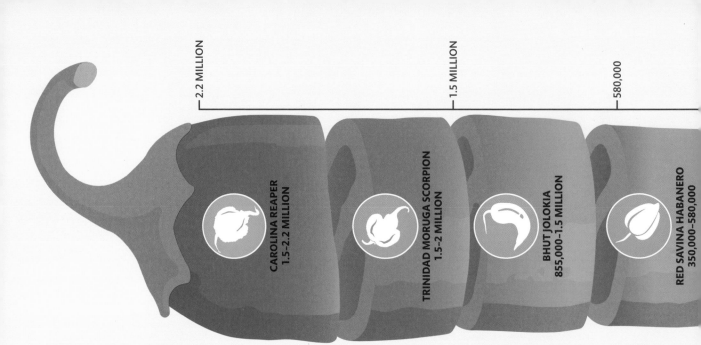

2.2 MILLION

1.5 MILLION

580,000

CAROLINA REAPER
1.5–2.2 MILLION

TRINIDAD MORUGA SCORPION
1.5–2 MILLION

BHUT JOLOKIA
855,000–1.5 MILLION

RED SAVINA HABANERO
350,000–580,000

SCOVILLE HEAT UNITS (SHU)

350,000   100,000   50,000   30,000   10,000   0

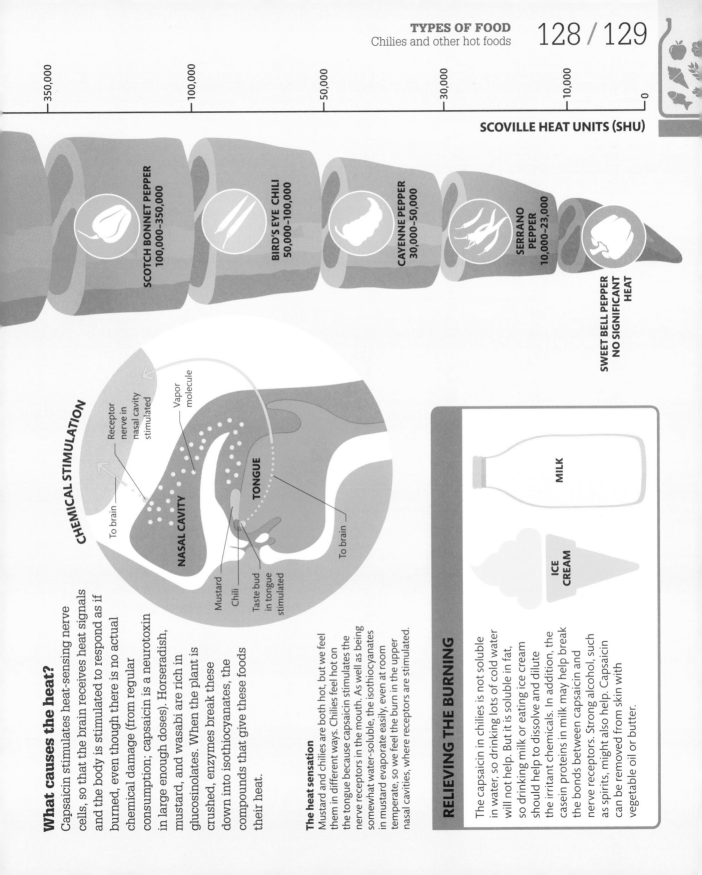

SCOTCH BONNET PEPPER
100,000–350,000

BIRD'S EYE CHILI
50,000–100,000

CAYENNE PEPPER
30,000–50,000

SERRANO PEPPER
10,000–23,000

SWEET BELL PEPPER
NO SIGNIFICANT HEAT

What causes the heat?

Capsaicin stimulates heat-sensing nerve cells, so that the brain receives heat signals and the body is stimulated to respond as if burned, even though there is no actual chemical damage (from regular consumption; capsaicin is a neurotoxin in large enough doses). Horseradish, mustard, and wasabi are rich in glucosinolates. When the plant is crushed, enzymes break these down into isothiocyanates, the compounds that give these foods their heat.

The heat sensation

Mustard and chilies are both hot, but we feel them in different ways. Chilies feel hot on the tongue because capsaicin stimulates the nerve receptors in the mouth. As well as being somewhat water-soluble, the isothiocyanates in mustard evaporate easily, even at room temperate, so we feel the burn in the upper nasal cavities, where receptors are stimulated.

CHEMICAL STIMULATION

Receptor nerve in nasal cavity stimulated

Vapor molecule

To brain

NASAL CAVITY

TONGUE

Mustard

Chili

Taste bud in tongue stimulated

To brain

RELIEVING THE BURNING

MILK

ICE CREAM

The capsaicin in chilies is not soluble in water, so drinking lots of cold water will not help. But it is soluble in fat, so drinking milk or eating ice cream should help to dissolve and dilute the irritant chemicals. In addition, the casein proteins in milk may help break the bonds between capsaicin and nerve receptors. Strong alcohol, such as spirits, might also help. Capsaicin can be removed from skin with vegetable oil or butter.

Spices

Spices are parts or extracts of dried seeds, fruits, roots, or bark—in contrast to herbs, which are the flowers, leaves, or stems from plants. Spices have been used for centuries for flavoring, coloring, and preserving food, and are key to producing the unique taste of many regional dishes. They also have a long history as traditional health remedies.

DOES CLOVE OIL REALLY RELIEVE TOOTHACHE?

Yes, a drop of clove oil placed on the area next to the aching tooth may help to ease pain temporarily, but it will not cure the underlying cause of the pain.

What makes spices spicy?

The flavors of spices are mainly due to aromatic oils they contain. These may make up as much as 15 percent of the weight of a spice and mostly consist of various phytochemicals (see pp.110–11), particularly terpenes (also known as terpenoids) and phenols (or phenolics). Each spice typically contains a unique mixture of several different terpenes and phenols, and this is what gives each spice its characteristic flavor.

Flavor chemicals
Many different chemicals contribute to the flavor of spices, although in some spices a single one may be dominant, such as eugenol in cloves and anethole in star anise. Heating releases more of the chemicals, although too much heat can destroy them.

Molecule of eugenol (a phenol)

Molecule of anethole (a terpene)

CLOVE

HEAT

STAR ANISE

Spices and health

With a history of use in traditional medicine, spices have attracted many health claims. However, most of these claims have not been rigorously assessed. Some chemicals in spices—certain phenols and terpenes—do seem to have beneficial health effects in laboratory tests, but there is little supporting evidence from studies carried out on people.

THE STAMENS OF **70,000 CROCUSES** ARE NEEDED TO PRODUCE **1LB (450G)** OF **SAFFRON**

Cinnamon
Claims for regulating blood pressure, lowering blood fat levels, and reducing the risk of blood clots are unproven.

Ginger
Some evidence that it may help to relieve nausea; claims for anticancer and antimigraine properties are unproven.

Nutmeg
Some evidence for antimicrobial, anti-inflammatory, and pain-relieving properties. Large doses of raw nutmeg have a psychoactive effect.

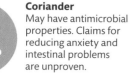

Coriander
May have antimicrobial properties. Claims for reducing anxiety and intestinal problems are unproven.

Mustard
Substances derived from mustard are used medically to treat cancer, but the anticancer effect of mustard itself is unproven.

Turmeric
Laboratory studies suggest it may have antimicrobial, anticancer, and anti-inflammatory properties.

Spicy cuisines

Although some spices, such as pepper and cardamom, are used very widely, many regional cuisines are associated with specific spices or spice mixtures. For example, star anise and Sichuan pepper are characteristic of traditional Sichuan cusine. Spice mixtures, such as ras el hanout, curry powder, garam masala, and Cajun seasoning, often vary in composition from place to place or even from one maker to another.

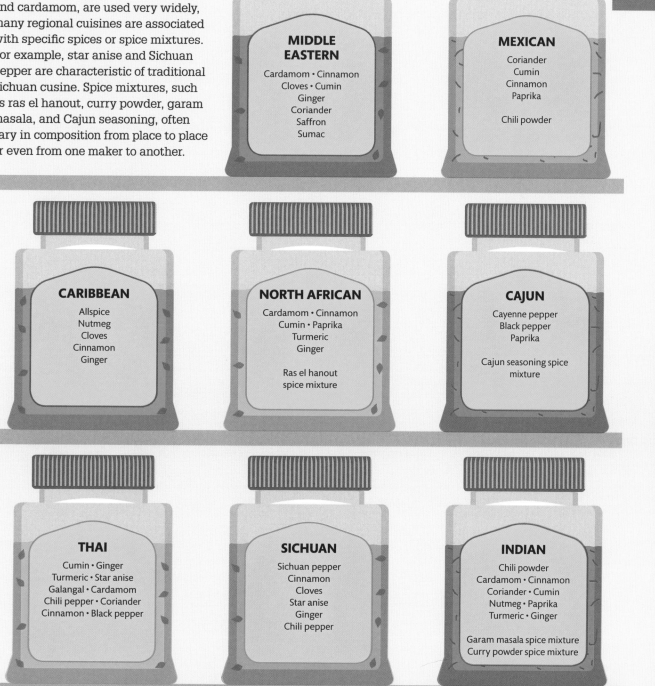

MIDDLE EASTERN

Cardamom · Cinnamon
Cloves · Cumin
Ginger
Coriander
Saffron
Sumac

MEXICAN

Coriander
Cumin
Cinnamon
Paprika

Chili powder

CARIBBEAN

Allspice
Nutmeg
Cloves
Cinnamon
Ginger

NORTH AFRICAN

Cardamom · Cinnamon
Cumin · Paprika
Turmeric
Ginger

Ras el hanout
spice mixture

CAJUN

Cayenne pepper
Black pepper
Paprika

Cajun seasoning spice
mixture

THAI

Cumin · Ginger
Turmeric · Star anise
Galangal · Cardamom
Chili pepper · Coriander
Cinnamon · Black pepper

SICHUAN

Sichuan pepper
Cinnamon
Cloves
Star anise
Ginger
Chili pepper

INDIAN

Chili powder
Cardamom · Cinnamon
Coriander · Cumin
Nutmeg · Paprika
Turmeric · Ginger

Garam masala spice mixture
Curry powder spice mixture

Herbs

Long valued for their medicinal properties, herbs are also packed with flavorful aromatics that can elevate dishes and add depth of flavor. Meats are particularly enhanced by the right seasoning.

Nutrients in herbs

Herbs evolved their flavor compounds as defensive chemicals, but this does not affect how we consume them, as we only use tiny amounts. This does limit the benefits we can glean from the excellent range of nutrients of many herbs, making them mainly of interest for their flavor.

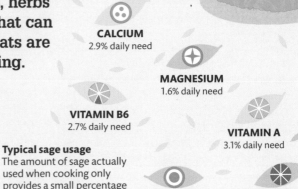

2 TSP SAGE
(0.05 oz/1.4g)

CALCIUM
2.9% daily need

MAGNESIUM
1.6% daily need

VITAMIN B6
2.7% daily need

VITAMIN A
3.1% daily need

Typical sage usage
The amount of sage actually used when cooking only provides a small percentage of a person's daily needs, except for vitamin K.

IRON
2.8% daily need

VITAMIN K
32% daily need

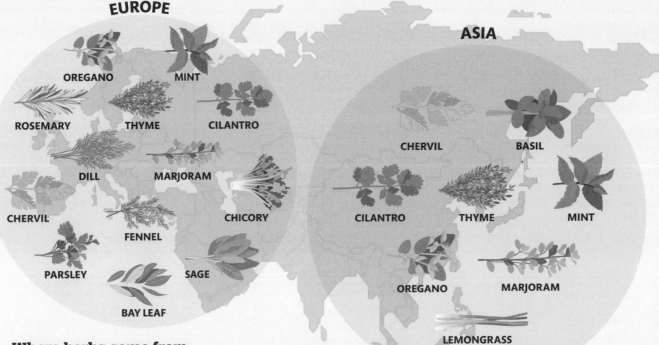

EUROPE

OREGANO
MINT
ROSEMARY
THYME
CILANTRO
DILL
MARJORAM
CHERVIL
CHICORY
FENNEL
PARSLEY
SAGE
BAY LEAF

ASIA

CHERVIL
BASIL
CILANTRO
THYME
MINT
OREGANO
MARJORAM
LEMONGRASS

Where herbs come from

Most herbs used around the world, and particularly in European cuisines, belong to either the mint family (such as basil and sage) or the carrot family (such as dill and fennel). Many herbs often associated with European or Asian cuisines originated elsewhere, and in general herbs seem to have spread worldwide early in human history. Cilantro, for instance, is a native of the Middle East but is now the most widely consumed fresh herb in the world.

Herbal zones of influence
Herbs have been carried and traded since early human history, making it hard to determine their wild origins. Early use was medicinal, but they were certainly being used for flavor by the ancient Greeks and Romans.

Medicinal culinary herbs

Herbs get their aroma and flavor from terpenes and phenols, which are also potent antioxidants and anti-inflammatories. Given the long history and widespread contemporary use of herbal medicine, and the known health benefits of some of the compounds they contain, it is hardly surprising that many culinary herbs are said to have health benefits. There are, however, very few robust, high-quality trials backing up many of the more remarkable claims made by some nutritionists.

AN INTENSE DISLIKE OF CILANTRO HAS BEEN LINKED TO A SPECIFIC GENE IN SOME PEOPLE

HERB	HEALTH CLAIMS
Oregano	Antimicrobial and rich in antioxidants; may help to loosen mucus, treat respiratory illness, and calm indigestion
Mint	May have antimicrobial, antiviral, antioxidant, anti-allergenic, and antitumour actions; may calm nausea, gas, and hiccups
Peppermint	In addition to the possible benefits of mint, above, clinical trials show that peppermint reduces intestinal spasms in irritable bowel syndrome
Sage	Leaves are used to reduce sweating, especially in women experiencing menopausal hot flushes and night sweats
Basil	May reduce blood cholesterol and other blood lipids; may reduce risk of cardiovascular disease; antioxidant, anticancer activity
Lemongrass	Antioxidant, antimicrobial, and antifungal; may aid digestion
Thyme	Believed to be a respiratory health booster; may relieve arthritis and diarrhea; may combat yeast and parasite infections; may reduce high blood pressure and high blood cholesterol; may be effective against acne
Rosemary	Anti-inflammatory; antimicrobial; may improve cardiovascular function
Fennel	Reduces bad breath; may relieve indigestion, bloating, and colic
Dill	May reduce heartburn, colic, and gas
Chicory	May relieve digestive problems, headaches, and menopausal symptoms; may be effective against some kidney and liver problems
Parsley	High in antioxidants; may relieve urinary infections and constipation
Cilantro	High in antioxidants; may aid digestive problems and improve appetite

Fresh or dried?

In general, phytonutrients degrade when heated and dried, but herbs respond surprisingly well to being dried. In particular, herbs from hot, dry zones, such as oregano, rosemary, and thyme, cope well because they are adapted to arid conditions. Not all drying is equal, however. Sun or oven drying will break down many nutrients, but aromatics are actually preserved by freeze and microwave drying. In fact, research shows that freeze-drying increases the concentrations of available terpenes and antioxidants by slowing the degradation process.

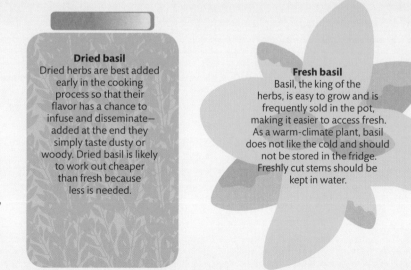

Dried basil
Dried herbs are best added early in the cooking process so that their flavor has a chance to infuse and disseminate—added at the end they simply taste dusty or woody. Dried basil is likely to work out cheaper than fresh because less is needed.

Fresh basil
Basil, the king of the herbs, is easy to grow and is frequently sold in the pot, making it easier to access fresh. As a warm-climate plant, basil does not like the cold and should not be stored in the fridge. Freshly cut stems should be kept in water.

Salt

The stuff of life, salt is integral to the biochemistry of all living things. We value its preservative effects and crave the flavors it adds and enhances—but are we eating too much, hidden in everyday foods?

Why do we need it?

Salt is composed of sodium and chloride ions. The chloride ions may be used to make stomach acid, but it is the sodium that is more widely important to the body. All cells in the body use sodium, and it is particularly important for maintaining the fluid balance of cells and tissues, and for nerve signaling. Because sodium is the more widely used component of salt, scientists and guidelines tend to talk about sodium content or sodium levels, rather than salt. Too much sodium can lead to high blood pressure, bone loss, and other negative health effects.

Role of salt in the body

Sodium ions are used in the cellular systems that shift water and other substances in and out of cells, and for generating charges across cell membranes (allowing nerve impulses to be transmitted around the body).

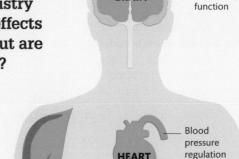

KEY
- Sodium
- Chloride

- BRAIN — Nervous system function
- HEART — Blood pressure regulation
- MUSCLE — Muscle contraction
- Stomach acid manufacture
- STOMACH
- KIDNEY
- KIDNEY — Water balance

Where does it come from?

Salt is recovered from seawater by evaporation, or mined or extracted in solution from deposits in rock. Rock and sea salt are generally large crystals or flakes of relatively unprocessed salt, while table salt is milled and processed to remove impurities and has anti-caking agents added to make it flow freely.

MORE THAN 200 MILLION TONS OF SALT ARE PRODUCED GLOBALLY EVERY YEAR

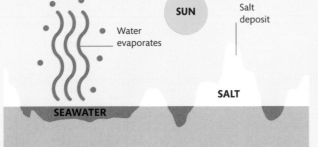

SUN

Water evaporates

Salt deposit

SALT

SEAWATER

Sea salt

Seawater in shallow ponds is evaporated by sunshine and wind. As it becomes more concentrated, it is shifted closer to the harvesting facility. At about 25 percent salinity, salt begins to crystallize.

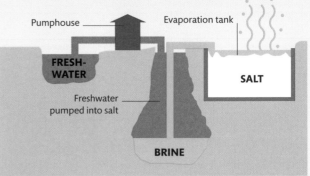

Pumphouse

Evaporation tank

FRESH-WATER

SALT

Freshwater pumped into salt

BRINE

Rock salt

Rock salt can be mined directly by cutting or with explosives, or can be dissolved to create very concentrated brine that is pumped to the surface to sit in evaporation ponds from which the salt is recovered.

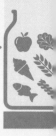

How much sodium do we need?

Most official recommendations for maximum daily sodium intake are around 2g per day. The 2015–2020 Dietary Guidelines for Americans recommend less than 2.3g of sodium per day, or around one teaspoon of salt. The actual average daily intake in the developed world exceeds 3.4g, increasing risk of high blood pressure (see pp.212–13) and associated health problems such as stroke.

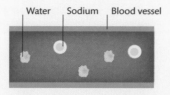

Water   Sodium   Blood vessel

HEALTHY BLOOD PRESSURE

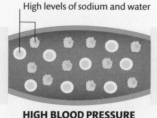

High levels of sodium and water

HIGH BLOOD PRESSURE

Sodium and blood pressure
Prolonged high salt intake causes high levels of sodium in the blood. As a result, the kidneys remove less water from the blood, causing high blood pressure.

Sodium in the diet

Sodium occurs naturally in certain foods, such as celery, beets, and milk. More often it is added during processing, cooking, and even during meal times. Hidden sources of sodium include processed foods, with preprepared meals especially high in sodium. Canned soup, for instance, contains the same concentration of salt as your blood plasma (around 1 percent salinity), and some processed foods may contain as much salt as seawater (3 percent). Another hidden source is the baking soda in baked goods.

A day's sodium intake
Given the high levels of hidden sodium in everyday foods, sodium intake quickly mounts up in the course of a day—unless you're careful.

WHY DO COOKS PREFER SEA SALT?

Though most types of salt are chemically similar (98–99.7 percent sodium chloride), chefs prefer the crystals and flakes in sea salt for finishing dishes, since they are easier to pinch and add texture.

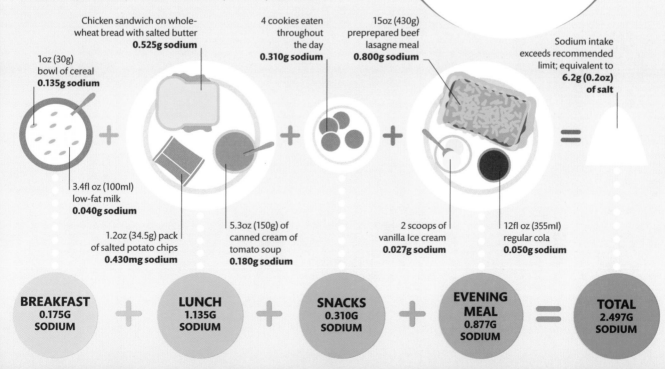

1oz (30g) bowl of cereal
0.135g sodium

Chicken sandwich on whole-wheat bread with salted butter
0.525g sodium

4 cookies eaten throughout the day
0.310g sodium

15oz (430g) preprepared beef lasagne meal
0.800g sodium

Sodium intake exceeds recommended limit; equivalent to **6.2g (0.2oz) of salt**

3.4fl oz (100ml) low-fat milk
0.040g sodium

1.2oz (34.5g) pack of salted potato chips
0.430mg sodium

5.3oz (150g) of canned cream of tomato soup
0.180g sodium

2 scoops of vanilla Ice cream
0.027g sodium

12fl oz (355ml) regular cola
0.050g sodium

BREAKFAST
0.175G SODIUM

+

LUNCH
1.135G SODIUM

+

SNACKS
0.310G SODIUM

+

EVENING MEAL
0.877G SODIUM

=

TOTAL
2.497G SODIUM

Fats and oils

Demonized in the public perception of healthy eating, the true story of fats and oils is complex and contradictory; essential to life and to good food, oils and fats can be superfoods if used properly. The main types of fat found in food are saturated and unsaturated fats. Most fats and oils contain both types.

Sources of fats and oils

Oils are fats that are liquid at room temperature, although the terms are often used interchangeably (see p.29). Those that you get through your food are called dietary fat. Although all fat contains the same number of calories—255kcal/oz (9kcal/g)—some sources are better for you than others. Oils from fish and plants are generally healthier than animal fats, because they contain more unsaturated fatty acid chains. But not all unsaturated fatty acids are the same either. Omega-3 fats are a type of polyunsaturate that tends to be anti-inflammatory, while omega-6 fats have the opposite effect.

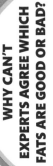

WHY CAN'T EXPERTS AGREE WHICH FATS ARE GOOD OR BAD?

Science in this area rarely offers clearcut answers; the best advice is to eat a varied diet rich in seafood, seeds, and small amounts of meat and dairy.

Saturated fats

Saturated fats have been linked for some time with a higher risk of cardiovascular disease (see pp.214–215), but this is now considered controversial. Coconut oil, butter, cheese, and red meat all contain high levels of saturated fat.

COCONUT OIL

SUNFLOWER OIL

Polyunsaturated fats

Unsaturated fat is found mainly in vegetable oils. Most popular oils, including sunflower, sesame, and corn oil, are dominated by omega-6 fatty acids. Linseed is a rare exception that provides plenty of omega-3.

Monounsaturated oils

Foods rich in monounsaturates such as olive, canola, sesame, and safflower oil are associated with lower levels of bad cholesterol and reduced risk of stroke and heart disease.

1 Olives
The riper the olive, the more oil it will yield, but flavor deteriorates, so choosing when to harvest is a compromise between the two factors.

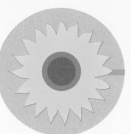

Stone rollers grind the olives to a paste

Olive press

Paste is collected

2 Milling
The olives are crushed to release oil. The resulting paste is "malaxed" or mixed to allow oil droplets to coalesce.

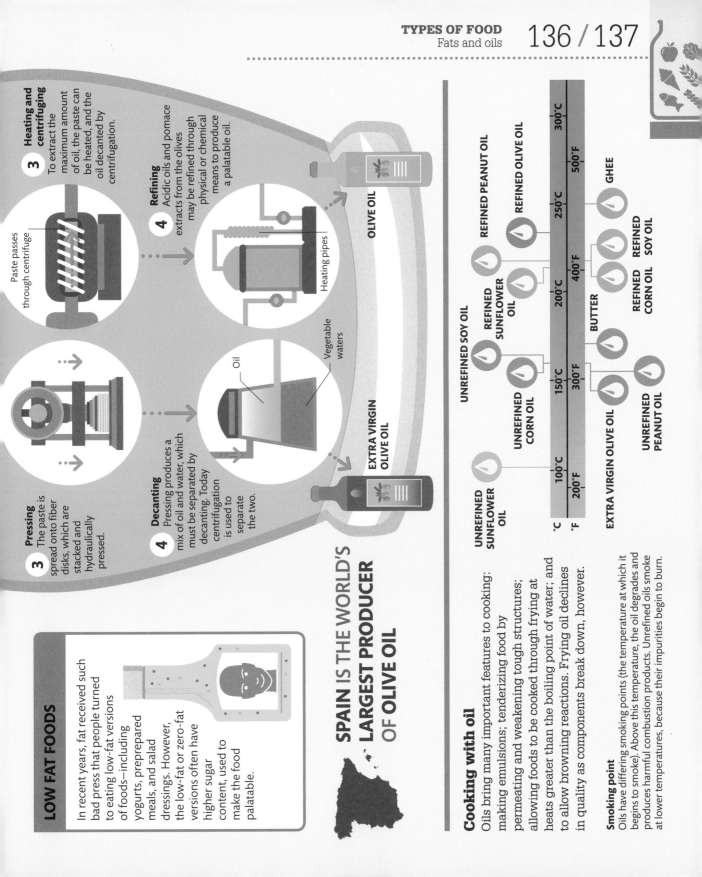

3 Heating and centrifuging
To extract the maximum amount of oil, the paste can be heated, and the oil decanted by centrifugation.

Paste passes through centrifuge

4 Refining
Acidic oils and pomace extracts from the olives may be refined through physical or chemical means to produce a palatable oil.

Heating pipes

OLIVE OIL

3 Pressing
The paste is spread onto fiber disks, which are stacked and hydraulically pressed.

4 Decanting
Pressing produces a mix of oil and water, which must be separated by decanting. Today centrifugation is used to separate the two.

Oil

Vegetable waters

EXTRA VIRGIN OLIVE OIL

LOW FAT FOODS

In recent years, fat received such bad press that people turned to eating low-fat versions of foods—including yogurts, preprepared meals, and salad dressings. However, the low-fat or zero-fat versions often have higher sugar content, used to make the food palatable.

SPAIN IS THE WORLD'S **LARGEST PRODUCER** OF OLIVE OIL

Cooking with oil

Oils bring many important features to cooking: making emulsions; tenderizing food by permeating and weakening tough structures; allowing foods to be cooked through frying at heats greater than the boiling point of water; and to allow browning reactions. Frying oil declines in quality as components break down, however.

Smoking point
Oils have differing smoking points (the temperature at which it begins to smoke). Above this temperature, the oil degrades and produces harmful combustion products. Unrefined oils smoke at lower temperatures, because their impurities begin to burn.

°C	100°C	150°C	200°C	250°C	300°C
°F	200°F	300°F	400°F	500°F	

UNREFINED SUNFLOWER OIL

UNREFINED SOY OIL

REFINED SUNFLOWER OIL

REFINED PEANUT OIL

REFINED OLIVE OIL

UNREFINED CORN OIL

BUTTER

GHEE

REFINED CORN OIL

REFINED SOY OIL

EXTRA VIRGIN OLIVE OIL

UNREFINED PEANUT OIL

Sugar

Sugars are simple carbohydrates (see pp.22–23), and although they are present in most foods, they can be obtained in pure form from natural sources such as honey, or by refining the sweet juice of sugarcane, sugar beets, or corn. The human body has no need for refined sugars, since it can get its glucose by breaking down more complex carbohydrates.

IS BROWN SUGAR HEALTHIER?

Brown sugar contains molasses, which is refined out of white sugar. Molasses contains vitamins and minerals, but they are present in only tiny amounts in brown sugar and won't make a significant contribution to your daily needs.

Common sugars

Around 80 percent of the world's sugar is produced by boiling down sugarcane juice. Filtering and purification result in white sugar, mainly composed of sucrose, that can be dried to make granules or powder. Further boiling and the addition of dark, sticky impurities called molasses results in brown sugar. Some syrups are made by splitting sucrose into glucose and fructose.

Sucrose is the main sugar in maple syrup and refined sugars, from muscovado to confectioners' sugar. It is made of a glucose and a fructose molecule joined. The body digests it to half glucose, half fructose.

SUCROSE

All digestible carbohydrates in the diet are ultimately broken down by the body into glucose molecules, which are hexagonal rings. Glucose is present in honey, or can by bought in pure form as glucose syrup, made from the starch in corn or potatoes.

GLUCOSE

Fructose occurs naturally in fruit and honey, but as an added sugar, it may be encountered in jam, inverted sugar syrups, and high-fructose corn syrup.

FRUCTOSE

SWEETENER	TIMES SWEETER THAN SUCROSE	ANY DRAWBACKS?
Saccharin (artificial)	300	Saccharin was found to cause bladder cancer in rats, but this effect is absent in humans and it is considered safe.
Aspartame (artificial)	160–200	Some people identify aspartame as the cause of their headaches, but tests have found no evidence for this.
Sucralose (artificial)	600	Sucralose is calorie free and does not affect blood sugar. It has no known drawbacks, but it is little studied.
Sorbitol (natural)	0.6	Sorbitol is not calorie free. However, it is slowly absorbed and does not cause blood sugar spikes.
Stevia (natural)	250	Stevia is an extract of the plant *Stevia rebaudiana*. The only known drawback is a sometimes bitter aftertaste.

Sugar substitutes

Several compounds many times sweeter than sucrose have been discovered. Some are natural, some are synthetic. They have low or no calories and little or no direct effect on blood sugar. Although most research suggests they are safe, some recent studies show that artificial sweeteners can alter gut flora, affecting blood sugar and the risk of obesity and diabetes.

Sugar demand went up as people became more affluent due to industrialization

YEAR

1700   1750   1800   18

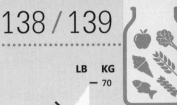

The sugar boom

In ancient and medieval times, most people relied on honey (itself a mixture of glucose and fructose) as a sweet treat. Sugarcane cultivation spread as far as the Caribbean and Brazil, but the resulting sugar remained a luxury for very few. Our exposure to refined sugar in the diet rocketed, however, when the Industrial Revolution (1760–1840) created wealth in Europe and North America. Sugar became fashionable and, eventually, a human need.

Historical sugar consumption

Sugar demand boomed in Britain in the 19th century, as the fashion for sugar in tea, cakes, and sweets took off. In the US, consumption continued to rise after the 1970s, coinciding with the adoption of cheap high-fructose corn syrup by makers of processed foods and soft drinks.

MANY PEOPLE IN ANCIENT **ROME WERE POISONED BY LEAD ACETATE,** WHICH THEY USED AS AN ARTIFICIAL **SWEETENER**

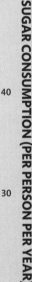

US CONSUMPTION

UK CONSUMPTION

US consumption kept rising to a peak in around 2000

UK consumption began falling from a peak in the mid-1970s

World War I disrupted trade, and sugar consumption briefly decreased

World War again reduced sugar availability and demand in 1939–45

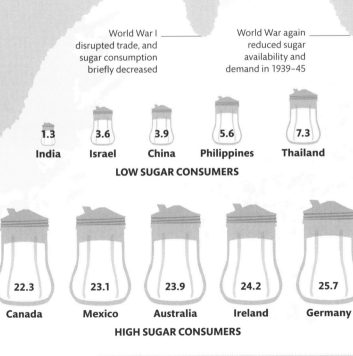

1.3	3.6	3.9	5.6	7.3
India	**Israel**	**China**	**Philippines**	**Thailand**

LOW SUGAR CONSUMERS

22.3	23.1	23.9	24.2	25.7
Canada	**Mexico**	**Australia**	**Ireland**	**Germany**

HIGH SUGAR CONSUMERS

Not all sugar lovers

Many historians credit India with the invention of refining sugar from cane more than 2,000 years ago, but Indians today eat very little added sugar per capita. People in many other Asian countries likewise do not share the West's sweet tooth.

Teaspoons per day

People in Europe, the Americas, and the Antipodes tend to be fans of sugar, eating typically five times more free (added) sugar than people in many parts of Asia.

LB   KG

SUGAR CONSUMPTION (PER PERSON PER YEAR)

70
140 — 60
130 — 50
100 — 40
80 — 30
60 — 20
40 —
20 — 10
0

1900   1950   2000

YEAR

Sugar highs and lows

Every cell in our body needs the sugar glucose for energy, and many different types of food can be broken down to provide this glucose. Eating a balanced diet gives us a steady supply, but sugary snacks can send blood sugar levels swinging wildly.

Regulating blood sugar

Our bodies function best when blood glucose levels are within a certain range. If levels increase too much, the pancreas releases insulin, encouraging fat and muscle cells to absorb glucose. Glucose not needed by cells immediately for energy is stored in the liver as glycogen or as fat in cells around the body. If blood glucose falls too low, another pancreatic hormone (glucagon) stimulates the liver to convert glycogen back into glucose. If this isn't enough, fat stores are used. In diabetes, cells don't produce or respond to insulin properly, so blood sugar levels can fluctuate greatly, producing various symptoms (see pp.216–17).

HYPERACTIVE KIDS?

Contrary to popular belief, children don't become hyperactive after eating sugary treats. Studies have shown that, rather than the child's actual behavior, it is the parents' perception of their child's behavior that changes after they are told their child has eaten sugar.

Riding a roller coaster

When we eat lots of sugary snacks, our body struggles to keep up, leading to a cycle of rising and falling blood sugar. Over years, this can cause a decrease in our sensitivity to insulin, leading to type 2 diabetes.

The sugary snack pushes blood glucose above normal levels as glucose floods into the bloodstream

SUGAR HIGH

Body maintains blood glucose within a normal range when provided with a balanced diet

IS SUGAR ADDICTIVE?

Sugar cravings are common, and there is evidence that some people may develop a psychological dependence on sugar. Whether it is physically addictive in the same way as alcohol is uncertain.

Sugary snack

SUGAR LOW

Blood sugar falls to the bottom of its normal range, which may stimulate us to eat a sugary snack

Food and blood sugar levels

To give an accurate idea of how different foods affect blood sugar levels, scientists have devised two measures, the glycemic index (GI) and glycemic load (GL). The GI of a food is a measure of how quickly it raises your blood sugar level (see p.91). However, it does not tell you the total amount of carbohydrate and so gives no indication of how high your blood sugar level could rise. The GL is designed to give a more accurate picture by taking into account both the GI of a food and the total amount of carbohydrate in the serving. In general, a GL of 10 or less is considered to be low, while 20 or more is high.

Glycemic index vs. glycemic load

Foods with a low GI may have a high GL, and vice versa. For example, watermelon has a high GI but, for a typical serving (4.2oz/120g), a low GL; chocolate cake has a relatively low GI, despite being a sweet food, but a much higher GL than watermelon for the same serving size of (4.2oz/120g).

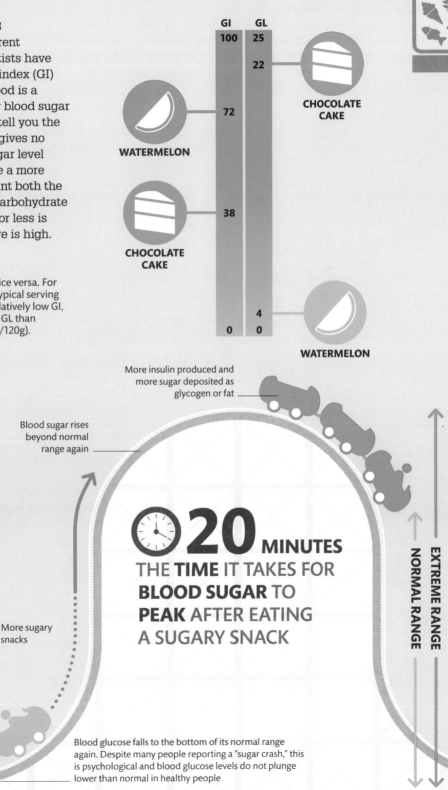

GI
100
72
38
0

GL
25
22
4
0

WATERMELON

CHOCOLATE CAKE

CHOCOLATE CAKE

WATERMELON

Excess glucose prompts production of insulin, which results in a rapid fall in blood sugar as glucose is taken up by muscle and fat cells and converted into glycogen or fat deposits

Blood sugar rises beyond normal range again

More insulin produced and more sugar deposited as glycogen or fat

BLOOD SUGAR LEVEL

More sugary snacks

🕐 **20** MINUTES
THE **TIME** IT TAKES FOR **BLOOD SUGAR** TO **PEAK** AFTER EATING A SUGARY SNACK

EXTREME RANGE
NORMAL RANGE

SUGAR LOW

Blood glucose falls to the bottom of its normal range again. Despite many people reporting a "sugar crash," this is psychological and blood glucose levels do not plunge lower than normal in healthy people

Affinity for desserts

Sugar and fat contain a lot of calories and we evolved to seek out these high-energy foods (see p.9). We like both individually, but combining the two (such as in cakes) activates the pleasure centers in our brains dramatically. Learned psychological associations between desserts and positive experiences, such as birthdays and romantic dinners, probably also contribute to the enjoyment.

Science of cake

For a light, fluffy texture, most cakes use chemical raising agents, such as baking powder. Before baking powder was invented, whipped egg whites or yeast were used; some recipes still rely on these.

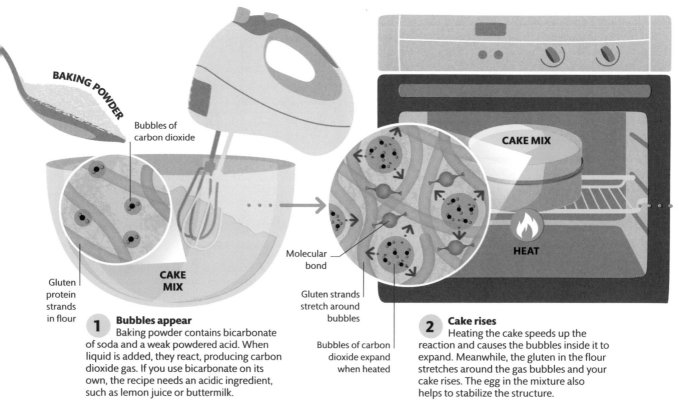

BAKING POWDER

Bubbles of carbon dioxide

CAKE MIX

CAKE MIX

HEAT

Gluten protein strands in flour

Molecular bond

Gluten strands stretch around bubbles

Bubbles of carbon dioxide expand when heated

1 Bubbles appear
Baking powder contains bicarbonate of soda and a weak powdered acid. When liquid is added, they react, producing carbon dioxide gas. If you use bicarbonate on its own, the recipe needs an acidic ingredient, such as lemon juice or buttermilk.

2 Cake rises
Heating the cake speeds up the reaction and causes the bubbles inside it to expand. Meanwhile, the gluten in the flour stretches around the gas bubbles and your cake rises. The egg in the mixture also helps to stabilize the structure.

Desserts

For many, there is no better way to end a special meal than with a decadent dessert. A surprising amount of science goes into creating our favorite treats; from ensuring the perfect rise on your cake to attempting to make healthier versions that taste just as good.

WHY DO I STILL HAVE ROOM FOR DESSERT?

We constantly seek variety, and the hormone ghrelin drives us to eat sweets despite feeling full. Sugar may even relax the stomach, to make room for more!

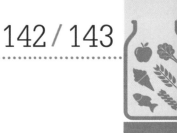

SPONGE CAKE

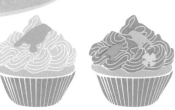

Gluten proteins become firmer, providing structure

3 Cake sets
As it cooks, the cake structure becomes firmer, trapping the bubbles within it and producing a light, airy texture. It is difficult to achieve this lightness in gluten-free cakes, because they don't have the stretchy protein to form the basis of the structure.

MELT-RESISTANT ICE CREAM

A protein that stabilizes mixtures of fat, water, and air bubbles is being tested and could produce a melt-resistant ice cream. It also prevents ice crystals from forming, ensuring your ice cream is silky and smooth, and may even allow low-fat desserts to taste as creamy as full-fat ones!

Healthy desserts?

Many "healthy dessert" options replace refined sugar or butter with "better" options, but they still tend to be high in overall sugars, fats, and calories. Raw, palaeo brownies (no sugar, no flour, and made with almond butter) will still cause weight gain if you eat too many. A truly healthy, nutritionally fulfilling dessert may only come in the form of fresh fruit with low fat, unsweetened yogurt, and a sprinkling of nuts and seeds.

SWAP	FOR	IS IT HEALTHIER?
Refined sugar	**Honey, maple syrup, coconut sugar**	Natural sugars can contain tiny amounts of beneficial nutrients, but they still raise blood sugar and provide lots of calories.
Cream	**Low-fat yogurt**	Substituting cream or butter with low-fat yogurt can cut the calories and saturated fat in your dessert substantially.
Sugar	**Sweeteners**	Sweeteners don't raise blood sugar—useful for people with diabetes. We don't know the effects of long-term consumption.
All-purpose flour	**Gluten-free flour**	Unless you suffer from an allergy or intolerance, there is no nutritional benefit from switching to gluten-free flour.

Chocolate

Chocolate is a big favorite around the world. Originally a bitter spicy drink invented in Central America, chocolate was drunk with sugar when it was brought to Europe in the 1500s. New processing methods create the solid bars we know today.

DOES CHOCOLATE HAVE CAFFEINE IN IT?

Yes, the small amount of caffeine in chocolate comes from the cocoa solids. It also contains other stimulants, such as theobromine.

How chocolate is made

Just like grape juice in wine-making, cocoa beans need to be fermented to develop their flavors before they are processed. Most chocolate contains other ingredients, too—milk chocolate has milk and sugar added, while white chocolate contains no cocoa solids, just the cocoa butter, along with milk, sugar, and often vanilla.

THE **SWISS** ARE THE **BIGGEST CONSUMERS OF CHOCOLATE WORLDWIDE**, EATING NEARLY **20 LB (9 KG) EACH YEAR**

Fresh cocoa beans are pale

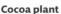

COCOA BEAN

COCOA POD

Cocoa plant
Cocoa pods are about the size of a football. The beans inside are surrounded by a white flesh with a sweet, acidic flavor. Making chocolate from the beans is a long and involved process.

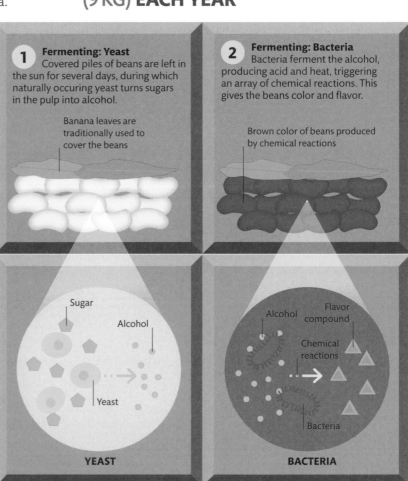

1 Fermenting: Yeast
Covered piles of beans are left in the sun for several days, during which naturally occuring yeast turns sugars in the pulp into alcohol.

Banana leaves are traditionally used to cover the beans

Sugar

Alcohol

Yeast

YEAST

2 Fermenting: Bacteria
Bacteria ferment the alcohol, producing acid and heat, triggering an array of chemical reactions. This gives the beans color and flavor.

Brown color of beans produced by chemical reactions

Alcohol

Flavor compound

Chemical reactions

Bacteria

BACTERIA

Chocolate and pleasure

When we eat chocolate our brain releases feel-good chemicals that give us a rush of pleasure. Studies have shown it is the sensory experience of chocolate we crave, not the stimulant compounds that chocolate contains. One of the most important factors in this experience, perhaps surprisingly, is not chocolate's taste but specifically its melting point.

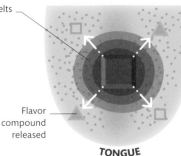

Chocolate melts

Flavor compound released

TONGUE

Melting bliss
Chocolate is one of the few foods that melts exactly at the temperature of your mouth. This allows the flavor to be released as the chocolate coats your tongue and mouth, heightening the sensory experience.

CHOCOLATE AND HEALTH

Antioxidants in cocoa have a number of health benefits, including temporarily reducing blood pressure. Unfortunately, most chocolate does not contain much cocoa, and the added sugar and fat is what makes chocolate unhealthy.

ANTIOXIDANTS

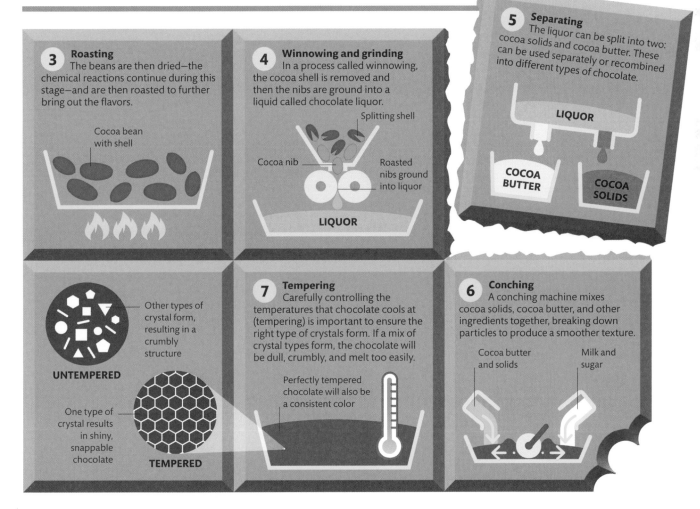

3 Roasting
The beans are then dried—the chemical reactions continue during this stage—and are then roasted to further bring out the flavors.

Cocoa bean with shell

4 Winnowing and grinding
In a process called winnowing, the cocoa shell is removed and then the nibs are ground into a liquid called chocolate liquor.

Splitting shell

Cocoa nib

Roasted nibs ground into liquor

LIQUOR

5 Separating
The liquor can be split into two: cocoa solids and cocoa butter. These can be used separately or recombined into different types of chocolate.

LIQUOR

COCOA BUTTER

COCOA SOLIDS

Other types of crystal form, resulting in a crumbly structure

UNTEMPERED

One type of crystal results in shiny, snappable chocolate

TEMPERED

7 Tempering
Carefully controlling the temperatures that chocolate cools at (tempering) is important to ensure the right type of crystals form. If a mix of crystal types form, the chocolate will be dull, crumbly, and melt too easily.

Perfectly tempered chocolate will also be a consistent color

6 Conching
A conching machine mixes cocoa solids, cocoa butter, and other ingredients together, breaking down particles to produce a smoother texture.

Cocoa butter and solids

Milk and sugar

Sweets

It may seem simple, but making sweets is a delicate process. Carefully controlling the temperature of a solution of sugar in water produces a huge range of different textures—from soft and chewy, to hard and brittle. The addition of butter, milk, or other ingredients expands the possibilities.

COTTON CANDY

Cotton candy is unusual in that it is made by melting sugar without dissolving it in water first. The hot molten sugar is sprayed through a fine, spinning nozzle. The force creates long strings, which cool instantly into an amorphous form, producing this fragile, melt-in-the-mouth confection.

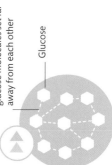

KEY

- Cooled slowly
- Cooled quickly
- Stirred while cooling

CRÈME CARAMEL

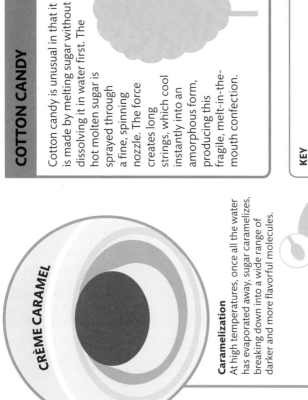

Caramelization
At high temperatures, once all the water has evaporated away, sugar caramelizes, breaking down into a wide range of darker and more flavorful molecules.

Sugar breaks down into different types of molecules

Cooling quickly
Heating the solution to a medium temperature and then cooling it rapidly does not allow crystals to form. Instead, this produces the clear, glassy appearance and hard, brittle texture of lollipops and boiled candy.

Rapid cooling means glucose molecules set far away from each other

Glucose

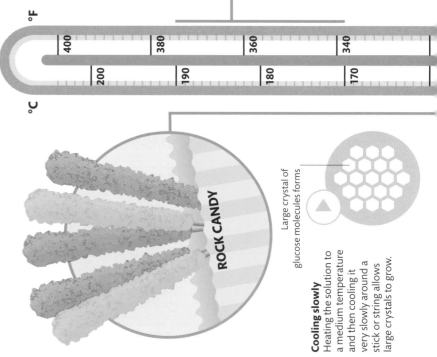

LOLLIPOPS

°F
400
380
360
340

°C
200
190
180
170

ROCK CANDY

Large crystal of glucose molecules forms

Cooling slowly
Heating the solution to a medium temperature and then cooling it very slowly around a stick or string allows large crystals to grow.

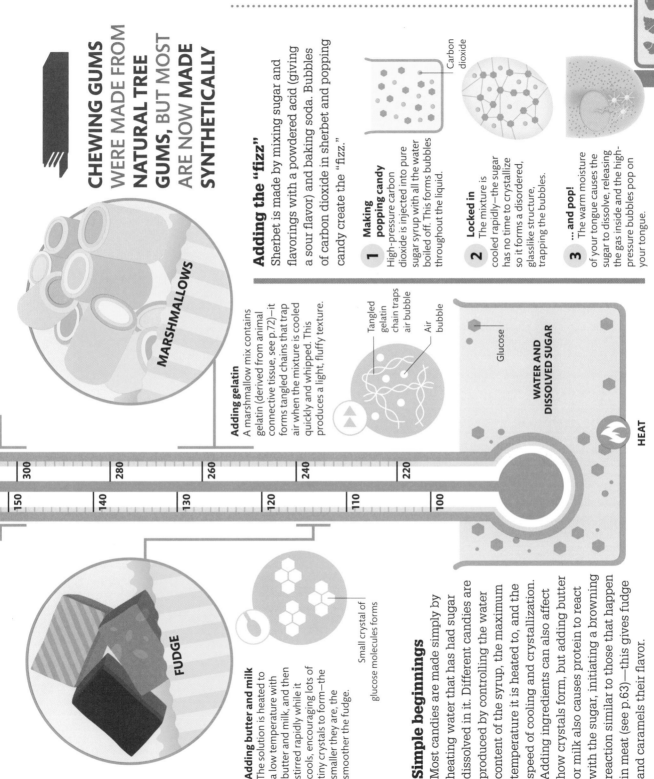

CHEWING GUMS WERE MADE FROM **NATURAL TREE GUMS,** BUT MOST ARE NOW MADE **SYNTHETICALLY**

MARSHMALLOWS

Adding gelatin
A marshmallow mix contains gelatin (derived from animal connective tissue, see p.72)—it forms tangled chains that trap air when the mixture is cooled quickly and whipped. This produces a light, fluffy texture.

Tangled gelatin chain traps air bubble

Air bubble

Adding the "fizz"

Sherbet is made by mixing sugar and flavorings with a powdered acid (giving a sour flavor) and baking soda. Bubbles of carbon dioxide in sherbet and popping candy create the "fizz."

Carbon dioxide

1 Making popping candy
High-pressure carbon dioxide is injected into pure sugar syrup with all the water boiled off. This forms bubbles throughout the liquid.

2 Locked in
The mixture is cooled rapidly—the sugar has no time to crystallize so it forms a disordered, glasslike structure, trapping the bubbles.

3 ...and pop!
The warm moisture of your tongue causes the sugar to dissolve, releasing the gas inside and the high-pressure bubbles pop on your tongue.

300
280
260
240
220
150
140
130
120
110
100

WATER AND DISSOLVED SUGAR

Glucose

HEAT

FUDGE

Small crystal of glucose molecules forms

Adding butter and milk
The solution is heated to a low temperature with butter and milk, and then stirred rapidly while it cools, encouraging lots of tiny crystals to form—the smaller they are, the smoother the fudge.

Simple beginnings

Most candies are made simply by heating water that has had sugar dissolved in it. Different candies are produced by controlling the water content of the syrup, the maximum temperature it is heated to, and the speed of cooling and crystallization. Adding ingredients can also affect how crystals form, but adding butter or milk also causes protein to react with the sugar, initiating a browning reaction similar to those that happen in meat (see p.63)—this gives fudge and caramels their flavor.

Alternative foods

With growing pressure on our main food sources, the need for alternatives is increasing. Possibilities for alleviating this pressure include making more use of existing but underused foods and developing entirely new sources of food.

Underutilized foods

A comparatively small number of plants and animals provide most of the world's food, but there are many more species that are eaten only in some areas or cultures but could be more widely used. In some cases, this may mean overcoming cultural norms about what things are considered acceptable to eat and what are viewed as disgusting—grubs, in many Western countries, for instance—or "cute," such as pet animals.

Mammals and birds
Horses, kangaroos, ostriches, songbirds, guinea pigs, and dogs are eaten in some cultures, but viewed with suspicion in others. Rats and mice are staple foods in some parts of Southeast Asia and Africa.

Worms and grubs
Worms and grubs are highly nutritious. They are often low in fat and are valued as a protein source in some cultures, a well-known example being the Australian witchetty grub.

Insects
Insects are already eaten by a large number of people (see pp.246–47), and their excellent efficiency in making protein makes them an atttractive option for even more widespread use.

Pulses and tubers
Even though pulses and tubers are already widely eaten, there are many other species that are nutrient-rich and could be valuable food sources, including African yam beans and oca tubers.

Cultured meat

The increasing global population has created a demand for more food, including more meat. Meat from animals requires a lot of resources, such as land, feed, and water, and may not be a sustainable long-term solution (see pp.228–29). One potential answer may be to grow meat in cultures, using muscle stem cells from animals as starter cells. The first edible example of cultured meat—a laboratory-grown sample—was announced publicly in 2013. But the technical challenge of making "test-tube meat" on a large scale has not yet been overcome and so this is unlikely to solve the short-term demands for more meat.

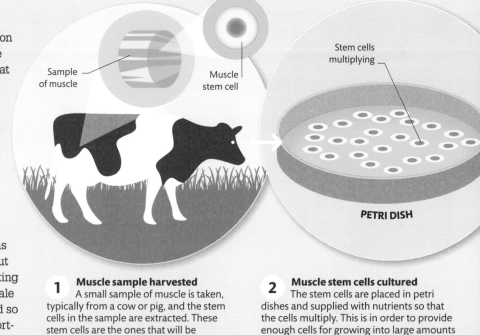

Sample of muscle

Muscle stem cell

Stem cells multiplying

PETRI DISH

1 Muscle sample harvested
A small sample of muscle is taken, typically from a cow or pig, and the stem cells in the sample are extracted. These stem cells are the ones that will be cultured and grown into meat.

2 Muscle stem cells cultured
The stem cells are placed in petri dishes and supplied with nutrients so that the cells multiply. This is in order to provide enough cells for growing into large amounts of meat in a bioreactor.

New foods

Any new food needs certain characteristics if it is to become a practical addition to the human diet: it must be safe, a good source of nutrients, economic to produce, and, ideally, have a small ecological footprint. A good starting point is to try to adapt existing foods, such as lupin beans and algae, although scientists are also trying to grow meat from animal muscle (see below).

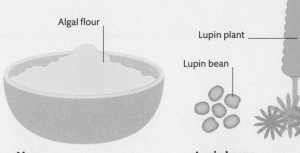

Algal flour

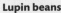

Lupin plant

Lupin bean

Algae
Large algae—seaweeds—are popular food items in Asia, but some microscopic algae have also been cultivated and used to make foods such as algal flour.

Lupin beans
Lupin beans are already part of some cuisines but they have also been used as the raw material to produce synthetic vegetable protein foods, such as lupin meat and flour.

COULD WE USE FIBER AS FOOD?

Although we cannot digest fiber, scientists have found a way to convert cellulose (a major component of fiber) into starch that we can digest and so could potentially be used as food.

20,000
THE NUMBER OF **EDIBLE PLANT SPECIES** WORLDWIDE

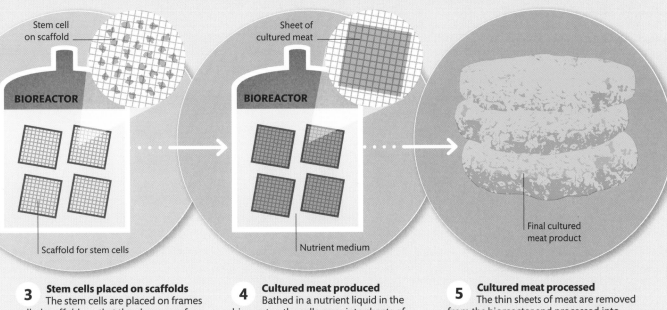

Stem cell on scaffold

BIOREACTOR

Scaffold for stem cells

Sheet of cultured meat

BIOREACTOR

Nutrient medium

Final cultured meat product

3 **Stem cells placed on scaffolds**
The stem cells are placed on frames called scaffolds so that they have a surface on which to grow. The scaffolds, which are biodegradable and edible, are then placed in a bioreactor.

4 **Cultured meat produced**
Bathed in a nutrient liquid in the bioreactor, the cells grow into sheets of meat. The sheets are very thin (about 1mm/0.04 inches) and need processing into larger, edible pieces.

5 **Cultured meat processed**
The thin sheets of meat are removed from the bioreactor and processed into thicker slices. Additives, such as colorings, flavourings, and fat, are mixed in to make the meat look and taste like natural meat.

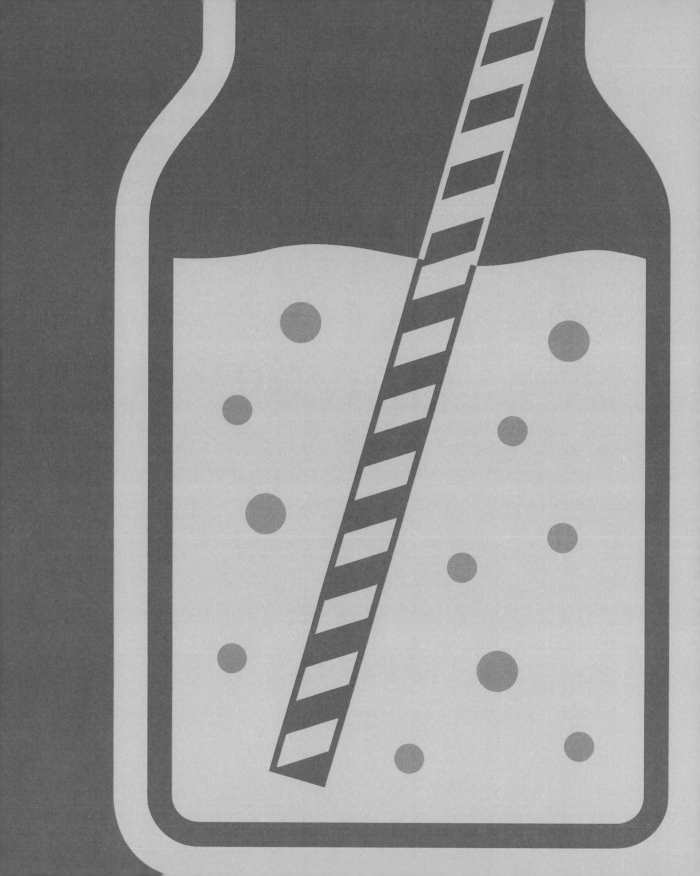

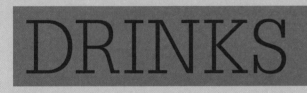

DRINKS

Drinking water

Clean, safe water from the faucet is one of the great achievements of civilization. Bottled water has become increasingly popular, but there are concerns about its environmental impact and no concrete evidence that it has health benefits.

WHAT ARE ELECTROLYTES?

In food science, electrolytes refers to dissolved minerals or salts. The body needs electrolytes such as sodium, potassium, and chloride for normal functioning of its tissues and cells.

Treatment of tap water

The purpose of water treatment is to remove dirt, debris, toxic chemicals, and microbes to produce water safe for human consumption. The details of the treatment process vary from region to region, depending on water standards, but it typically involves the stages shown here.

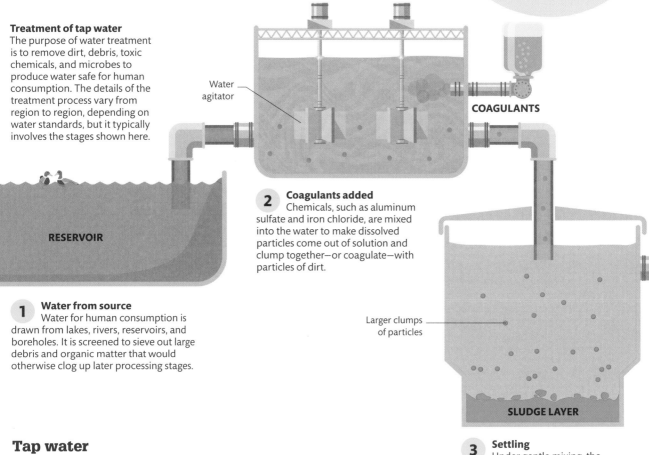

Water agitator

COAGULANTS

RESERVOIR

Larger clumps of particles

SLUDGE LAYER

1 **Water from source**
Water for human consumption is drawn from lakes, rivers, reservoirs, and boreholes. It is screened to sieve out large debris and organic matter that would otherwise clog up later processing stages.

2 **Coagulants added**
Chemicals, such as aluminum sulfate and iron chloride, are mixed into the water to make dissolved particles come out of solution and clump together—or coagulate—with particles of dirt.

3 **Settling**
Under gentle mixing, the coagulated particles cluster together to form large clumps, a process known as flocculation. These clumps settle out to the bottom of the tank (sedimentation), where they form a layer of sludge that can be removed and treated for use as fertilizer.

Tap water

In developed countries, tap water is thoroughly treated to remove dirt, microbes, and toxic contaminants. It is also rigorously tested to ensure it remains safe to drink and cook with; in fact, the testing may be to a higher standard than that for some bottled waters. In addition to ensuring safety, water treatment may also include adjusting the acidity or alkalinity of the water, so that it does not corrode pipes. Tap water may have certain substances added to improve health—for instance, fluoride to reduce tooth decay—but any such additives vary according to local regulations.

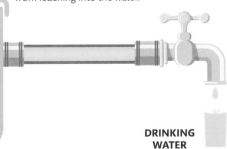

Mineral water

Mineral waters were traditionally drunk at their natural sources, such as spas or wells. Now, they are more commonly bottled at the source and distributed for sale. They often have high levels of dissolved minerals, although these do not necessarily confer health benefits, and they must have a consistent composition and be safe to drink without any treatment. Spring water also originates from a natural source, but its composition may vary and it may be filtered or treated.

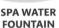
Mineral-rich water from natural spring

Spa water
Many spas historically developed around natural springs, where the mineral water was believed to be beneficial for health, both when drunk and also when bathed in.

SPA WATER FOUNTAIN

Bottled water

Bottled water is not necessarily from a spring or other natural source. Many bottled waters essentially come from the tap, and some are not treated in any way. Bottled water is typically sold in plastic bottles, and there are concerns about the environmental impact of the packaging: the bottles need a lot of energy and other resources to make, and they also create a lot of waste.

Energy in a bottle
Only a fraction of the energy cost of producing water in a plastic bottle comes from treating and bottling the water. The vast majority is used in making the bottle and transporting it for sale.

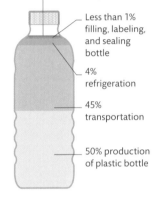

Less than 1% treatment at plant

Less than 1% filling, labeling, and sealing bottle

4% refrigeration

45% transportation

50% production of plastic bottle

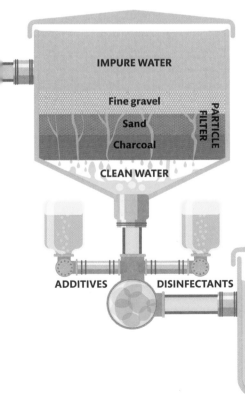

IMPURE WATER

Fine gravel

Sand

Charcoal

PARTICLE FILTER

CLEAN WATER

ADDITIVES   **DISINFECTANTS**

STORAGE TANK

DRINKING WATER

4 Filtration
The water is then passed through beds of increasingly fine gravel, sand, and charcoal to remove remaining particles and microbes.

5 Disinfection and storage
Chemicals are added to the water to make sure it is not acid or alkaline and to destroy any remaining microbes. The water is then stored, ready for distribution.

35 BILLION
THE NUMBER OF PLASTIC **WATER BOTTLES THROWN AWAY EVERY YEAR** IN THE **US** ALONE

6 Public water supply
Water is distributed to homes and businesses through public water pipes. Water that will pass through lead pipes sometimes has additives that prevent lead from leaching into the water.

From berry to bean

Coffee is an infusion of ground, roasted beans that come from inside the berries of shrubs belonging to the *Coffea* group of plants. Once the berries have ripened on the bush, they are picked and the pulpy flesh must be removed from the beans within. Sometimes they are left to dry and ferment in the sun before the pulp is removed; another method is to remove most of the pulp first and then ferment the bean. They are then washed and dried.

Coffee

Every day, more than two billion cups of coffee are drunk by people all around the world. It is valued for its stimulant properties, and for its complex flavors and aromas.

1 Harvesting
When a coffee plant is five years old or more, its berries can be harvested. They are picked when they have ripened from green to red.

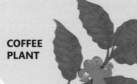

COFFEE PLANT

2 Processing
The ripe berries are processed to remove the outer skin, pulp, and parchment. The end result is raw green beans.

Parchment

Bean

Pulp

BEANS PROCESSED

3 Roasting
The green beans are roasted (typically in a large drum) to bring out the characteristic coffee aroma and taste.

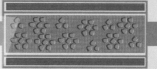

DRUM ROASTING

How much caffeine?

Although tea leaves contain more caffeine than coffee beans (2–3 percent against 1–2 percent), in brewing, much more caffeine is extracted from coffee than from tea. A typical cup of coffee may contain about 50–100mg of caffeine, compared to 20–50mg for a cup of tea. Different methods of brewing can radically alter the amount of caffeine that is extracted from ground coffee.

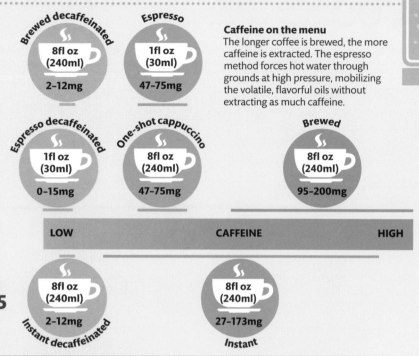

Brewed decaffeinated
8fl oz (240ml)
2–12mg

Espresso
1fl oz (30ml)
47–75mg

Caffeine on the menu
The longer coffee is brewed, the more caffeine is extracted. The espresso method forces hot water through grounds at high pressure, mobilizing the volatile, flavorful oils without extracting as much caffeine.

Espresso decaffeinated
1fl oz (30ml)
0–15mg

One-shot cappuccino
8fl oz (240ml)
47–75mg

Brewed
8fl oz (240ml)
95–200mg

LOW	CAFFEINE	HIGH

Instant decaffeinated
8fl oz (240ml)
2–12mg

Instant
8fl oz (240ml)
27–173mg

10 MILLION TONS OF COFFEE WERE PRODUCED IN 2015

HOW CAFFEINE AFFECTS THE BODY

Caffeine is the most widely consumed psychoactive substance (one that alters mental processes) in the world. The most notable effects of caffeine occur after consumption of low-to-moderate amounts (50–300mg—the recommended daily limit is 400mg). They include increased alertness, energy, and ability to concentrate. Large amounts can lead to negative effects, such as anxiety and insomnia.

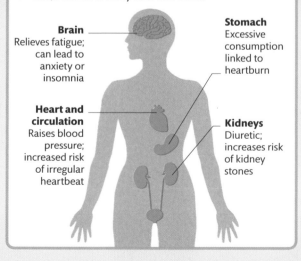

Brain
Relieves fatigue; can lead to anxiety or insomnia

Stomach
Excessive consumption linked to heartburn

Heart and circulation
Raises blood pressure; increased risk of irregular heartbeat

Kidneys
Diuretic; increases risk of kidney stones

How instant coffee is made

Instant coffee is coffee that has been brewed and then dried to a powder so that it can be reconstituted simply by adding water. There are two methods for doing this: either the liquid coffee is sprayed into a hot, dry atmosphere through a tiny nozzle to give a superfine mist, which quickly dries into powder, or liquid coffee is frozen and then freeze-dried, with the water turning directly from ice to gas.

Freeze-dried coffee
All types of instant coffee lose flavor and caffeine during manufacture, but freeze-drying preserves more of the aroma compounds.

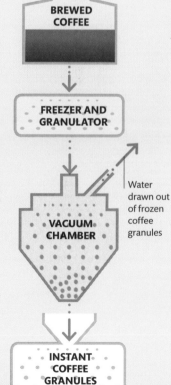

BREWED COFFEE

FREEZER AND GRANULATOR

VACUUM CHAMBER

Water drawn out of frozen coffee granules

INSTANT COFFEE GRANULES

Tea

The world's most popular brew has a rich history, stretching back thousands of years, and an equally rich store of nutrients. There are many types of tea, from black to white.

The main varieties
Tea varieties are determined by the maturity of the leaves when picked, and the degree and duration of their processing.

DOES TEA HAVE LESS CAFFEINE THAN COFFEE?

Although tea has a higher caffeine content than coffee, usually less makes it into the tea infusion—50mg per cup of tea compared to 175mg per cup of coffee.

WHITE
Buds or young leaves are steamed to deactivate enzymes and prevent more than light fermentation, then dried.

YELLOW
Mature leaves are pan fired, lightly rolled and dried, allowed to partially ferment after heating, and then dried some more.

GREEN
Mature leaves are steamed or pan fired to deactivate enzymes, so that no fermentation occurs, then rolled and dried.

BLACK
A fully fermented tea, made from mature leaves that are withered, rolled and left to ferment (or oxidize) for several hours before firing and drying.

OOLONG
Said to be semi-fermented, this tea is made from withered mature leaves that are bruised and fermented for a short time, before being pan fired and dried.

PU-ERH
Also known as dark tea, pu-erh tea, like yellow tea, undergoes secondary fermentation after heating and rolling, though for longer.

HERBAL TEAS

Herbal teas are made from the infusion of herbs, spices, or fruit extracts in hot water. To distinguish it from a "true" tea, a herbal tea may also be referred to as a tisane, or infusion. Taken hot or cold, they do not contain caffeine.

Types of tea
Tea most commonly refers to an infusion of dried leaves of a camellia bush (*Camellia sinensis*, not the garden variety). The basic preparation of dried mature leaves is green tea. Freeing enzymes in the cells of the tea leaves produces darker teas, transforming simple phenols into more complex ones—a process commonly but mistakenly called fermentation.

38
PERCENT OF **TEA** IS GROWN IN **CHINA**, THE **LARGEST PRODUCER** OF TEA IN THE WORLD

What is in a cup of tea?

Green tea is rich in colorless, bitter, but not astringent phenols called catechins. In the production of black tea, enzymes released during rolling and bruising of the leaves and oxidation convert most of the catechins into theaflavins, which give black tea its slightly bitter, astringent flavor. Tea also contains caffeine, theanine, flavonoids, saponins, vitamins, and minerals.

Green tea
The color of green tea comes from the chlorophyll in the leaves. This is preserved because the leaves undergo little processing, and it is not masked by dark phenols.

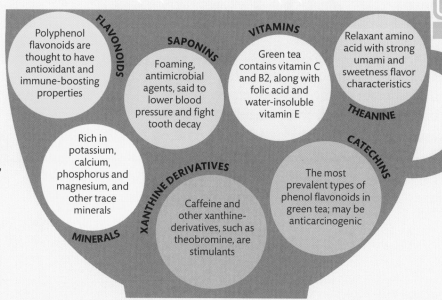

FLAVONOIDS
Polyphenol flavonoids are thought to have antioxidant and immune-boosting properties

SAPONINS
Foaming, antimicrobial agents, said to lower blood pressure and fight tooth decay

VITAMINS
Green tea contains vitamin C and B2, along with folic acid and water-insoluble vitamin E

THEANINE
Relaxant amino acid with strong umami and sweetness flavor characteristics

MINERALS
Rich in potassium, calcium, phosphorus and magnesium, and other trace minerals

XANTHINE DERIVATIVES
Caffeine and other xanthine-derivatives, such as theobromine, are stimulants

CATECHINS
The most prevalent types of phenol flavonoids in green tea; may be anticarcinogenic

Water, steeping times, and temperatures

Brewing the perfect cup of tea is an art and a science. The final brew should be slightly acidic—with a pH close to 5—so it is best to start with water that is neutral, and with a moderate mineral content. Mineral water may be better suited than tap water in many regions. While larger flavor compounds emerge slowly, and at higher temperatures, in green tea, cooler water limits the extraction of bitter and astringent compounds.

Optimum conditions
Different types of tea are best prepared using particular water temperatures and brewing times.

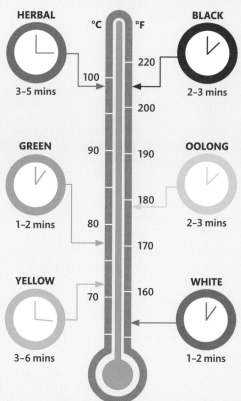

HERBAL
3–5 mins

°C   °F

100   220

200

GREEN
1–2 mins

90   190

180

80   170

YELLOW
3–6 mins

70   160

BLACK
2–3 mins

OOLONG
2–3 mins

WHITE
1–2 mins

Cooling down

A hot drink can actually help you to cool down on a hot day, by increasing the amount you sweat. Although the drink raises your core temperature, the net effect is heat loss.

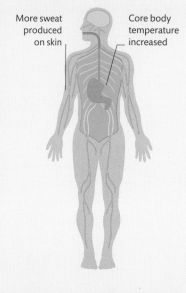

More sweat produced on skin

Core body temperature increased

Fruit juice and smoothies

One of the hottest diet fads is the extracting and blending of healthy ingredients to make easy-to-consume drinks. Although juices and smoothies have much to recommend them, the hype masks some potential downsides.

Fruit and vegetables versus juice

While juice is often touted as offering the health benefits of fruit and vegetables, in fact, juices differ significantly from the whole foods from which they are made. In addition to removing the beneficial insoluble fiber from fruit and vegetables, juicing removes their texture and, especially in vegetables, strips away the structure that can actually have a cleansing action on teeth. In fruit juice, all the sugar from a large amount of fruit is concentrated into a much smaller volume, resulting in a very high sugar content. The sugars are liberated and immediately available to bacteria in the mouth that contribute to tooth decay.

Solid or liquid?

A small glass of orange juice contains almost all the fruit sugar (fructose) of three medium-sized oranges—more oranges than most people would eat. Furthermore, it contains only a very small fraction of the fiber content.

KEY

- Portion of fruit eaten whole
- Portion of fruit in a glass of juice
- Sugar (oz/g)

IS FRESHLY SQUEEZED JUICE BETTER THAN JUICE FROM CONCENTRATE?

There is no difference in the nutritional value of juice from concentrate. If sugar has been added, however, it will raise calories and the risk of tooth decay.

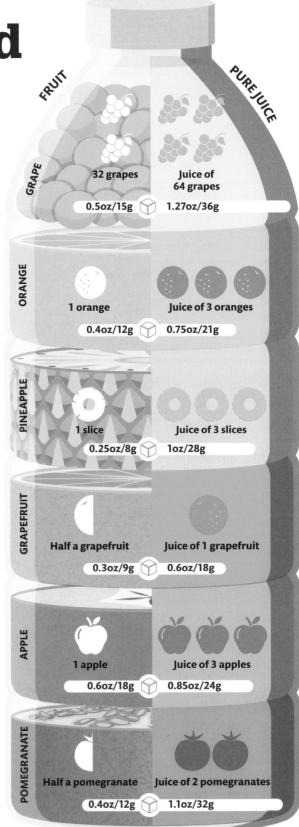

FRUIT | **PURE JUICE**

GRAPE
- 32 grapes — 0.5oz/15g
- Juice of 64 grapes — 1.27oz/36g

ORANGE
- 1 orange — 0.4oz/12g
- Juice of 3 oranges — 0.75oz/21g

PINEAPPLE
- 1 slice — 0.25oz/8g
- Juice of 3 slices — 1oz/28g

GRAPEFRUIT
- Half a grapefruit — 0.3oz/9g
- Juice of 1 grapefruit — 0.6oz/18g

APPLE
- 1 apple — 0.6oz/18g
- Juice of 3 apples — 0.85oz/24g

POMEGRANATE
- Half a pomegranate — 0.4oz/12g
- Juice of 2 pomegranates — 1.1oz/32g

More nitrates
Green smoothies are high in nitrates, which can help to dilate the body's blood vessels and reduce blood pressure.

Sugar spike
Blending ingredients increases their glycemic index, meaning that the body absorbs their sugars more quickly. Adding greens to smoothies can counteract this.

More fruit and vegetables
Smoothies can help us to meet the five-a-day target of fruit and vegetables, but are better used as a complement rather than to replace whole meals.

PROS

Smoothies
Smoothies are blended whole ingredients, often promoted as health foods, because unlike juices, they retain the fiber of the whole food. In practice, there are nutritional pros and cons. On the one hand, they can encourage the intake of fruits and vegetables, and blending can help to break down cell walls, releasing more nutrients. On the other hand, they can lead to the rapid intake of large amounts of sugar. Store-bought smoothies may even contain added sugar.

CONS

Tooth decay
A flood of fruit sugars and the lack of beneficial texture increase the risk of tooth decay. Rinsing your mouth with water can help you avoid this.

More phytochemicals
Using whole fruit and vegetables in a smoothie helps to boost fiber intake and that of phytochemicals attached to fiber.

Smoothie sense
The faults in smoothies can be counteracted by the way you make them. Adding greens, such as spinach or celery, can not only accentuate the benefits, but also reduce the drawbacks, such as blood-sugar spikes.

Kidney stones
Green smoothies can be high in compounds called oxalates, which increase the risk of kidney stone formation.

Fruit juice versus soft drinks
Fruit juices may not be much healthier than soft drinks or energy drinks. They contain comparable levels of sugar and can take daily sugar intake to levels that contribute to obesity and diabetes, especially in children.

Sugar content of drinks
Energy drinks can contain amazing quantities of sugar. While a typical can of soda contains around seven spoonfuls, orange juice is not that far behind.

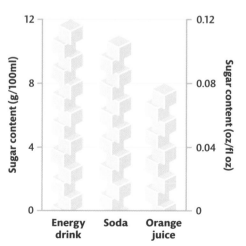

Sugar content (g/100ml): 0, 4, 8, 12
Sugar content (oz/fl oz): 0, 0.04, 0.08, 0.12

Energy drink | Soda | Orange juice

BLENDED SOUPS

At least one study backs up the claim that soups can fill you up more than solid foods taken with water. This implies that blended soups stay in the stomach longer, inhibiting the release of ghrelin, the "hunger hormone," so that appetite is suppressed.

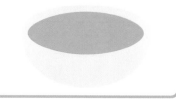

Carbonated drinks

Many people enjoy carbonated drinks as a regular part of their diet. Although they are mostly water, they contain a significant quantity of sugar and have been implicated in a number of health problems.

What is in soda?

Typically, a carbonated drink starts as a "simple syrup" of sugar and water. The other ingredients are then added in a specific order to give what is called the "finished syrup." This is diluted with water, carbonated, and bottled (or canned). For some bottled drinks, carbonation is done after bottling, just before the bottle is sealed.

Under pressure

Putting the fizz in a drink is achieved by bubbling carbon dioxide gas through the liquid under high pressure, so that the carbon dioxide dissolves. When the pressure is released, the carbon dioxide forms gas bubbles again.

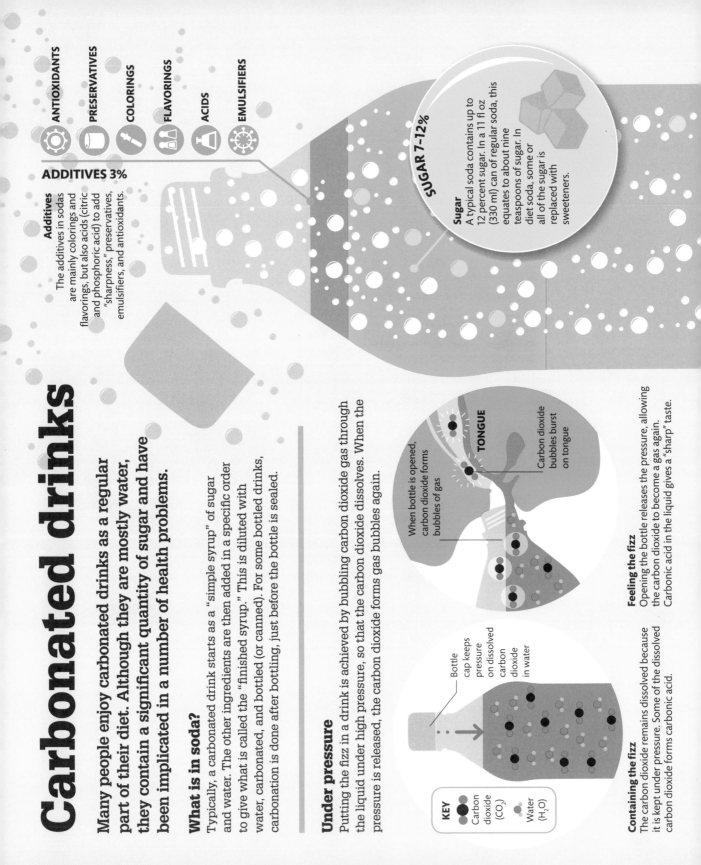

ADDITIVES 3%

ANTIOXIDANTS
PRESERVATIVES
COLORINGS
FLAVORINGS
ACIDS
EMULSIFIERS

Additives
The additives in sodas are mainly colorings and flavorings, but also acids (citric and phosphoric acid) to add "sharpness," preservatives, emulsifiers, and antioxidants.

SUGAR 7–12%

Sugar
A typical soda contains up to 12 percent sugar. In a 11 fl oz (330 ml) can of regular soda, this equates to about nine teaspoons of sugar. In diet soda, some or all of the sugar is replaced with sweeteners.

Containing the fizz
The carbon dioxide remains dissolved because it is kept under pressure. Some of the dissolved carbon dioxide forms carbonic acid.

Bottle cap keeps pressure on dissolved carbon dioxide in water

KEY
Carbon dioxide (CO_2)
Water (H_2O)

When bottle is opened, carbon dioxide forms bubbles of gas

TONGUE

Carbon dioxide bubbles burst on tongue

Feeling the fizz
Opening the bottle releases the pressure, allowing the carbon dioxide to become a gas again. Carbonic acid in the liquid gives a "sharp" taste.

Supersizing drinks

The introduction of cheap sugar alternatives in the 1970s led to an increasing supersizing of soft drinks. Previously, drinks came in 6.5fl oz (190mL) bottles, but the standard can now contains 110fl oz (330mL). As a result, people are often consuming significantly more calories in drinks than they could possibly eat.

Movie theater-sized portion is equivalent to three standard cans

LARGE SIZE CARBONATED DRINK
32fl oz (940mL)

364 CALORIES

Butter not included in calories

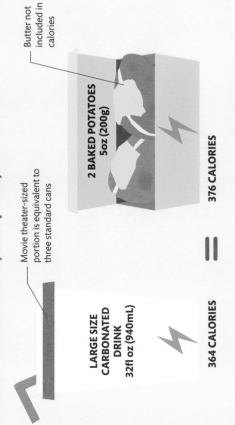

2 BAKED POTATOES
5oz (200g)

376 CALORIES

TRUCKS TRANSPORTING
SODA HAVE TO DISPLAY THE
HAZARD WARNING SYMBOL
FOR HIGHLY CORROSIVE MATERIAL

Rotting the teeth

It is not only the sugar in sodas that is bad for you; they also contain three acids—citric, carbonic, and phosphoric. These all have an average pH of 2.5, which is slightly stronger than stomach acid. These acids erode the enamel of teeth, exposing them to microbial attack and subsequent decay.

Tooth staining and decay
The sugar in soda contributes to the buildup of plaque, which can lead to staining and decay.

Water

WATER 85%

Water makes up most of a soft drink. Usually taken from the city water supply, the water is filtered and treated to remove solid particles and microbes before adding sugar and additives. After this, the liquid is carbonated.

TOXIC TONICS

Sodas began as health tonics, based on the widespread belief that carbonated spa waters were healthy. Cola drinks began as a mixture of wine and cocaine until Prohibition in 1886, when the wine was replaced by soda water. Cocaine remained until 1904, when its addictive qualities became a matter of concern.

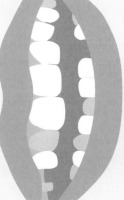

Energy drinks

Manufacturers' claims have driven the explosive growth of the energy drink market. Positioned at the intersection between soft drinks and supplements, energy drinks struggle to back up their boasts.

Types of energy drinks

Energy drinks are soft drinks that claim to boost energy levels. They usually have high levels of caffeine and sugar, and may contain electrolytes (mineral ions, such as sodium, normally dissolved in the blood). Many feature amino acids, herbal extracts, and other ingredients claimed to have health benefits. The market has diversified to include sugar-free varieties and concentrated versions in the form of shots and gels. Drinking them with alcohol increases the risk of overindulgence and dehydration.

CAN PROTEIN SHAKES REPLACE MEALS?

Protein shakes can be an effective meal replacement as part of a balanced diet, but they lack the essential vitamins and minerals of a complete meal.

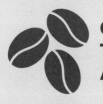

GUARANA SEEDS HAVE TWICE AS MUCH CAFFEINE AS COFFEE BEANS

The verdict
Packed with caffeine and usually full of sugar, energy drinks are not regulated. They can contain 200 milligrams or more of caffeine per serving (a very strong cup of coffee might contain 180 milligrams), and may contain as many as 400 calories.

ENERGY DRINK

Main ingredients:

 Stimulants

Sugar

Water

Effects and drawbacks
Simple sugars can give an immediate surge in blood sugar levels and caffeine can mask feelings of fatigue, but any energy-boosting effects are short-lived and typically precede a crash. Negative impacts include weight gain, headaches, and anxiety.

Real benefits?
Sports drinks differ in electrolyte levels formulated for before, during, and after exercise. However, other than endurance athletes, people are unlikely to run low on electrolytes or exhaust energy stores, so sports drinks rarely perform better than water.

SPORTS DRINK

Main ingredients:

Electrolytes

Sugar

Water

Claimed benefits
Formulated to replace electrolytes lost in sweat, and replenish energy stores depleted by long exercise, sports drinks are supposed to improve stamina and prevent athletes from exhausting their carbohydrate-based energy stores.

Stimulating the body

Energy drinks often contain caffeine, taurine, guarana, ephedrine (restricted in some countries), or ginseng—all included as stimulants. Caffeine works by stimulating adrenaline release and by blocking the "fatigue" signal produced by adenosine—a chemical made when the body's metabolism releases energy. Ephedrine is also a stimulant but one with dangerous side-effects including high blood pressure and heartbeat irregularities.

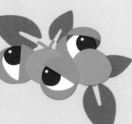

Guarana
Seeds of the guarana plant contain more caffeine than coffee beans, but supposedly release it more slowly. They also contain cardiac stimulants theobromine and theophylline.

CAFFEINE AND SPORTS

Caffeine can increase muscle endurance and speeds up the production of glycogen—the body's carbohydrate energy store. High adrenaline levels boost blood flow to the heart and muscles and stimulate energy production. Adrenaline may also reduce perceived levels of pain and fatigue.

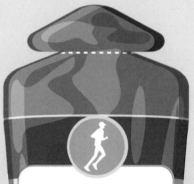

Brain

Heart

Muscle

Do they work?
Designed to help build muscle mass, protein shakes provide the amino acids necessary to build up muscles. In reality, only high-level body-builders need more than can easily be obtained in the diet. Excessive levels of protein may cause kidney damage and bone loss.

PROTEIN SHAKE

Main ingredients:
- Protein powder
- Flavorings
- Sweeteners

What is on offer
Protein shakes are drinks made from protein-rich supplements, most often from whey (milk proteins left behind by cheese making), but also from casein in milk, soy, egg, hemp, rice, and pea. They are high in calories.

Conclusion
As with sports drinks, gels are unlikely to benefit anyone other than endurance athletes, such as marathon runners. For everyone else, they provide empty calories, with implications for weight gain and diabetes risk.

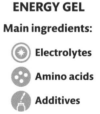

ENERGY GEL

Main ingredients:
- Electrolytes
- Amino acids
- Additives

Product breakdown
Highly concentrated into syrupy gels, these provide portable forms of energy supplement, intended for endurance athletes on the go who need to minimize the weight they are carrying. They may also contain caffeine and other stimulants.

Alcohol

All alcoholic drinks contain ethanol—the chemical name for the simplest form of alcohol. Most forms of alcohol are made by fermenting grains (for beer, see pp.172–73) or grapes (for wine, see pp.170–71). More pure forms of alcohol are produced by distillation.

IS ALCOHOL A POISON?

In sufficient amounts, alcohol slows down brain function, irritates the stomach, dehydrates you, and lowers your body temperature and blood sugar levels. So yes, it is a poison.

Volatile compounds such as ethanol evaporate

2 **Evaporating alcohol**
Ethanol boils at 173°F (78.4°C) so it evaporates, leaving water behind. Other chemicals in the mix, including highly toxic methanol, are also volatile so evaporate, too.

BOILER

3 **Condensing**
In the pot distillation process, the different components condense as the evaporate passes through a system of cooling pipes.

Cooling pipe

CONDENSER

Distillation

Alcohol is made initially through the fermentation of sugary plant juices. Distillation is used to produce a more pure form of alcohol. The various components of a mixture boil at different temperatures, so as the mix is heated, some components boil off before others. If these can be captured and condensed separately, it is possible to obtain alcohol of 95–98 percent purity.

Distillate collects

Methanol
This lightest of alcohols comes off first. Distillers throw this away because it is poisonous.

4 **Distillate**
The distiller must draw off and discard lighter volatile compounds (congeners), which pass through the condenser first. In small quantities, these congeners provide flavor. The distillate is diluted for consumption (see pp.166–67).

Ethanol
The principle alcohol in all alcoholic drinks.

Butanol
This gives some spirits their oily nature, as its structure is similar to those of fatty acids.

COLLECTING VESSEL

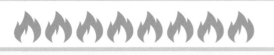

1 **Heating the ferment**
Grapes (to produce brandy, for example) or grain (to make whiskey) are first fermented to produce alcohol. Once the fermentation has finished, the ferment is heated inside the distillation plant or still.

How much in a drink?

Guidelines as to what counts as moderate drinking, and particularly what constitutes a standard drink, vary by country. In the US, one standard drink contains 0.6fl oz (14g) of alcohol, while in Austria it is 0.3fl oz (6g) and in Japan 0.85fl oz (19.75g). In the UK, official guidelines refer to units (one unit is about 0.35fl oz, or 8g, of alcohol).

PURE ALCOHOL

Calorie count

At 7 calories per gram, alcohol contains almost as many calories as pure fat. Most drinks contain sugars, too, which add to the calorie count. The drinks below each contain 0.6fl oz (14g) alcohol—a standard US drink.

5fl oz (150ml)
12% alcohol
125 calories

12fl oz (355ml)
5% alcohol
155 calories

Many of the calories in beer come from unfermented sugars

Red wine can be up to 16% alcohol, and even more calories

1.5fl oz (44ml)
40% alcohol
95 calories

6.5fl oz (192ml)
5% alcohol
150 calories

Alcohol and calorie content depends on the ratio of alcohol to mixer

BEER **SPIRITS** **WINE** **SPIRITS AND MIXER**

Is alcohol ever healthy?

There is a paradox around alcohol and health. Alcohol increases the risk of liver disease and a range of cancers, but studies have shown a correlation between moderate alcohol consumption and improved heart health. Some experts are sceptical, others point to beneficial effects of antioxidants or nitrous oxide boosting blood flow. There may even be a link to less anxiety and more sociability, with associated health benefits.

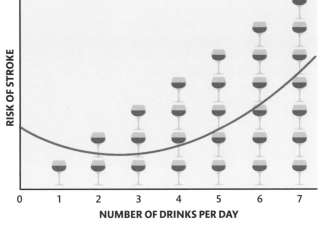

RISK OF STROKE

0 1 2 3 4 5 6 7
NUMBER OF DRINKS PER DAY

The case of stroke

Small amounts of alcohol may have a protective effect on the heart. One study in 2007 showed how the risk of stroke (purple line) correlated with alcohol intake—with a moderate consumption having a protective effect. However, more recently other studies have raised doubts over this.

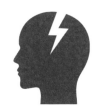

MODERATE ALCOHOL INTAKE MAY **REDUCE STROKE RISK**

Spirits

Ever since ancient and medieval pioneers first practiced the art of distillation, the production of spirits has been an alchemical process capable of transforming base ingredients into concentrated alcohol.

Spirit or liqueur?

Spirits are alcohol (ethanol) products made by the distillation of a fermented mash (see p.164). While beer may contain as little as 3 percent alcohol by volume (ABV), spirits have an alcohol content of more than 20 percent and are generally at least 40 percent. A liqueur is a sweetened, and often flavored, spirit.

Popular spirits

Spirits differ according to the source of their original fermented sugars, as well as by the purity of the distillate before it is diluted. Coloured impurities in the distillate (congeners) provide flavor.

ALCOHOL IS THE CAUSE OF **5 PERCENT OF ALL CANCERS** WORLDWIDE

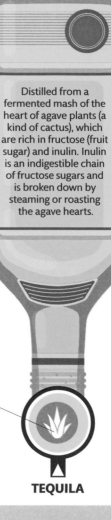

Distilled from a fermented mash of the heart of agave plants (a kind of cactus), which are rich in fructose (fruit sugar) and inulin. Inulin is an indigestible chain of fructose sugars and is broken down by steaming or roasting the agave hearts.

Spirits distilled from grape wine. The two most famous brandies—Cognac and Armagnac, named after their French regions of origin—are made from white wine.

Blue agave is the species commonly used in tequila

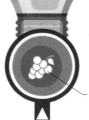

Fermented grape juice yields brandy when distilled

BRANDY

TEQUILA

Drinking dangers

Although some data suggests one or two drinks a day can benefit heart health (see p.165), even moderate drinking could be a cause of cancer. Alcohol has been linked with nine cancers, including mouth and throat, liver, breast, and bowel. The chief suspect is acetaldehyde, a breakdown product of alcohol.

Mouth cancer

Oral cancer cases increase with alcohol consumption (1 unit = $\frac{1}{3}$fl oz, or 10ml, of pure alcohol, or one modest drink). When it comes to cancer, there is no safe drinking limit.

NO ALCOHOL

One extra case

10.5 UNITS PER WEEK

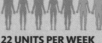

Three extra lifetime cases per 1,000 people

22 UNITS PER WEEK

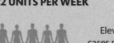

Eleven extra cases per 1,000

44 UNITS PER WEEK

ARE SPIRITS MORE HARMFUL THAN WINE OR BEER?

All forms of alcohol are harmful, being broken down into toxic substances in the liver. Spirits are more strongly linked with mouth cancer, especially in smokers.

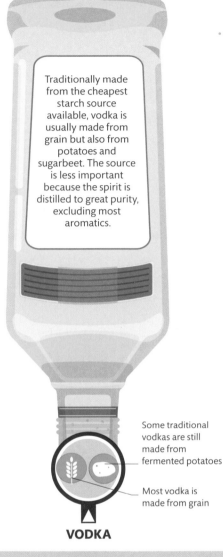

Traditionally made from the cheapest starch source available, vodka is usually made from grain but also from potatoes and sugarbeet. The source is less important because the spirit is distilled to great purity, excluding most aromatics.

Some traditional vodkas are still made from fermented potatoes

Most vodka is made from grain

VODKA

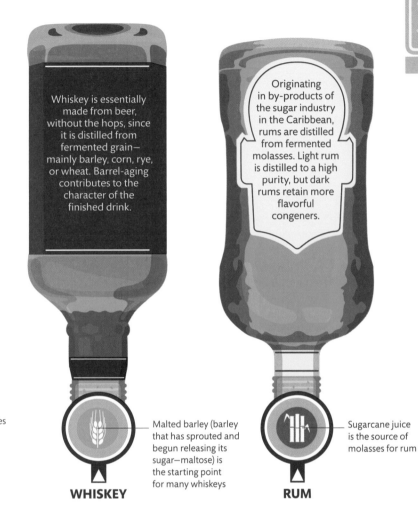

Whiskey is essentially made from beer, without the hops, since it is distilled from fermented grain—mainly barley, corn, rye, or wheat. Barrel-aging contributes to the character of the finished drink.

Malted barley (barley that has sprouted and begun releasing its sugar—maltose) is the starting point for many whiskeys

WHISKEY

Originating in by-products of the sugar industry in the Caribbean, rums are distilled from fermented molasses. Light rum is distilled to a high purity, but dark rums retain more flavorful congeners.

Sugarcane juice is the source of molasses for rum

RUM

Alcohol abuse

Alcohol and its breakdown products (such as acetaldehyde) are toxic to many different organs and tissues of the body. Long-term overuse of alcohol over a decade or more can damage most systems of the body and seriously increase the risk of cancer (see opposite), liver disease, stroke, heart disease, brain damage, neurological damage, depression, seizures, gout, pancreatitis, and anemia. In all, over 60 diseases have been linked to alcohol abuse.

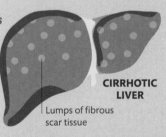

CIRRHOTIC LIVER

Lumps of fibrous scar tissue

Liver damage
Alcoholic cirrhosis of the liver is where alcohol breakdown products damage the liver, causing it to regrow with scar tissue and fatty deposits that limit its ability to function. Cirrhosis can be fatal.

EXPLOITING DENSITY

The strongest, most alcoholic drinks float on water, since water is denser than ethanol. Heavier ingredients, however, such as coffee, make most drinks heavier than water. Skilled bartenders exploit different drink densities to create layered cocktails.

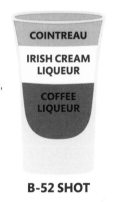

COINTREAU

IRISH CREAM LIQUEUR

COFFEE LIQUEUR

B-52 SHOT

Alcohol and the body

Alcohol gets into the body very fast. Unlike most food and drink, it is absorbed into the bloodstream within minutes. It takes the liver about one hour to process one unit of alcohol, forming a highly toxic compound as it breaks it down for elimination.

Effects of alcohol on the body

As alcohol hits the stomach, around 20 percent begins to cross into the bloodstream right away. It is quickly passed to the liver, brain, and pancreas, where it starts to break down. The rest is absorbed through the gut. Alcohol is first broken down into acetaldehyde, then acetate, and is finally eliminated as carbon dioxide and water. Acetaldehyde is highly toxic and causes damage to cells, especially those of the liver, which can become irreparably damaged.

Genes and alcohol

Some ethnic groups have genetic variations that prolong the endurance of acetaldehyde in the body. This can cause unpleasant nausea and flushing, but may also have the effect of putting them off drinking. Genetics can also play a part in whether someone is predisposed to become an alcoholic.

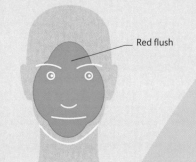

Red flush

MOUTH

STOMACH

CIRCULATORY SYSTEM

LIVER

Taking it in
Contact with strong alcohol can damage the cells lining the mouth, throat, and esophagus, promoting cancers in these areas, especially among smokers.

Upset stomach
Alcohol stimulates the stomach to produce large quantities of acid that can irritate the lining of the stomach and lead to ulcers over time.

Warm feelings
Alcohol makes the blood vessels widen, making you feel warm. It also causes a temporary drop in blood pressure and pulse rate. Small vessels can also break.

Fatty liver
Repeated use leads to inflammation and scarring of liver cells. Fat becomes deposited between the cells, making it hard for the liver to work properly.

Under the influence
Alcohol is a psychoactive drug. In small doses it acts as a depressant, but reduces inhibitions and anxiety to produce feelings of euphoria. At higher doses it causes intoxication, stupor, and unconsciousness.

IT TAKES ABOUT **THREE HOURS** FOR YOUR BODY TO **BREAK DOWN** THE **ALCOHOL** IN A **LARGE** (8.5 FL OZ/250 ML) **GLASS OF WINE**

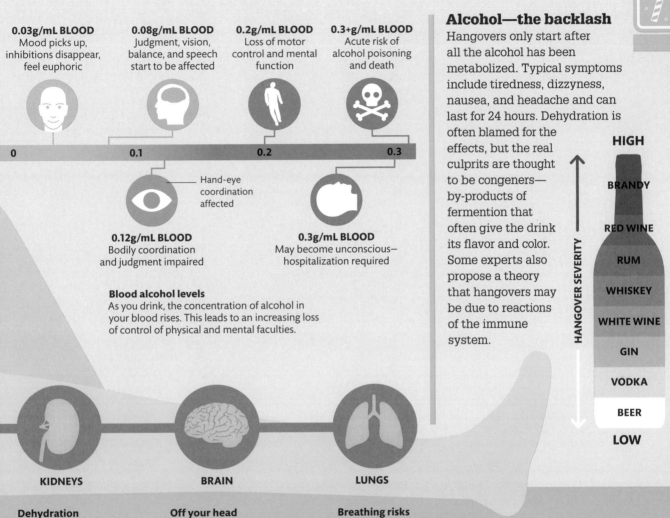

0.03g/mL BLOOD
Mood picks up, inhibitions disappear, feel euphoric

0.08g/mL BLOOD
Judgment, vision, balance, and speech start to be affected

0.2g/mL BLOOD
Loss of motor control and mental function

0.3+g/mL BLOOD
Acute risk of alcohol poisoning and death

0   0.1   0.2   0.3

Hand-eye coordination affected

0.12g/mL BLOOD
Bodily coordination and judgment impaired

0.3g/mL BLOOD
May become unconscious—hospitalization required

Blood alcohol levels
As you drink, the concentration of alcohol in your blood rises. This leads to an increasing loss of control of physical and mental faculties.

Alcohol—the backlash

Hangovers only start after all the alcohol has been metabolized. Typical symptoms include tiredness, dizzyness, nausea, and headache and can last for 24 hours. Dehydration is often blamed for the effects, but the real culprits are thought to be congeners—by-products of fermentation that often give the drink its flavor and color. Some experts also propose a theory that hangovers may be due to reactions of the immune system.

HANGOVER SEVERITY

HIGH
BRANDY
RED WINE
RUM
WHISKEY
WHITE WINE
GIN
VODKA
BEER
LOW

KIDNEYS

BRAIN

LUNGS

Dehydration
Alcohol increases urine production as soon as 20 minutes after being drunk. Excess drinking can lead to thirst and dehydration.

Off your head
Some alcohol is broken down by the brain, which is instantly affected. Control of mental and physical functions becomes progressively harder.

Breathing risks
Drinking increases the risk of inhaling vomit and also affects nitric oxide levels, both of which make the lungs more susceptible to infection.

Alcoholism
Overuse of alcohol can tip a social drinker into becoming an alcoholic. The body develops a physical tolerance to alcohol and it becomes psychologically difficult to stop drinking. Giving up produces withdrawal symptoms that can be as bad as those of drinking.

WHY DOES CHAMPAGNE MAKE YOU DRUNK SO FAST?

The bubbles in champagne helps the body absorb alcohol into the bloodstream more quickly, as do carbonated mixers with spirits.

CRUSHER

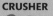

RED GRAPES

Fermentation vessel is warm, encouraging the release of chemicals from the skins and seeds

1 **Grapes crushed**
To release juice, grapes are first crushed and the stems removed. The squashed grapes, with skins and seeds, are poured out.

FERMENTING TANK

2 **Warm fermentation**
Yeast ferments the crushed grapes, converting its sugar to alcohol. Winemakers may add a cultured yeast, or they may rely on the yeast on the grape skins.

PRESS

3 **Pulp pressed**
The crushed, fermented grapes flow into the wine press, which applies pressure to release further color and flavor from the grapes.

Wine from the fermenting tank, known as free-run juice, is mixed with a little fluid from the press

Richly colored press wine pours from the press and is added to the free-run juice to improve appearance and flavor

CHEMICALS IN WINE

Procyanidins
A kind of tannin that makes young reds bitter, procyanidins may act on artery linings to improve cardiovascular health.

Resveratrol
This phytochemical has been shown in rodents to lower blood sugar and fight cancer (in high doses).

Flavonols
Shown to have antioxidant and anti-cancer actions in animals, although the dose in red wine is very low.

Anthocyanins
The human body metabolizes these antioxidants quickly, so if active, they must be effective in trace amounts.

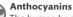

Is red wine better for you?

Interest in the possible health benefits of moderate wine drinking reached a high in the 1990s. It was then that US journalists noted that the population of France was longer lived and more free of coronary heart disease than those of other countries with high-fat diets, such as the UK and US. Attention focused on red wine, because unlike white, it is made by fermenting whole grapes, skins and all, and contains a range of chemicals such as tannins, flavonoids, and pigments called anthocyanins. Scientists are still investigating the therapeutic actions of many of these.

Wine

In recent decades, wine has gained publicity for its potential benefits to health. Some experts claim a glass of red a day lowers the risk of heart disease and other cardiovascular problems. So what is it about wine that is healthy, and is red better?

Secret ingredients
The red wine making process fills your glass with extracts of grape skins and seeds. It is not clear which of these, if any, benefits human health. One chemical called resveratrol has a range of benefits in lab mice, but only in doses impossible to achieve by drinking wine. Procyanidins in high-tannin wines might be more promising candidates.

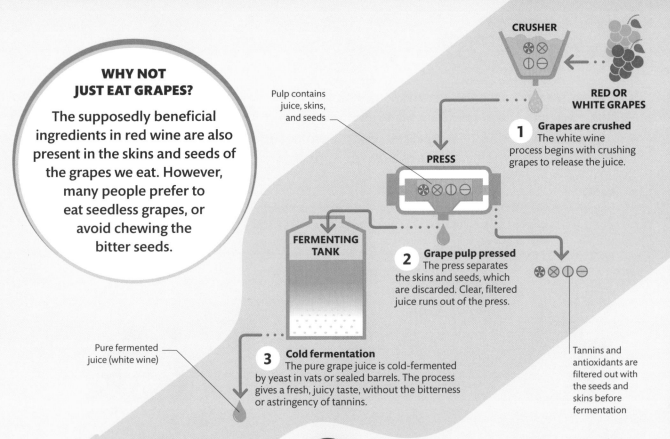

WHY NOT JUST EAT GRAPES?

The supposedly beneficial ingredients in red wine are also present in the skins and seeds of the grapes we eat. However, many people prefer to eat seedless grapes, or avoid chewing the bitter seeds.

CRUSHER

RED OR WHITE GRAPES

Pulp contains juice, skins, and seeds

PRESS

1 Grapes are crushed
The white wine process begins with crushing grapes to release the juice.

2 Grape pulp pressed
The press separates the skins and seeds, which are discarded. Clear, filtered juice runs out of the press.

FERMENTING TANK

Pure fermented juice (white wine)

3 Cold fermentation
The pure grape juice is cold-fermented by yeast in vats or sealed barrels. The process gives a fresh, juicy taste, without the bitterness or astringency of tannins.

Tannins and antioxidants are filtered out with the seeds and skins before fermentation

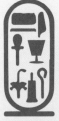

WINE IS AN INGREDIENT IN THE **OLDEST KNOWN RECIPES FOR MEDICINE**, DOCUMENTED IN **2200** BCE, ON **PAPYRI IN EGYPT**

A little of what you like
In white wine, the skins and seeds are removed before fermentation so white lacks the phytochemicals of red wine. However, experts are learning that the health benefits of red wine may have been overstated, and some studies find, paradoxically, that it is actually the alcohol in wine that is healthy (see pp.166–67). If true, white-wine drinkers could also benefit from a glass a day.

IT'S ONLY A GLASS

Wine measures vary from place to place and according to trends, so it can be difficult to know that you drinking in moderation. A large glass can be one-third of a 750ml (25fl oz) bottle, containing 200 calories, or more, in the form of sugar and alcohol. Alcohol content has increased in recent years, as modern production involves leaving fruit to ripen longer on the vine, so it becomes more sugary, resulting in more alcoholic wine with more calories.

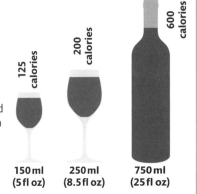

125 calories
150ml (5fl oz)

200 calories
250ml (8.5fl oz)

600 calories
750ml (25fl oz)

Beer

Probably the first alcoholic drink created by humans, beer is the world's most widely produced and consumed alcoholic beverage. This is reflected in the enormous variety of beers now available.

Brewing

Brewing relies on mobilizing the sugars in grain. This is usually begun by malting—letting the grain sprout, so that it converts its stored starch to the sugar, maltose. Brewers add flavors to the ground grain, such as hops (a flower that imparts bitter or zesty tastes), and the brew is then fermented with yeast. The finished beer can be left with some yeast to continue to mature in a cask, or it is stored, yeast-free, in bottles or kegs.

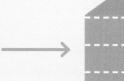

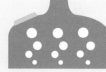

1 Producing the mash
Milled, malted grain and hot water are mixed to produce the mash. Enzymes in the grain convert its starches into sugar.

2 Lautering
The initial extraction fluid—wort—is drawn off, and then the solid remains of the malt are sparged, or washed, to release remaining sugars.

3 Boiling
The wort is boiled for up to two hours to deactivate enzymes, and to bring out bitterness. Hops are added at this stage.

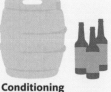

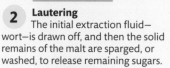

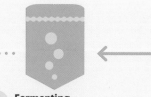

6 Conditioning
The beer is matured with a second fermentation to develop flavor and carbonation, and cleared of detritus before packaging.

5 Fermenting
Yeast is added to the wort and the mixture is fermented for four to five days, during which sugars are converted to alcohol and carbon dioxide.

4 Centrifuging
The wort is cooled in a heat exchanger and then put in a centrifuge to remove coagulated proteins and spent hops.

IN 2014, 9.25 GALLONS (35 LITERS) OF BEER WERE PRODUCED FOR EVERY ADULT ON EARTH

BEER BELLY

Although beer contains antioxidants, B vitamins, and minerals, it is also high in calories due to sugar and alcohol content, and is often consumed with fatty foods, leading to weight gain.

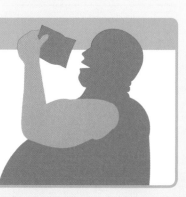

Main beer varieties
The two basic Western types of beer are ales, made using yeasts that ferment at the top of the brew, and lagers, fermented at the bottom. Top fermentation is quicker and results in more color, flavor, and fruitiness.

Light lager
Light lager is brewed using less malt, but by converting more of the sugar from which it is fermented, to give a beer with about the same alcohol content, fewer calories, but less body and flavor.

Lager
Bottom fermented in cold conditions, originally in casks stored away in cool cellars ("lager" is German for "storing"), lager is a clean, crisp tasting beer with about four to five percent alcohol.

Wheat beer
Often known as white beer, these top-fermented beers use a high proportion of wheat compared to barley, and tend to be foamier, hazier, tart, and fruity.

Ale
Top fermented, with a robust, hoppy, fruity character, ales are more colorful and cloudy than lager. Although they taste stronger, they generally have similar alcohol content to lager.

Stout
Stout is a type of ale, in which unmalted barley is sometimes used to create more browning and rich flavors. Noted for its dark color and for retaining its head, stout has three to six percent alcohol.

Types of beer

Beer has been around so long that many different types and methods have evolved around the world. Brewers often use the main staple crops available, so while European and North American beers are made from barley or wheat, many people in Africa and Asia brew their beer from millet, sorghum, or rice. In some parts of South America and Africa, when making beers from corn or cassava root, some beer makers aid the brewing process with their own saliva enzymes, contributed by chewing the crop.

GETTING A HEAD

A head of foam helps to release a beer's aroma and flavor. Beer develops foam because it is carbonated and relatively high in proteins, which prevent the air bubbles from popping. Generating and retaining the foam depends on variables such as the acidity and alcohol content of the beer, and even the type of glass used.

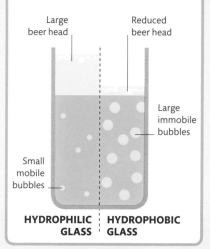

Large beer head

Reduced beer head

Large immobile bubbles

Small mobile bubbles

HYDROPHILIC GLASS

HYDROPHOBIC GLASS

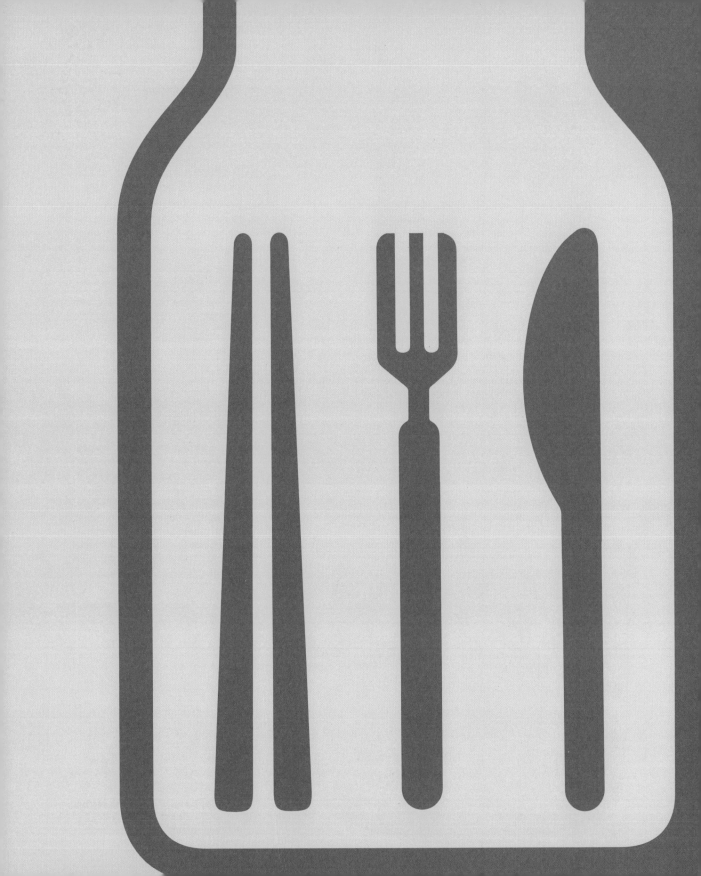

DIETS

Balanced diet

We all know that we should eat a healthy, balanced diet, but what exactly does that mean? It turns out guidelines differ around the world.

Government guidelines

Many countries' governments provide nutritional guidelines to help their people make good food choices. These are based on scientific research but are adapted to create an achievable diet in each country. After all, there would be little point recommending a diet so wildly different from the national average that nobody even tries to stick to it. While most countries recommend a diet based on whole grains and plenty of fruit and vegetables, with limited sugar, salt, and fat, guidelines differ from country to country. Some give more precise suggestions than others for the different sources of protein, and the proportions of dairy foods suggested vary dramatically.

US GUIDELINES ADVISE LESS THAN 10 TEASPOONS OF SUGAR A DAY, NOT THE CURRENT AVERAGE OF 22

Water intake
The UK recommends 6–8 drinks per day. Water, tea, coffee, milk, and sugar-free soft drinks all count. Fruit juice's high sugar content means only one small glass should be consumed daily.

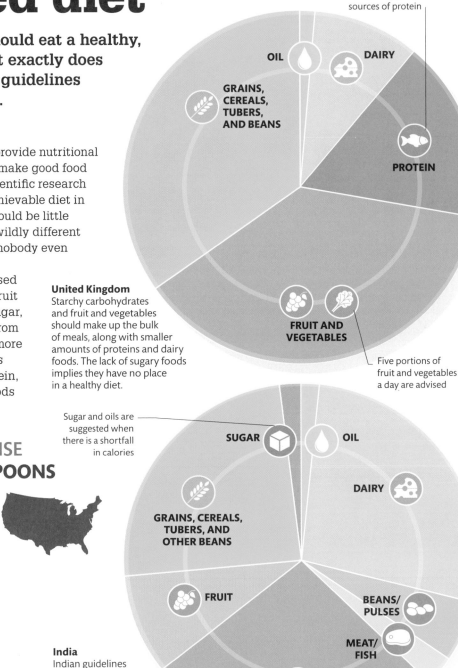

Beans, pulses, and fish are suggested sources of protein

OIL

DAIRY

GRAINS, CEREALS, TUBERS, AND BEANS

PROTEIN

United Kingdom
Starchy carbohydrates and fruit and vegetables should make up the bulk of meals, along with smaller amounts of proteins and dairy foods. The lack of sugary foods implies they have no place in a healthy diet.

FRUIT AND VEGETABLES

Five portions of fruit and vegetables a day are advised

Sugar and oils are suggested when there is a shortfall in calories

SUGAR

OIL

DAIRY

GRAINS, CEREALS, TUBERS, AND OTHER BEANS

FRUIT

BEANS/ PULSES

MEAT/ FISH

VEGETABLES

India
Indian guidelines suggest a diet rich in grains, dairy foods, and vegetables. Much of the protein comes from pulses, with a smaller amount coming from meat. Variety is important in the Indian diet.

Homegrown or locally sourced vegetables are recommended

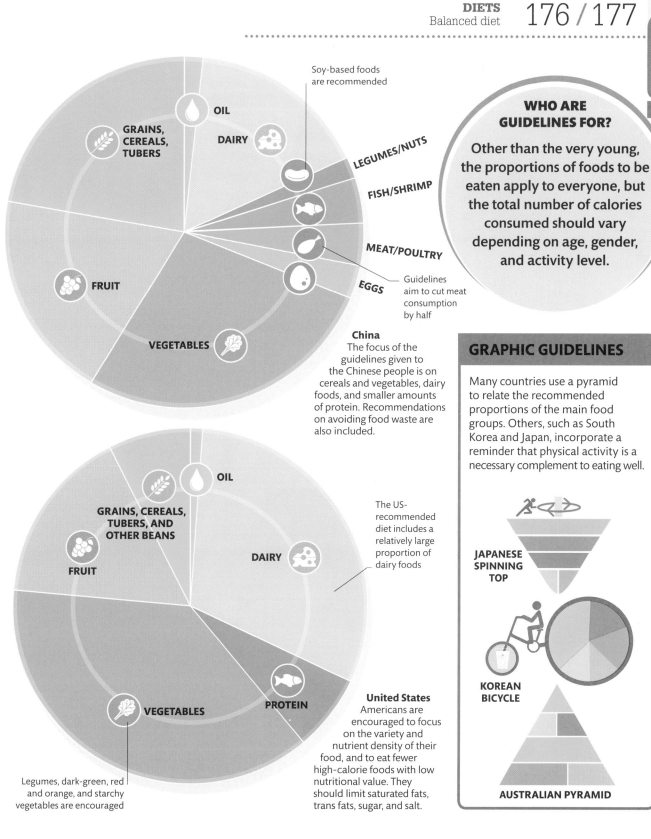

Soy-based foods are recommended

OIL

GRAINS, CEREALS, TUBERS

DAIRY

LEGUMES/NUTS

FISH/SHRIMP

MEAT/POULTRY

Guidelines aim to cut meat consumption by half

EGGS

FRUIT

VEGETABLES

WHO ARE GUIDELINES FOR?

Other than the very young, the proportions of foods to be eaten apply to everyone, but the total number of calories consumed should vary depending on age, gender, and activity level.

China
The focus of the guidelines given to the Chinese people is on cereals and vegetables, dairy foods, and smaller amounts of protein. Recommendations on avoiding food waste are also included.

GRAPHIC GUIDELINES

Many countries use a pyramid to relate the recommended proportions of the main food groups. Others, such as South Korea and Japan, incorporate a reminder that physical activity is a necessary complement to eating well.

JAPANESE SPINNING TOP

KOREAN BICYCLE

AUSTRALIAN PYRAMID

OIL

GRAINS, CEREALS, TUBERS, AND OTHER BEANS

DAIRY

The US-recommended diet includes a relatively large proportion of dairy foods

FRUIT

VEGETABLES

PROTEIN

United States
Americans are encouraged to focus on the variety and nutrient density of their food, and to eat fewer high-calorie foods with low nutritional value. They should limit saturated fats, trans fats, sugar, and salt.

Legumes, dark-green, red and orange, and starchy vegetables are encouraged

Do we need supplements?

Many people take multivitamins or other supplements as part of their daily routine, but do we really need them? Health experts disagree.

YES

Many experts argue that supplements are beneficial, at least for some people, and even if you aren't in one of the groups that will benefit, taking them won't do you any harm. They can be thought of as a "safety net," ensuring good nutrition.

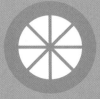

No harm
There is no evidence that taking multivitamin supplements causes harm, as long as they don't provide significantly more than the recommended intake of each nutrient.

Benefits to specific groups
Certain groups have been found to benefit from particular vitamin supplements—particularly A, C, and D in children, and folic acid in pregnant women. These effects don't show up in large population studies.

Acts as a backup
Even healthy diets can lack one nutrient or another occasionally. Vitamin supplements may act as a "safety net," preventing accidental deficiency. People who take them do show fewer nutritional inadequacies, but this may be because they also tend to eat healthily.

Boosts a poor or restricted diet
Many people have a limited or poor diet, whether because of beliefs, illness, access to food, or simply being fussy eaters. In these cases, a multivitamin can help to ensure adequate intake of vital compounds.

Can be tailored to specific needs
Males, females, and people of different ages and activity levels have different nutritional needs. Tailored supplements are matched to the requirements of the group to which you belong. This may be easier than dietary changes to ensure complete nutrition.

Vitamin D
Vitamin D helps our bodies to absorb calcium, and is a key factor in bone health. While we receive a small amount of vitamin D from the food we eat, most is made in our skin when it is exposed to ultraviolet (UV) radiation in sunlight. However, not everyone can get enough sunlight, and many people at higher latitudes may benefit from supplements.

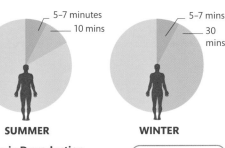

SUMMER — 5–7 minutes / 10 mins

WINTER — 5–7 mins / 30 mins

Vitamin D production
How much vitamin D the body makes can vary with age, weight, and skin type (darker skin requires more sunlight), as well as levels of UV exposure. The amount of sunlight our skin receives is affected by our latitude and the seasons.

KEY
Sun exposure time necessary for daily vitamin D dose.

- Tropical
- Temperate

IS NATURAL ALWAYS GOOD?

Not all "natural" products are safe and beneficial. Many herbal supplements, and even vitamins, can produce unpleasant side effects or interact with prescribed medications.

Multivitamins

Supplements offering multiple nutrients range from minimal to comprehensive. Many contain far more than the recommended dose of some vitamins, while they miss out others. Sometimes vitamins aren't absorbed or processed as effectively when they are not taken in combination with the foods in which they naturally occur.

TABLET WITH 24 INGREDIENTS

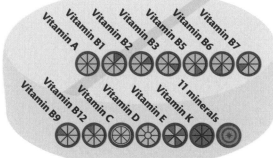

70 PERCENT OF PATIENTS WHO USE SUPPLEMENTS OR OTHER ALTERNATIVE THERAPIES DO NOT TELL THEIR DOCTOR

FOLIC ACID

Folic acid, also known as vitamin B9, is found in pulses, dark-green leafy vegetables, and citrus fruits. Pregnant women are advised to take lots of folic acid, as it helps to reduce the risk of spina bifida (defects in the spinal cord and vertebral column) in babies. However, as getting enough folic acid from even the healthiest diet may be difficult, supplements are recommended for all women in the early stages of pregnancy and even those trying to conceive.

NO

Many experts aren't convinced that supplements are a good idea for everyone. They point to the lack of evidence for their benefit in most people, the possibility of harm from high-dose formulas, and their expense.

No benefits in general population
Large studies of healthy people have not found consistent evidence that multivitamins are beneficial. Specifically, they have been found to have no effect on cardiovascular disease in the general population, or on memory in older adults.

Harmful
Some multivitamins contain huge doses of each vitamin, which may be harmful. For example, excess iron, selenium, and vitamin A can be toxic, so it is good practice to keep all supplements out of sight and reach of children.

Overdoses cannot be processed
If you take large doses of a vitamin or mineral, even if it is harmless, if the amount is more than the body needs, the body will treat it as waste and excrete it. Water-soluble vitamins cannot be stored for later use.

Not tightly regulated
Many vitamins are regulated as foods or supplements, not drugs. So while safety must be proven, composition and quality can vary dramatically. Also, there is often no guarantee you are getting exactly what's on the label.

Expensive
Multivitamins can be expensive, and in many cases the money might be better spent on supplementing the diet with more fresh fruit and vegetables, which also contain beneficial fiber.

Eating patterns

There is no scientific basis for recommending the three-meals-a-day pattern that is common in so much of the world. Scientists are trying to discover whether eating differently could make us healthier.

DO NIGHTSHIFTS AFFECT NUTRITION?

Shift workers are at higher risk of obesity, type 2 diabetes, and other illnesses. This may be due to reduced sleep leading to higher calorie intake, or time-shifted activities directly affecting the body's daily rhythm.

Breakfast like a king?

Breakfast is often described as the most important meal of the day, but is it? People who eat breakfast do tend to have lower BMIs (that is, they have lower body fat—see p.190), and those who skip it tend to have a higher risk of obesity, heart disease, and other related disorders, possibly because of the extra unhealthy snacks consumed when hunger hits midmorning. But recent studies contradict this and suggest that breakfast-skippers still eat fewer calories overall and suffer no ill effects. Skipping breakfast also extends the fasting period, which may be beneficial (see pp.200–01).

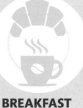

BREAKFAST

Large breakfast
Eating a large breakfast may help you resist snacking before lunch, but it isn't clear whether this will help you consume fewer calories overall.

6:00   8:00   10:00   12:

Light breakfast
Having a small breakfast, or skipping it completely, extends the overnight fast, which may be beneficial. However, it might also encourage you to make less healthy food choices when you do eat.

BREAKFAST

Snack
While it is easy to eat a lot of unhealthy foods as snacks and then gain weight, there is no evidence that healthy, portion-controlled snacks are bad.

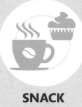

SNACK

Snacking

It is difficult to establish whether eating little and often between meals is better for your health than restricting eating to set mealtimes. What is certain is that snack foods are often high in calories and low in micronutrients. There are good snack options, however—fruit and nuts contribute to a better diet.

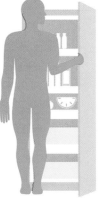

Raiding the fridge
Midnight fridge raids and other snacking habits have grown, as traditional social eating customs have become less common in many countries.

SPANISH RHYTHMS

In Spain and the Spanish-speaking Americas, people follow a markedly different pattern from three meals a day. The midday meal is the largest, but *cena* (dinner) is eaten so late (sometimes midnight) that people eat extra small meals, such as *merienda*, to bridge the gap. Tapas can also be eaten in the period before dinner.

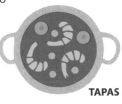

TAPAS

MORE THAN 53 PERCENT OF AMERICANS SKIP BREAKFAST AT LEAST ONCE A WEEK, AND 12 PERCENT ALWAYS SKIP IT

Dine like a pauper?

An old folk saying tells us to eat a light evening meal. Eating certainly affects the body clock—a set of processes occurring all over the body every 24 hours. Body-clock processes in the liver and fat cells may be disrupted by eating late in the day and may compete with the body's master rhythm. This may explain why meals at night paired with daytime sleep affect the body's control of blood pressure and sugar level.

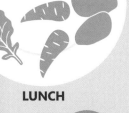

Large midday meal
There is some evidence that consuming more of your calories earlier in the day helps reduce feelings of hunger, making weight loss easier.

LUNCH

Light evening meal
Studies in mice found that their control of blood sugar varies over the day. This could mean that light meals are better when we are less active later in the day.

DINNER

2:00   **4:00**   **6:00**   **8:00**   **10:00**

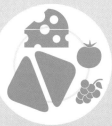

Light lunch
Distracted eating, such as a desk lunch, may lead to weight gain. Not paying attention as you eat means you are likely to overeat, or snack later on.

LUNCH

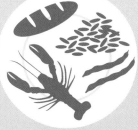

Large evening meal
Dinner times have shifted later as working and living patterns have changed. It seems this may be damaging to health, confusing the body's natural rhythms.

DINNER

Weight-gaining regime

While most of us strive to keep body fat down, sumo competitors rely on a low center of gravity to win wrestling bouts, so their daily regime of eating and activity is aimed specifically at developing a bulky physique. Wrestlers' days start with training done on an empty stomach, then they sleep at midday after an enormous meal. Scientists can't confirm why, but the sumo regime does succeed in causing weight gain.

8:00 A.M. FOOD PREP

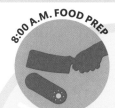

11:00 A.M. BIG MEAL

12 P.M. LONG NAP

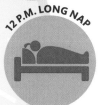

5:00 A.M. TRAINING

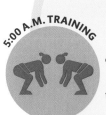

Sumo rules
Sumo competitors belong to "stables" where their eating patterns are strictly controlled. They prepare their own hearty, protein-rich stew called chakonabe and eat it with huge quantities of rice. A long nap after lunch aims to encourage the body to store calories as fat.

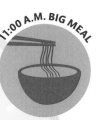

Western diets

The term "Western" diet has come to mean the processed-food-dominated diet that is now common across the world, but that originated in the US and Europe.

Western customs

At most Western meals, each person is served a plate of food, which they are expected to clear. Meals are based around protein (usually meat), with accompaniments of vegetables and carbohydrates. The main course is often followed by a sweet dessert, and sugary drinks are often consumed. Recently, trends have moved away from shared family meals to snacks and preprepared foods eaten on the go or in front of the television.

Western pattern diet

The modern Western diet is high in saturated fat, salt, sugar, and omega-6 fats (see p.136), and low in omega-3 and fiber. It has been linked to increased rates of obesity, heart disease, type 2 diabetes, and colon cancer. Some studies also suggest that it might contribute to other cancers, inflammatory diseases such as asthma and allergies, and autoimmune diseases.

HIGH ←	WESTERN PATTERN DIET	→ LOW

RED MEAT · **HIGH-FAT DAIRY** · **FRUIT** · **VEGETABLES**

PROCESSED FOOD · **SALT** · **FISH** · **LEGUMES** · **OILS**

SUGARY DRINKS · **SWEETENED FOOD** · **LOW-FAT DAIRY** · **WHOLE GRAINS**

LOW ←	WESTERN PRUDENT DIET	→ HIGH

Good versus bad diet
Not every Westerner eats badly. The "prudent" diet includes less red meat, processed foods, sugar, and salt, and focuses on whole grains, vegetables, fruit, and oils. Examples include the Mediterranean diet (see opposite) and the vegetarian diet of the Seventh Day Adventists, which provide wide-ranging health benefits.

One plate each
Portions are served at the start of the meal, and it is often considered rude not to finish the plate of food. This can make it difficult to respond to the body's fullness cues as the meal progresses.

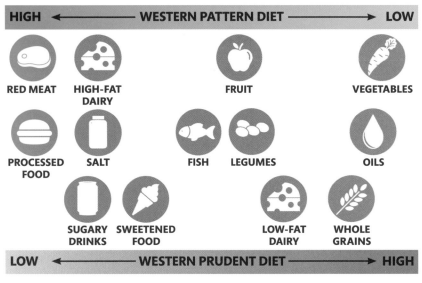

WATER

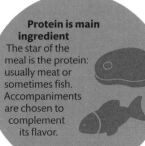

Protein is main ingredient
The star of the meal is the protein: usually meat or sometimes fish. Accompaniments are chosen to complement its flavor.

Vegetables as accompaniments

Vegetables are often viewed as a necessary but boring side dish to the protein, and are served plainly boiled or steamed. Different types are usually cooked separately.

Mediterranean food pyramid

Mediterranean meals are based around whole grains, beans, vegetables, and olive oil. Fish, fruit, dairy foods, and wine are consumed moderately, and meat and sugary dishes are considered occasional treats.

MEAT

CHEESE
YOGURT
WINE
FISH
FRUIT

WHOLE GRAINS
BEANS AND VEGETABLES
OLIVE OIL

BREAD

SPOON

WINE GLASS

FORK

KNIFE

The Mediterranean diet

The traditional diet followed by some people in the Mediterranean region, and elsewhere, is characterized by experts as "Mediterranean" and regarded as one of the world's healthiest. Studies suggest that it lowers the risk of type 2 diabetes, high blood pressure, heart disease, stroke, and Alzheimer's disease. Olive oil consumption is key in reducing inflammatory responses, reducing blood cholesterol levels, and protecting the brain.

INUIT DIET

Traditional diets of the Inuit and other Arctic peoples were rich in fish and sea mammals. However, since there was very little opportunity to enrich the diet with plant foods, it was one of the world's most restricted diets. Polar populations could survive because eating organ meat and chewing whale skin provided just enough vitamins.

SEAL

NARWHAL

Staple is bread or potatoes

Bread and potatoes are the most traditional carbohydrates, although rice and pasta are also common. These form an important part of the meal.

Cold drink

The drinks served with a meal are usually cold—wine, water, carbonated soft drinks, and juice are all common. Sugary drinks can add a lot of hidden calories to the meal.

WORLD **TYPE 2 DIABETES** CASES ARE PREDICTED TO **DOUBLE BY 2030**

Eastern diets

Eastern diets vary hugely, from the sushi of Japan to the curries of India. But they share a love of spices and strong flavors, and a reduced focus on meat, compared to most Western cuisines.

Asian customs

Despite their differences, Asian cuisines share clear similarities that make them distinct from Western cooking. One is the focus on vegetables as a main component of a meal, rather than as an accompaniment. Another is the reliance on rice as the staple grain. The flavors and ingredients are often chosen for balance, with pairings between dissimilar flavors—sweet and sour, salty and hot—more common than in Western cooking.

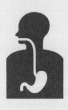

UNLIKE IN OTHER CULTURES, THE **CHINESE SERVE SOUP** AT THE **END OF A MEAL**, AS IT IS THOUGHT TO AID **DIGESTION**

Vegetable dishes
Vegetables are served as a dish in their own right, cooked and seasoned with care and valued as a dish of equal status to those featuring fish or meat. They do not simply accompany the protein part of the meal.

CHOPSTICKS

RICE DISH

TEA

SHARED VEGETABLE DISH

SOUP

IS GREEN TEA REALLY GOOD FOR ME?

At very high doses, green tea's active compound is antioxidant, anti-inflammatory, and antimicrobial, and is thought to help regulate weight, burn fat, and control blood sugar levels.

Hot drink or broth
Fluids form an important part of the meal, in the form of broth, soup, sauce, or tea. Cold drinks are less common, in some cases possibly due to an Indian Ayurvedic teaching that cold drinks slow and dilute digestive juices, although science does not support this.

Rice or noodles
Meals are usually based around rice or noodles, since rice is easily grown in most Asian countries. White (or polished) rice is favored, despite its lower nutritional value than brown rice, which has the husk left on.

SHARED VEGETABLE DISH

MAIN DISH OR BOWL

POT OF TEA

SHARED FISH DISH

Bowl filled repeatedly
It is common for individuals to take food from shared plates into their own bowl as many times as they like throughout the meal. In many cultures, it is polite to leave some food, indicating that you have eaten your fill and that the host has met your needs.

OKINAWAN DIET

Many residents of the Japanese islands of Okinawa stay slim and healthy to the age of 100 or older. Their low-calorie diet, high in fruit and vegetables (including their staple purple sweet potato) and low in refined grains, saturated fat, salt, and sugar, is thought to be the reason, along with an active, community-based lifestyle.

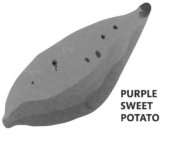

PURPLE SWEET POTATO

Higher risk group

Some Asian ethnicities, including south Asians, are more likely to develop cardiovascular disease than others, even when risk factors, such as smoking and diet, are taken into account. As Western food becomes more popular in the East, and more Asian people move to North America and Europe, obesity and its related problems are on the rise in these high-risk populations.

It's in the genes
The incidence of heart disease suggests people from south Asia are more susceptible to the dangers of a Western diet. This leads experts to suspect something in their DNA code affects how they respond to high-fat, low-fiber food.

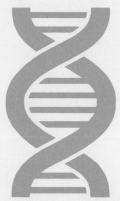

Religious and ethical diets

Many people, in all parts of the world, make diet choices based not just on taste and health, but on their ethical or religious beliefs. Whether we follow a doctrine-defined set of laws, or a few self-imposed guidelines, we each express our individual convictions through the types of food and drink we consume.

Religion-based diets

Food and dining practices play an important part in most religions, both as expressions of religious piety and group identity. While religions share some similar practices, most have their own set of laws that dictate what types of food and drink they may, and may not, consume. Guidelines for food preparation, including animal slaughter, are also followed. For some religions, particular days of the week and times of the year also have special dietary significance.

JAINISM

Jains follow an ancient Indian religion with the principle of nonviolence at its core. They go out of their way to avoid harming any living creature and eat a very strict lacto-vegetarian (egg-free) diet. They also exclude onions, garlic, and root vegetables that are necessarily killed when harvested.

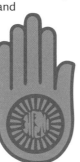

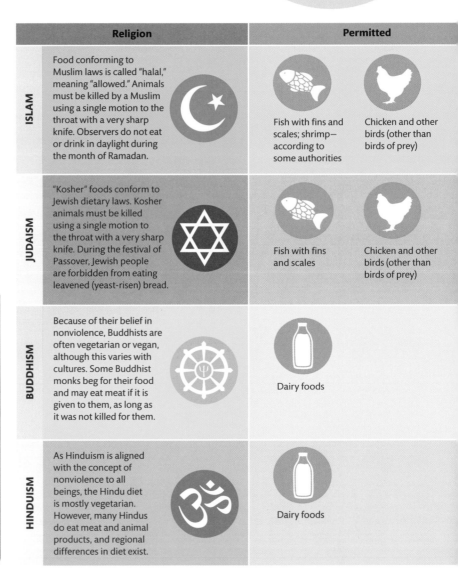

Religion			Permitted	
ISLAM	Food conforming to Muslim laws is called "halal," meaning "allowed." Animals must be killed by a Muslim using a single motion to the throat with a very sharp knife. Observers do not eat or drink in daylight during the month of Ramadan.		Fish with fins and scales; shrimp—according to some authorities	Chicken and other birds (other than birds of prey)
JUDAISM	"Kosher" foods conform to Jewish dietary laws. Kosher animals must be killed using a single motion to the throat with a very sharp knife. During the festival of Passover, Jewish people are forbidden from eating leavened (yeast-risen) bread.		Fish with fins and scales	Chicken and other birds (other than birds of prey)
BUDDHISM	Because of their belief in nonviolence, Buddhists are often vegetarian or vegan, although this varies with cultures. Some Buddhist monks beg for their food and may eat meat if it is given to them, as long as it was not killed for them.		Dairy foods	
HINDUISM	As Hinduism is aligned with the concept of nonviolence to all beings, the Hindu diet is mostly vegetarian. However, many Hindus do eat meat and animal products, and regional differences in diet exist.		Dairy foods	

Ethical diets

Our ethical beliefs can affect what foods we choose to eat and how we source them. Most vegetarians don't eat meat because they believe killing animals for food is unethical. Similarly, many people express ethical concerns about issues surrounding food production when choosing food.

Animal welfare
Some people avoid factory-farmed meat or eggs, or other meat or animal products that they consider to have been produced inhumanely.

Environment
People address issues concerning land use and global warming by avoiding red meat, which does the most environmental damage.

Sustainability
Avoiding some foods—such as types of fish—can slow the depletion of these resources, allowing stocks to recover.

Waste
People that have ethical concerns about food waste include so-called "freegans" who live off discarded food.

Permitted		Forbidden			

Animals with cloven hooves that chew the cud (cows, goats, sheep, deer)	Permitted animals slaughtered according to halal principles	Animals not slaughtered according to halal principles	Pigs, shellfish, fish without scales	Blood	Alcohol
Animals with cloven hooves that chew the cud (cows, goats, sheep, deer)	Permitted animals slaughtered according to kosher principles	Animals not slaughtered according to kosher principles	Pigs, shellfish, fish without scales	Blood	Wine or grape products from non-Jewish producers / Meat and dairy products eaten together
Vegetables, fruit, and most plant-based foods		Most animals	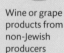 Pungent foods with strong flavors, such as garlic and ginger	Alcohol	
Vegetables, fruit, and most plant-based foods		Most animals	Eggs	Beef (extra prohibition even for meat eaters)	Pork (extra prohibition even for meat eaters)

Vegetarians and vegans

Vegetarian and related diets are usually chosen because of concerns over animal welfare, the environmental impact of eating meat, or for their health benefits. Less strict are pescatarians, who eat fish, and "flexitarians" who occasionally include meat or fish in their diet.

Nutrients

It is possible to get all necessary nutrients from a wholefood vegetarian diet, but vegans will need to consume some processed and fortified products to get everything their body needs. The only reliable, natural sources of vitamin B12, for example, are meat and animal products, and there is very little vitamin D in vegan products, other than fortified options.

Different varieties

Vegetarians don't eat meat or fish, but many eat animal products such as eggs and dairy. In India, eggs aren't seen as vegetarian, but dairy foods are encouraged. Vegans choose not to eat any products that come from animals, including honey.

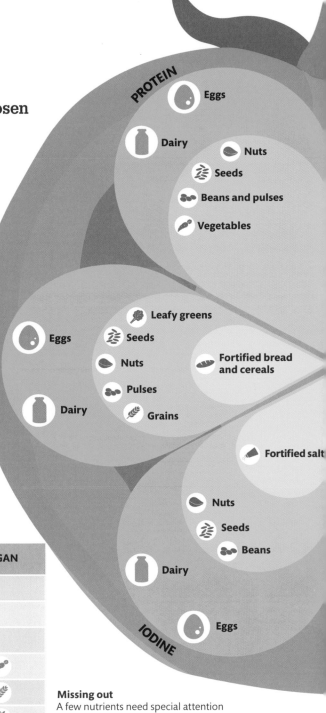

PROTEIN
- Eggs
- Dairy
- Nuts
- Seeds
- Beans and pulses
- Vegetables

IRON
- Eggs
- Dairy
- Leafy greens
- Seeds
- Nuts
- Pulses
- Grains
- Fortified bread and cereals

IODINE
- Fortified salt
- Nuts
- Seeds
- Beans
- Dairy
- Eggs

FOOD TYPES	VEGETARIAN (WESTERN)	VEGETARIAN (INDIAN)	VEGAN
Eggs	●		
Dairy	●	●	
Honey	●	●	
Vegetables	●	●	●
Grain	●	●	●
Fruit	●	●	●
Nuts and seeds	●	●	●
Beans and pulses	●	●	●

Missing out

A few nutrients need special attention in a vegetarian diet. The forms of iron and zinc found in plants are harder to absorb than those in meat, so more must be consumed, and it is difficult to get enough essential omega-3 fatty acids without eating fish.

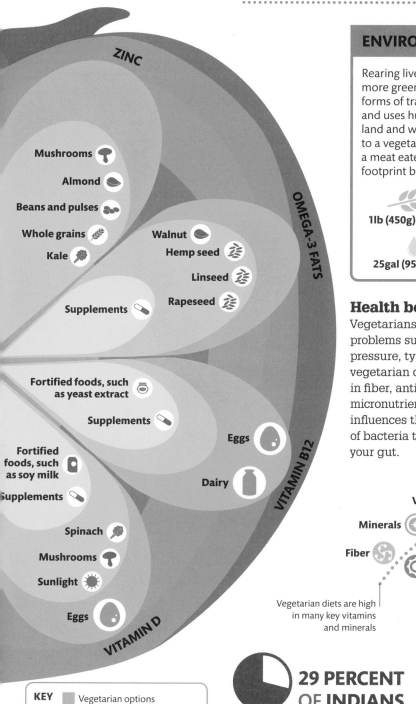

ZINC

Mushrooms

Almond

Beans and pulses

Whole grains

Kale

OMEGA-3 FATS

Walnut

Hemp seed

Linseed

Rapeseed

Supplements

Fortified foods, such as yeast extract

Supplements

Eggs

Dairy

VITAMIN B12

Fortified foods, such as soy milk

Supplements

Spinach

Mushrooms

Sunlight

Eggs

VITAMIN D

KEY

Vegetarian options

Vegan and vegetarian options

Fortified foods and supplements to a vegan diet

ENVIRONMENT

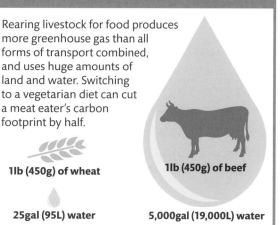

Rearing livestock for food produces more greenhouse gas than all forms of transport combined, and uses huge amounts of land and water. Switching to a vegetarian diet can cut a meat eater's carbon footprint by half.

1lb (450g) of wheat

25gal (95L) water

1lb (450g) of beef

5,000gal (19,000L) water

Health benefits

Vegetarians have a reduced chance of obesity and problems such as heart disease, high blood pressure, type 2 diabetes, and cancer. A healthy vegetarian diet is lower in saturated fat and higher in fiber, antioxidants, phytochemicals, and other micronutrients. It also influences the varieties of bacteria that inhabit your gut.

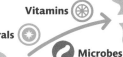

Vitamins

Minerals

Microbes

Fiber

Antioxidants

Vegetarian diets are high in many key vitamins and minerals

Fiber feeds the good bacteria in your gut, which help keep your digestive system healthy

LARGE INTESTINE

29 PERCENT OF INDIANS ARE VEGETARIAN, VERSUS 3 PERCENT OF AMERICANS

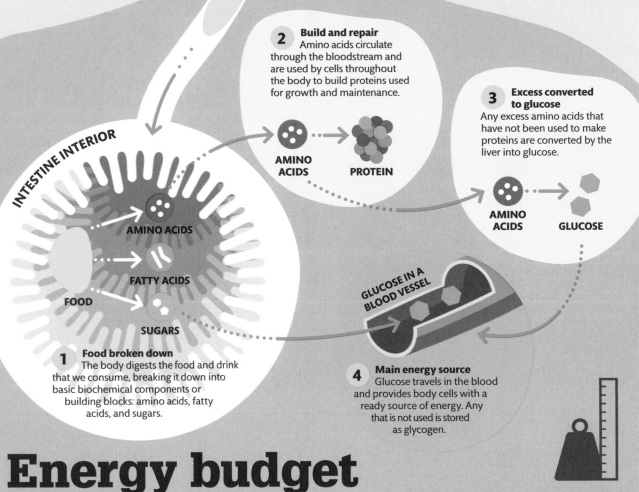

FOOD

Metabolism
Metabolism refers to our body's vital chemical processes, including extracting energy from food and using it to build molecules and repair our cells. Around 40–70 percent of the energy we burn each day goes into these basic metabolic functions—the proportion depends on how physically active we are.

INTESTINE INTERIOR

AMINO ACIDS

FATTY ACIDS

FOOD

SUGARS

2 Build and repair
Amino acids circulate through the bloodstream and are used by cells throughout the body to build proteins used for growth and maintenance.

AMINO ACIDS

PROTEIN

3 Excess converted to glucose
Any excess amino acids that have not been used to make proteins are converted by the liver into glucose.

AMINO ACIDS

GLUCOSE

GLUCOSE IN A BLOOD VESSEL

1 Food broken down
The body digests the food and drink that we consume, breaking it down into basic biochemical components or building blocks: amino acids, fatty acids, and sugars.

4 Main energy source
Glucose travels in the blood and provides body cells with a ready source of energy. Any that is not used is stored as glycogen.

Energy budget
The way in which our body processes energy may be understood in terms of an energy budget. How much energy we put in—through our food—and how much we expend—our levels of activity—determine what we have left over—our fat stores.

YOUR BODY MASS INDEX (BMI) IS SIMPLY YOUR WEIGHT IN KG DIVIDED BY THE SQUARE OF YOUR HEIGHT IN METERS

BURNING FAT TO KEEP WARM

Recently, scientists have discovered that some adults have stores of brown fat that burns to keep us warm. Previously, they thought only babies had brown fat. They have also discovered beige fat, which can change to an energy-burning state when the environment changes, such as when the temperature drops. Finding ways to maintain this burnable fat in the long term could lead to treatments for obesity.

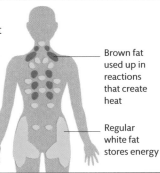

Brown fat used up in reactions that create heat

Regular white fat stores energy

DOES HAVING A SLOW METABOLISM MAKE YOU PUT ON WEIGHT?

No difference has been found between the metabolisms of overweight and slim people. If anything, metabolic rate increases as your body size increases.

Losing weight

When we deprive it of food, our body exploits its stores of energy. First, it uses all available glucose in the blood. Glucose is replenished as the liver breaks down its glycogen store. When glycogen runs out, the body turns to its fat stores. So the only way to lose weight is to remain in an energy deficit—using more calories than you take in—for a prolonged period. Do this too strictly for long, however, and muscles waste, as the body breaks them down to liberate amino acids for energy.

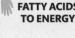

GLUCOSE AND GLYCOGEN TO ENERGY

FATTY ACIDS TO ENERGY

AMINO ACIDS TO ENERGY

Glucose burning
If the body has a good supply of glucose, it will use this as its primary source of energy until it runs out.

Fat burning
If the body does not have enough glucose to burn, it will next turn to its fat stores for energy.

Protein burning
When starved, the body will take the extreme measure of using amino acids for energy.

Putting on weight

When we consume more calories than we expend through metabolism and exercise, we store the extra energy, first as glycogen, then as fat. Fat is stored under the skin (subcutaneous) and around our organs in our abdominal cavity (visceral). It is visceral fat that leads to obesity-related diseases. White fat cells also secrete hormones and hormonelike molecules, which affect food intake (see pp.14–15) and insulin secretion and sensitivity (see pp. 216–17).

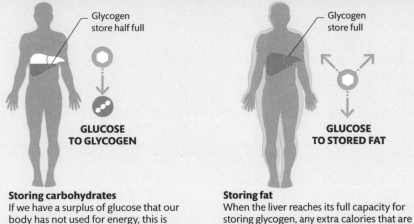

Glycogen store half full

GLUCOSE TO GLYCOGEN

Glycogen store full

GLUCOSE TO STORED FAT

Storing carbohydrates
If we have a surplus of glucose that our body has not used for energy, this is taken up by our liver cells and stored as a complex carbohydrate called glycogen.

Storing fat
When the liver reaches its full capacity for storing glycogen, any extra calories that are consumed are converted to fat and placed in stores throughout the body.

Diet and exercise

It's commonly thought that exercise keeps us slim, but recent research seems to be casting doubt. While exercise is good for you in many ways, an extra trip to the gym may not actually do that much for your waistline.

Effects of exercise

Exercise can help with weight loss, and particularly weight maintenance, but it doesn't have as large an effect as might be expected. In the short term, exercise seems to boost our basal metabolic rate (BMR—the amount of energy used daily at rest). It may do this by increasing muscle mass, since muscle burns more calories at rest than fat does. However, new studies suggest that once we reach a certain sustained high level of exercise, our body may compensate by actually reducing our basal metabolic rate.

KEY

Calories

Exercise

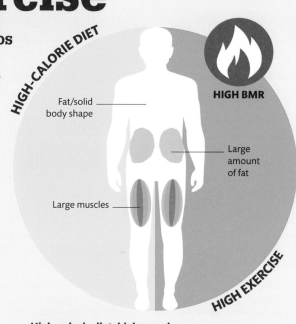

High-calorie diet, high exercise
If you exercise a reasonable amount, you are likely to have strong muscles and a high basal metabolic rate. However, if you also eat a high-calorie diet you can still store fat and become overweight.

High intensity exercise

High-intensity interval training (HIIT) seems to reduce body fat more than other exercise, but why is not clear. One study found that for the same calories burned, HIIT reduced nine times more subcutaneous fat than regular exercise. Paradoxically, it also increased fitness for both aerobic (sustained, low-intensity) and anaerobic (high-intensity) exercise.

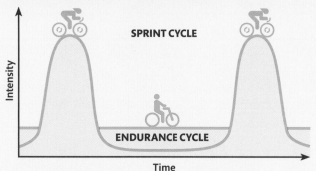

Peaks of intensity
HIIT involves working at full power for short periods—for example, cycling all-out for just 10 seconds, then resting before repeating the intense burst.

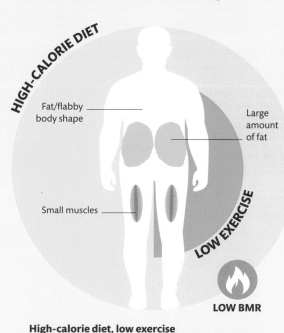

High-calorie diet, low exercise
Taking in a lot more calories than you burn leads to rapid weight gain and fat accumulation. If you don't take much exercise, you are likely to have undeveloped muscles and a low basal metabolic rate.

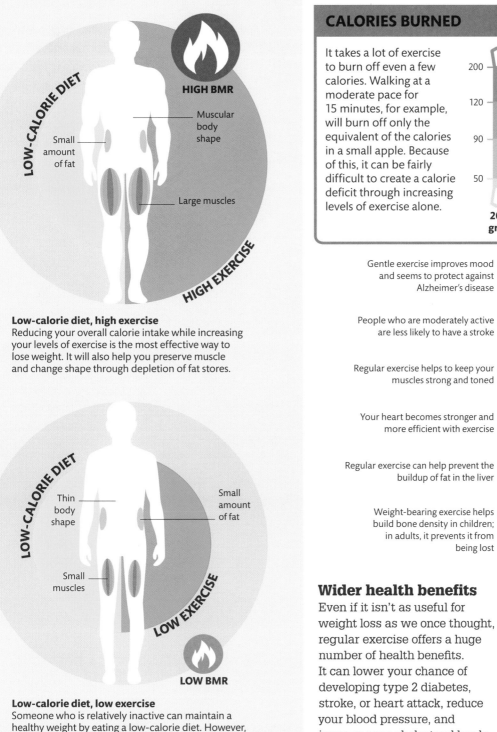

LOW-CALORIE DIET

HIGH BMR

Small amount of fat

Muscular body shape

Large muscles

HIGH EXERCISE

Low-calorie diet, high exercise
Reducing your overall calorie intake while increasing your levels of exercise is the most effective way to lose weight. It will also help you preserve muscle and change shape through depletion of fat stores.

LOW-CALORIE DIET

Thin body shape

Small amount of fat

Small muscles

LOW EXERCISE

LOW BMR

Low-calorie diet, low exercise
Someone who is relatively inactive can maintain a healthy weight by eating a low-calorie diet. However, they will be missing out on the many health benefits exercise offers.

CALORIES BURNED

It takes a lot of exercise to burn off even a few calories. Walking at a moderate pace for 15 minutes, for example, will burn off only the equivalent of the calories in a small apple. Because of this, it can be fairly difficult to create a calorie deficit through increasing levels of exercise alone.

200

120 — Dancing

90 — Cycling

50 — Walking

10 mins

200 calorie granola bar

Gentle exercise improves mood and seems to protect against Alzheimer's disease

ALZHEIMER'S MOOD

STROKE

People who are moderately active are less likely to have a stroke

Regular exercise helps to keep your muscles strong and toned

MUSCLE

Your heart becomes stronger and more efficient with exercise

LUNGS

HEART

Regular exercise can help prevent the buildup of fat in the liver

Weight-bearing exercise helps build bone density in children; in adults, it prevents it from being lost

LIVER

BONES

Wider health benefits
Even if it isn't as useful for weight loss as we once thought, regular exercise offers a huge number of health benefits. It can lower your chance of developing type 2 diabetes, stroke, or heart attack, reduce your blood pressure, and improve your cholesterol levels, independent of weight loss.

Calorie counting

Counting the calories in the food we eat is a basic strategy of weight management. While a "calorie-controlled" diet may be a useful way to monitor our intake, we shouldn't make food choices on calorie content alone. For optimum health, we must still eat a balanced diet containing all food groups.

DOES LOW-FAT MEAN LOW-CALORIE?

Low fat diets do tend to reduce calories overall, so can work for weight loss. But many low-fat products have more sugar and salt added, meaning they aren't always the healthier choice.

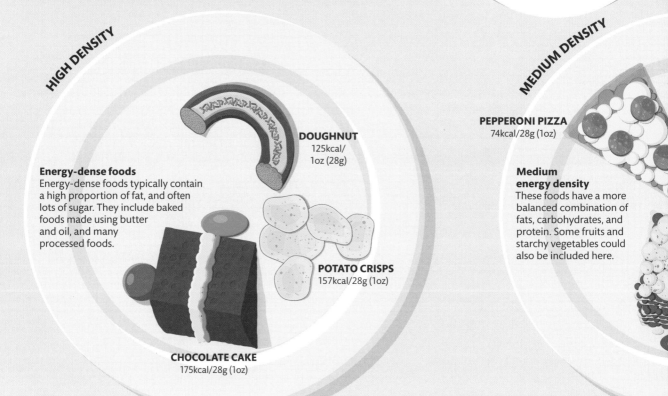

HIGH DENSITY

DOUGHNUT
125kcal/
1oz (28g)

Energy-dense foods
Energy-dense foods typically contain a high proportion of fat, and often lots of sugar. They include baked foods made using butter and oil, and many processed foods.

POTATO CRISPS
157kcal/28g (1oz)

CHOCOLATE CAKE
175kcal/28g (1oz)

MEDIUM DENSITY

PEPPERONI PIZZA
74kcal/28g (1oz)

Medium energy density
These foods have a more balanced combination of fats, carbohydrates, and protein. Some fruits and starchy vegetables could also be included here.

Energy density

The energy density of a food is the amount of energy it contains per unit of weight—usually expressed in calories per gram (kcal/g). Energy-dense foods provide more calories per gram than those with low energy density. A food's energy density is determined by its proportions of fat, carbohydrates, protein, fiber, and water. Fat contains 9kcal/g, carbohydrates and protein both contain 4kcal/g, and alcohol 7kcal/g. Fiber and water provide no energy—just structure and bulk.

SELF-IMPOSED RESTRAINT

A custom practiced by the people of Okinawa, Japan, *hara hachi bu* roughly translates as "eat until you are 80 percent full." The Okinawans are known for having the world's highest proportion of centenarians, and their approach to eating clearly plays a role in this. *Hara hachi bu* contrasts with the traditional Western custom of eating until the plate is completely empty.

What is a calorie?

A food calorie is a unit used to measure the energy in food. Although the calorie is widely used in the context of food, scientists now mainly use the joule as a unit of energy, and the kilojoule (kJ) for food quantities. One food calorie (kcal) converts to 4.184kJ. Depending on location, food labeling uses either one or both of these units.

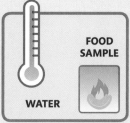

WATER
FOOD SAMPLE

Measuring calories
A food's calories are measured by burning a freeze-dried sample in oxygen. The calorific value is measured by how much a volume of water, surrounding the food, increases in temperature.

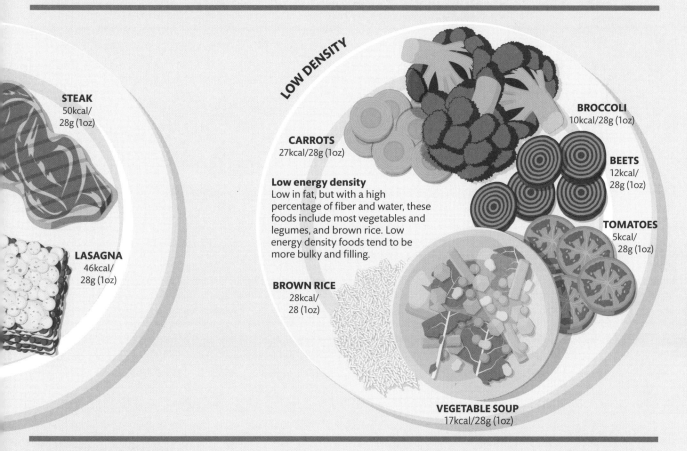

LOW DENSITY

STEAK
50kcal/ 28g (1oz)

LASAGNA
46kcal/ 28g (1oz)

CARROTS
27kcal/28g (1oz)

BROCCOLI
10kcal/28g (1oz)

BEETS
12kcal/ 28g (1oz)

Low energy density
Low in fat, but with a high percentage of fiber and water, these foods include most vegetables and legumes, and brown rice. Low energy density foods tend to be more bulky and filling.

TOMATOES
5kcal/ 28g (1oz)

BROWN RICE
28kcal/ 28 (1oz)

VEGETABLE SOUP
17kcal/28g (1oz)

Absorbing calories

Our bodies don't treat all foods equally. Some are harder to digest than others, which means we don't extract all the calories they contain. Furthermore, we are not all same, and one person's digestive system may extract more calories than another's from the same meal.

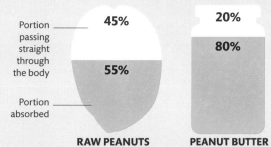

Portion passing straight through the body — 45%

55%

Portion absorbed

RAW PEANUTS

20%

80%

PEANUT BUTTER

Varied absorption
Many of the plant cells that make up nuts aren't broken down as they pass through our gut, meaning their nutrients remain locked up inside the indigestible cell walls. However, in nut butter, the processing has started the digestion process for you, so you extract more calories.

Low-carb diets

Proponents of "low-carb" diets claim that limiting our consumption of carbohydrates can help us to lose weight and avoid the side effects of eratically fluctuating blood-sugar levels.

How it works

In low-carb diets, instead of carbohydrates providing the main source of calories and energy, fats and proteins do. It is claimed that by keeping our blood sugar and insulin levels low, we can train our body to burn its stores of fat. Also, since low-carb diets are high in protein, and protein helps us to feel full for longer, this enables us to eat smaller portions, reduce snacking between meals, and cut down our overall calorie intake.

Fat burning
By reducing the levels of glucose in our bloodstream, we can force our body into using alternative sources of energy. A sustained lack of glucose can lead to ketosis, a state in which the body burns its stores of fat at a very high rate.

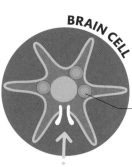

BRAIN CELL

Ketone body being used for energy in a brain cell

Ketone body produced from fatty acids in the liver

LIVER

What to eat?

Anyone planning to significantly reduce one of the main food groups needs a diet strategy that will compensate. While protein-rich foods and natural fats can replace carbohydrates as sources of energy, high-protein diets often lack fiber, which is essential for healthy digestion and maintaining good cholesterol levels. Including generous servings of vegetables such as broccoli, cauliflower, and lettuce in your diet can boost fiber intake, contribute micronutrients, and add bulk to meals.

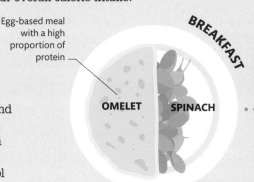

Egg-based meal with a high proportion of protein

BREAKFAST

OMELET   SPINACH

Daily diet
By combining protein-rich foods with bulky low-carb vegetables it is relatively easy to eliminate carbohydrate-rich foods such as pasta, bread, rice, and sugary foods from each meal of the day.

2 State of ketosis
Unlike other tissues, the brain can't use fatty acids as an energy source. So when blood glucose is low, the liver converts fatty acids into ketone bodies—molecules that provide energy for brain cells.

Fatty acid released into bloodstream

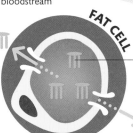

FAT CELL

Stored fatty acid

Fatty acid being used for energy in muscle cell

MUSCLE CELL

1 Releasing fatty acids
When blood glucose levels are maintained at a healthy level, insulin levels remain low. This allows the release of fatty acids from fat cells into the bloodstream, which are then used for energy in most cells.

LOW-CARB DIETS CAN HELP PEOPLE WITH **DIABETES** IN THE SHORT-TERM CONTROL OF **BLOOD-SUGAR LEVELS**

WHAT IS THE CONSENSUS ON LOW-CARB DIETS?

Although most medical organizations recognize the effectiveness of low-carb diets for weight loss, very few, if any, recommend them as a long-term health strategy.

LIMITED FOODS

Some low-carb diets are very restrictive, and as well as cutting out foods that are obviously rich in carbohydrates, such as pasta and bread, they limit the intake of many other foods, at least at first. These include all fruit and sweet-tasting vegetables such as peas and corn. Potatoes and other starchy vegetables including squash, carrots, parsnips, beets, and lentils are restricted, as are whole grains including quinoa and oats. However, many of these foods are key sources of fiber, vitamins, and minerals, which are essential in a healthy diet.

BEET

SQUASH

LUNCH

TUNA

SALAD

Low-calorie, low-carb salad makes up the bulk of the meal

SNACK

CHEESE

NUTS

High-protein, high-fat snacks are eaten instead of wheat-based snacks

DINNER

Dinner lacks high-carb foods such as pasta and potatoes

CHICKEN BREAST

BROCCOLI

CAULIFLOWER

High-protein diets

Low-carb diets are, by definition, often also high-protein diets. Moderate high-protein diets increase protein intake above the standard recommended amount—around 15 percent of total calories. They continue to allow other food groups, including carbohydrates. More extreme high-protein diets dramatically restrict carbohydrate intake. Some also encourage high fat intake.

	Benefits	Drawbacks
MODERATE HIGH-PROTEIN DIETS	• Protein helps you feel full for longer so you may be less likely to snack between meals • A high-protein diet during weight loss can help you lose fat rather than muscle • Protein takes more energy to digest, so some of the calories will be burned off	• Research is mixed as to whether these diets will help you lose weight • Protein-containing foods, including meats, are often more expensive • Eating too much animal protein may increase your risk of developing heart disease and some cancers
EXTREME HIGH-PROTEIN DIETS	• Protein keeps you full for longer so you are unlikely to become hungry • Lots of popular foods, including meat, cheese, and butter are unrestricted • Many extreme diets don't involve the need to count calories	• A very restrictive diet is difficult to stick to, especially when socializing • Cutting out food groups can lead to a lack of essential vitamins and minerals • Lack of fiber can cause constipation • Reliance on animal proteins may put you at risk of diseases including heart disease and some cancers • Cholesterol levels may increase • Kidney problems can become worse as the kidneys have to deal with more protein • May be ineffective if calories aren't restricted

High-fiber diet

Diets such as the F-Plan Diet became popular in the 1980s after Dr. Denis Burkitt connected the benefits of traditional rural African diets with their high fiber intake. The idea went out of fashion as the focus moved to reducing carbs, but it is now becoming popular again.

Benefits of a high-fiber diet

As a weight-loss plan, high-fiber diets reduce calories while increasing fiber. The diet focuses on eating plenty of vegetables and whole grains, so it fits with governmental guidelines on healthy eating and is recommended by many dieticians. No food is off limits, and the foods eaten can reduce the risk of obesity, diabetes, and other diseases related to insulin resistance. However, some people find high-fiber foods unappealing, which may make the diet difficult to stick to. If water intake isn't increased, it can cause short-term constipation.

IS FOOD WITH ADDED FIBER AS GOOD AS FOOD NATURALLY HIGH IN FIBER?

Producers may add fiber to cereals, bread, yogurt, and other products. Although the fiber is less varied than natural fiber, the beneficial health effects are almost the same.

What to eat
A high-fiber diet should contain lots of fruit and vegetables (including skins and peels, where possible), whole grains, nuts, seeds, beans, and pulses. By swapping to items like whole-wheat bread and high-fiber breakfast cereals, you can easily increase your fiber intake.

BREAKFAST

BRAN FLAKES

BANANA

A banana contains about $^1/_{10}$oz (2–3g) of fiber

LUNCH

WHOLE-WHEAT SANDWICH

Switch to whole-wheat bread for sandwiches

SNACK

Leave the skin on fruit to maximize fiber intake

APPLE

FIG

DRIED APRICOTS

PRUNES

PISTACHIOS

ONE STUDY FOUND THAT PEOPLE **LOST WEIGHT** SIMPLY BY ADDING **FIBER TO THEIR DIETS,** CHANGING **NOTHING ELSE!**

HIGH-FIBER FOODS

Well-known high-fiber foods range from 5 percent fiber by weight (broccoli) to 15 percent (lentils) and also include whole-wheat pasta, avocados, and peas. Eclipsing all of these, however, are chia seeds, which are 37 percent fiber, four-fifths of which is soluble. That is why when soaked in water, chia seeds dissolve into a gloopy gel—a useful consistency for desserts.

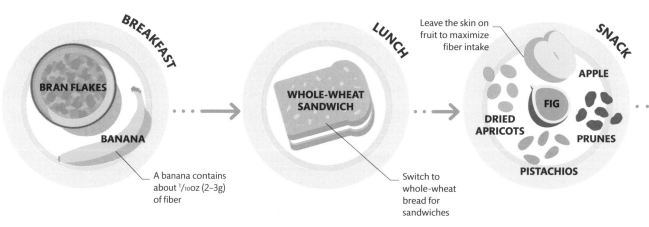

Chia seeds soaked in water form a gel

How does it work?

Fiber helps with weight loss in a range of ways. It isn't easily digested, so it doesn't provide many calories, but the bulk makes you feel full quickly. High-fiber foods also need a lot of chewing, so you eat more slowly, meaning your body can register you are full before you overeat. Fiber-rich foods also travel slowly through the stomach, keeping you full for longer, so it is easier to resist unhealthy snacks. Soluble fiber (see p.24) can even reduce blood sugar spikes after meals, which helps to avoid insulin resistance (see pp.216–17).

Keeping regular

Fiber helps keep your gut healthy by bulking out and softening your stool and reducing the time it takes to pass through the bowel. This can help reduce constipation. Fiber is also prebiotic, meaning it feeds beneficial gut bacteria. These bacteria produce byproducts that help keep our colon cells healthy and protect against bacteria that can make us ill by making the colon more acidic. The bacteria also produce vitamins B and K, which we can then absorb.

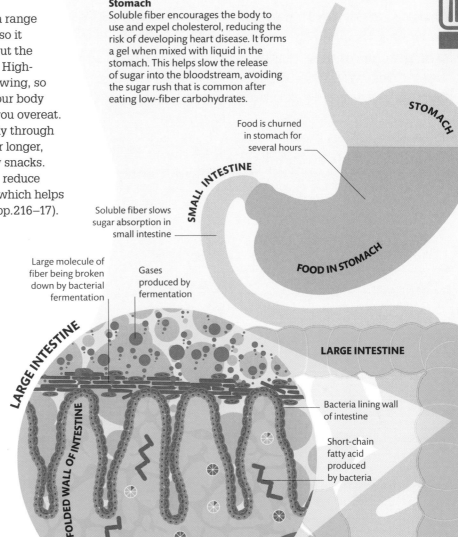

Stomach
Soluble fiber encourages the body to use and expel cholesterol, reducing the risk of developing heart disease. It forms a gel when mixed with liquid in the stomach. This helps slow the release of sugar into the bloodstream, avoiding the sugar rush that is common after eating low-fiber carbohydrates.

STOMACH

SMALL INTESTINE

Food is churned in stomach for several hours

Soluble fiber slows sugar absorption in small intestine

FOOD IN STOMACH

Broccoli provides vitamins as well as fiber

DINNER

FIVE BEAN CHILI WITH BULGAR WHEAT AND BROCCOLI

Large molecule of fiber being broken down by bacterial fermentation

Gases produced by fermentation

LARGE INTESTINE

LARGE INTESTINE

Bacteria lining wall of intestine

FOLDED WALL OF INTESTINE

Short-chain fatty acid produced by bacteria

BLOODSTREAM

Products of fermentation, including vitamins K and B, enter bloodstream

Colon
Fiber passes through the stomach and small intestine relatively unchanged, but in the colon, some types are fermented by bacteria. Although this produces embarrassing gas, it also generates beneficial products including some vitamins and short-chain fatty acids. Over time, the gut adapts to a higher-fiber diet and flatulence decreases.

Intermittent fasting

Fasting has traditionally been part of many religious diets, but recently it has started to gain more interest in scientific communities. In addition to helping with weight loss, it is thought that intermittent fasting has the potential to produce other health benefits.

Common fasting diets

Intermittent fasting diets involve sequenced periods of fasting and non-fasting. In the 5:2 diet, dieters eat normally on five days a week (feast days) but have a much reduced calorie intake on two nonconsecutive days (fast days). The alternate day diet involves eating whatever you like one day, then fasting the next. Diets that involve a restricted feeding window allow you to eat only during a set time period each day—usually of 8–12 hours.

SHOULD YOU EXERCISE ON FAST DAYS?

There is evidence to suggest that exercising while fasting helps the body burn more fat. However, it makes sense to limit yourself to moderate forms of exercise on fast days.

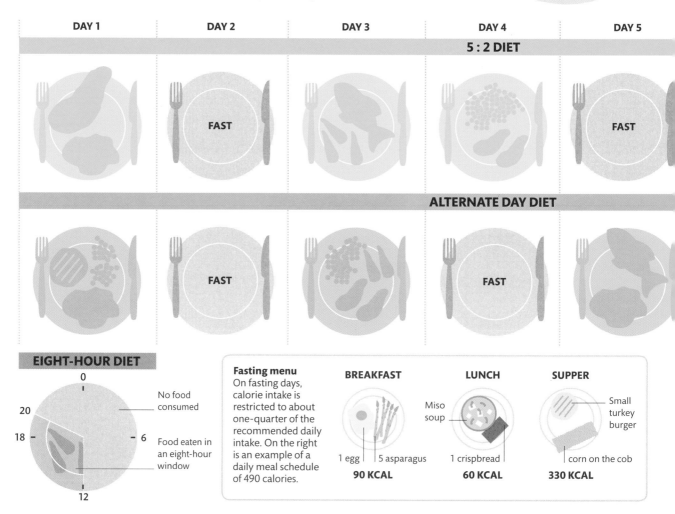

DAY 1	DAY 2	DAY 3	DAY 4	DAY 5

5 : 2 DIET

ALTERNATE DAY DIET

EIGHT-HOUR DIET

0

20

18

6

12

No food consumed

Food eaten in an eight-hour window

Fasting menu
On fasting days, calorie intake is restricted to about one-quarter of the recommended daily intake. On the right is an example of a daily meal schedule of 490 calories.

BREAKFAST
1 egg | 5 asparagus
90 KCAL

LUNCH
Miso soup
1 crispbread
60 KCAL

SUPPER
Small turkey burger
corn on the cob
330 KCAL

Is it good for you?

The evidence that suggests that intermittent fasting is good for weight loss comes mainly from animal studies (see below). If these results are applicable to humans, these fasting diets could be effective in countering obesity—and the health benefits of that are widely known. However, the very few human studies on fasting have had mixed results and we don't yet understand the potential negative impacts of fasting.

BENEFITS	DRAWBACKS
Simple rules and easy to follow	Possibility of extreme hunger, headaches, and tiredness on fast days
No special food or supplements are required	Risk of mood swings and irritability
Possible health benefits	Long-term effects not yet understood
Offers some flexibility—you don't need to fast on the same days each week	Risk of low blood pressure on fast days may make driving dangerous
Some people report increased energy	May not suit some people's lifestyles
Reduced food costs	Can be hard to keep it up over a long period
On fast days, frees up time usually spent planning meals	Some people believe that fasting can lead to an unhealthy obsession with food

DAY 6   **DAY 7**

FAST

Feast and famine
Of the variety of fasting regimes available, the three pictured here are among the most popular. Fasting involves considerable commitment, and may not suit some lifestyles, but the degree to which people fast varies. Some follow a 500kcal fasting regime (see left), but others commit to 300kcal a day, or even nothing but water.

Potential health benefits

There is growing evidence to support the health benefits of fasting in animals. Positive effects on blood pressure, insulin sensitivity, and the risk of some chronic diseases have led some scientists to believe that fasting has the potential to produce similar health benefits in humans.

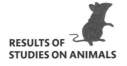

RESULTS OF STUDIES ON ANIMALS

Increased insulin sensitivity
Higher insulin sensitivity helps the body to process glucose in carbohydrates more efficiently, reducing the risk of obesity and diabetes.

Fighting cancers
When used both on its own, and alongside chemotherapy, fasting has been shown to slow the growth and spread of some cancers in mice.

Lower blood pressure
Fasting has been shown to reduce blood pressure in mice, and even maintain blood pressure levels when they were fed a high-calorie diet.

Helps brain diseases
Fasting has been shown to slow cognitive decline in mice with engineered versions of Alzheimer's and Parkinson's disease.

Improved brain health
Feeding mice a restricted-calorie diet has improved brain neuron regeneration and improved the cognitive abilities of older mice.

Reduced cancer risk
Fasting mice have been found to experience significant reductions in cell proliferation, considered an indicator for cancer risk.

Increased cell resistance
The heart and brain cells in fasting mice have become more resistant to the damage caused by heart attack and stroke.

Detoxing

A recent fad has seen ranges of items, including drinks, supplements, and even shampoos, being sold as "detox" agents that we can use to cleanse our bodies and eliminate toxins. However, there is no scientific evidence to back up such claims.

The detox claim

Detox proponents claim that by following a particular diet, or using certain products, we can help our body to flush-out toxins that have built up through our exposure to substances such as alcohol, caffeine, tobacco, fat, and sugar. Detoxing can therefore improve our health.

Detox methods

A whole industry has built up around an array of detox methods and products. These include diet regimes, fasting, food supplements, and even invasive procedures such as colonic irrigation.

CAN NATURAL PRODUCTS EVER DETOX?

Although there is very limited evidence from animal studies that cilantro may help to expel heavy metals, heavy metal poisoning is a serious problem that requires medical treatment.

GOJI BERRY

ACAI BERRY

TOXINS BUILD-UP

CELERY

LAXATIVES

FRUIT

DETOXED

SUPPLEMENTS

HERBAL TEA

BEETS

GARLIC

JUICE

SMOOTHIES

What are toxins?

Many substances can be harmful in large doses—even water. However, the body has an efficient system in place, featuring the liver and kidneys, which neutralizes or expels excess harmful chemicals daily. Toxins do not accumulate as detox advocates claim. There are a few exceptions, however. Some dangerous chemicals that dissolve in fat can build up in our fat stores over years. Exposure to these should be limited.

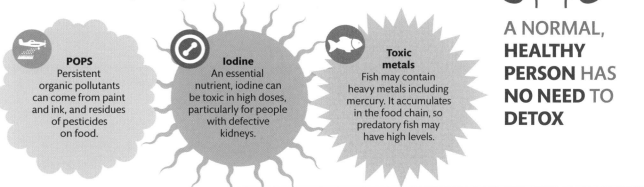

POPS
Persistent organic pollutants can come from paint and ink, and residues of pesticides on food.

Iodine
An essential nutrient, iodine can be toxic in high doses, particularly for people with defective kidneys.

Toxic metals
Fish may contain heavy metals including mercury. It accumulates in the food chain, so predatory fish may have high levels.

A NORMAL, **HEALTHY PERSON** HAS **NO NEED** TO DETOX

The reality of detoxing

Our bodies have sophisticated ways of removing most of the unwanted substances we ingest. Therefore, it is doubtful that the term "detoxing" has any real validity. The mainstream medical view is that the idea is little more than a marketing myth and a waste of time and money.

COLONIC IRRIGATION

Colonic irrigation is a potentially dangerous practice of inserting liquids (often herbal concoctions or even coffee) through the rectum into the colon, and holding it there before expelling it. Despite what its advocates claim, the colon does not need cleaning, and this practice can perforate its lining, leading to serious complications. People have even died from infections caused by colonic irrigation.

PRODUCT	CLAIM	REALITY
Herbal teas	Herbal teas help to flush toxins out of your system	They can have a diuretic effect, making you urinate more—giving the appearance of "flushing"
Supplements	Supplements boost your body's detoxing organs with scientifically developed vitamin formulas	While valuable in some cases of deficiency, there is no evidence for their detoxing properties
Superfoods	Some foods, such as garlic, help to decrease the buildup of toxins in the body	They may contain high amounts of vitamins and minerals that are essential to our general health
Detox patches	Detox patches draw toxins out through the skin	There is no evidence supporting the idea that toxins can be drawn out through the skin
Calorie restriction	Fasting or low-calorie diets will help you detox and lose weight	Denying your body the nutrients it needs to function can result in serious health problems
Laxatives	Laxatives can help to cleanse your colon	Regular use can lead to dependency—you may struggle to pass waste without them

Popular diets

With a 2014 WHO report finding 39 percent of adults worldwide overweight or obese, dieting has never been more popular or necessary. But with so many diets available, which are scientifically proven to be healthy and effective? For some, the consensus is clear, but for others, the jury is still out.

Lifestyle choices

The word "diet" is often used to talk about short-term changes or significant adjustments in eating habits for a set time frame. Weight loss can often be achieved in these ways, but the results are unlikely to stick if a long-term change in lifestyle is not made. Indeed, if the dieter simply returns to earlier habits, any weight lost will almost certainly be regained. For sustained weight loss and maintenance, healthy choices need to turn into lifelong behaviors.

BY 2025 GLOBAL OBESITY LEVELS MAY REACH 18 PERCENT IN MEN AND 21 PERCENT IN WOMEN

DO CRASH DIETS WORK?

While following a very low-calorie diet can lead to rapid weight loss, it is essentially impossible to lose more than about 3lb (1.5kg) of fat in one week, even if you could eat nothing.

Diet	What are its goals? How is it supposed to work?
Low-calorie	The basic equation for weight loss is to consume fewer calories than you use—counting calories can help ensure this happens.
Low-fat	Fat is high in calories, so reducing the amount eaten cuts total calories consumed and encourages weight loss. In the past, it was also thought to help cut cholesterol and heart disease risk.
Very low-calorie	By drastically reducing calorie intake, a very low-calorie diet is designed to promote rapid, short-term weight loss.
Low-carb	Low-carb diets claim carbohydrates are stored more easily as fat. Some reduce carbohydrates enough that the body starts burning fat reserves as it enters ketosis, leading to weight loss.
Low-GI (glycemic index)	The glycemic index measures how rapidly food raises blood sugar levels. Low-GI foods help you feel fuller longer, keeping your body from producing so much insulin (which promotes fat storage).
High-fiber	Fiber fills you up and keeps you full for a long time, reducing the amount you feel you need to eat. Much of it isn't digested, so it doesn't provide many calories.
Mediterranean	Mediterranean people live long and healthy lives. Many have tried imitating their diets in the hope of reaping the same benefits.
Paleolithic	Proponents claim that we haven't evolved since Paleolithic (Old Stone Age) times, so we can't process food produced by farming. By replicating our ancestors' diets, they claim we will be healthier.
Intermittent fasting	By restricting calorie intake to particular times of day, or days of the week, this approach is designed to lower the overall calorie intake and encourage fat burning and weight loss.
Clean eating	Based on a "whole food" approach, clean eating advises avoiding anything "processed" in order to eat a higher quality diet, feel fuller for longer, and be more mindful of the food being consumed.
Alkaline	Claims that some foods have an acid-producing effect, and the body has to work hard to bring its pH under control. Eating alkali-producing foods aims to ease this pressure and improve health.
Macrobiotic	This diet focuses on consuming a balance of foods that are locally produced, in keeping with the seasons. Rather than strict guidelines, the food eaten varies from person to person.
Blood-type	Advocates of this diet argue that our different blood types affect how we digest food. To optimize health, they say we should eat the right foods for our blood type.

Crash and burn

A persistently popular fad diet is the cabbage soup diet. Based on eating a low-calorie soup (and little else) for one week, many experts criticize it as a quick fix, with much of the weight lost being water, not fat. This is because reducing calorie intake leads the body to burn through glycogen stores for energy. Glycogen retains water, so using it also releases the "water weight," but this can be quickly regained.

CABBAGE SOUP

What does it consist of? What do people eat or avoid?	Is there evidence that it works?
No foods are off limits, but portions are controlled and low-energy-density foods are preferred.	Yes—reducing your calorie intake is a surefire way to lose weight, but it can be hard to stick to because you need to track everything you eat.
Dieters switch to low-fat versions of products such as cheese and yogurt, and eat lean cuts of meat. The consumption of high-fat foods, such as oils and spreads, is limited.	Low-fat products are often high in sugar and may not keep you full. While it is a way to cut calories, some fats (such as the unsaturated ones in olive oil and oily fish) are necessary for health.
Some or all meals are replaced with "nutritionally balanced," low-calorie, ready-made drinks, soups, or bars. Any other food eaten should be healthy and low in fat. Products can be very expensive.	Can lead to rapid weight loss at first, but products lack many of the benefits of normal food. Cannot be followed long-term, and doesn't change eating habits, so weight often returns when the dieting stops.
Bread, pasta, grains, and starchy vegetables are off limits. In some extreme cases, a lot of fruit and vegetables are banned at the start of the diet. Protein and fat are unlimited.	Limiting refined carbohydrates is sensible as they are energy-dense and easy to overeat, but cutting out fruit and vegetables is never wise. Can help short-term weight loss, but longer-term consequences are not clear.
Whole-grain products are promoted, because they have a generally lower GI than their white counterparts. Only carbohydrates have a GI rating, so fats and protein are not limited.	Low-GI isn't always healthy—fries, for example, are lower-GI than boiled potatoes. But this diet may be beneficial in preventing and treating obesity and related diseases, such as type 2 diabetes.
Whole-grain cereals, fruit and vegetables (especially with skins) are good sources of fiber. Processed foods generally aren't, and fats and protein don't contain fiber.	High-fiber diets can help with weight loss, and have lots of other health benefits, such as reducing the risk of certain cancers, decreasing cholesterol levels, and promoting good gut bacteria.
Traditional Mediterranean diets focus on fresh vegetables, whole grains, olive oil, garlic, and some fish, fruit, and wine. Sugar, red meat, and processed foods are limited.	There is some evidence olive oil is protective against a range of age-related diseases. The plant-based, high-fiber approach of the diet also makes it a good choice.
Most grains and dairy are out, but plenty of meat, leafy greens and nuts are consumed. Processed food, salt, and sugar are also avoided.	Eating less processed food and more vegetables is good, but there is no evidence that most of us have trouble processing cereals. Our ancestors did not have one specific diet, and we have adapted to more variety.
Followers eat normally part of the time and restrict calories dramatically on certain days or at certain times. On fast days, only 500 calories are allowed by some regimes, which is very limiting.	There is emerging evidence that fasting can benefit health. Many people lose weight on this diet, as the lack of restriction on non-fast days fits in with a busy lifestyle.
There is a focus on expensive "superfoods," such as chia seeds, goji berries, and organic kale. Normal sugar is out, but honey, maple syrup, and coconut sugar are fine, as are foods processed at home.	Some principles are sound (more fruit and vegetables, fewer refined carbohydrates, sugar, and salt) but some advice is illogical—the sugar in honey is just as bad for you as refined sugar.
Lemon water is recommended to make your body more alkaline. Fruit and vegetables are encouraged; meat, dairy, and most grains are out.	The pH of the blood is tightly controlled. Acidic blood would indicate a serious illness, and drinking lemon water will not help. However, the focus on fresh fruit and vegetables in this diet is good.
Whole grains, vegetables, and beans are encouraged. Dairy, eggs, meat, tropical fruits, and nightshade vegetables (including tomatoes and eggplants) are to be avoided.	Good for reducing food miles and meat consumption, but devotees miss out on some healthy foods. Its focus on vegetables and whole grains, with limited fat and sugar, might help you lose weight.
Based on ideas of when blood groups evolved and what was eaten by ancestors at those times. Type O should eat a "paleo"-style diet high in meat, while A should be vegetarian. B can consume more dairy.	There is no evidence that blood type affects the way we process food or that this diet improves health. The theories of when each blood group evolved have been disproven by genetic evidence.

Allergies

An allergy is the body's oversensitive immune response to a substance that should normally be harmless. Food allergies cause a variety of symptoms, ranging from the uncomfortable to the life-threatening.

How allergies work

In people with food allergies, exposure to specific proteins in particular kinds of food causes their body's immune system to react inappropriately. It triggers the release of chemicals into the bloodstream that aggravate or inflame different parts of the body. Food allergies may cause skin problems, such as itching and eczema, and digestion issues including nausea and diarrhea. Severe allergies may also cause asthmatic symptoms, or even a systemic reaction—anaphylaxis—that can be fatal.

 1–2 PERCENT OF ADULTS AND 8 PERCENT OF CHILDREN IN THE UK HAVE A FOOD ALLERGY

PEANUTS

ALLERGIES ON THE RISE

Food allergies are on the rise in developed countries, but scientists aren't sure why. One popular idea, known as the "hygiene hypothesis," suggests that the fact our children don't encounter as many pathogens, such as bacteria, as they used to has somehow affected the natural development of their immune systems. Another theory is that modern lifestyles—including diet, antibiotics, and hygiene—interfere with our gut flora. We know these microbes moderate our immune systems, so this interference may affect how our immune cells are primed, causing allergies.

BACTERIA

FIRST EXPOSURE

Protein in peanut ingested

STOMACH

INTESTINE

Amino acid absorbed into body

1 Protein absorbed
The trigger food—in this case peanuts—is ingested and the proteins in it are broken down into amino acids, which are absorbed through the gut. Exposure can also be through skin contact or inhalation.

IMMUNE CELL

NO SYMPTOMS

Antibody released by immune cell

2 Antibodies produced
If allergic to peanuts, the body's immune cells produce antibodies that are specific to the particular allergen. The antibodies travel in the bloodstream.

Antibody bound to mast cell

MAST CELL

3 Mast cells
The antibodies bind to the surface of white blood cells called mast cells, which become sensitized. At this stage there are no symptoms of an allergy, but the cells are primed for a second exposure.

SUBSEQUENT EXPOSURE

How allergies are diagnosed

A combination of a detailed patient history and either a skin prick test or blood test for food-specific antibodies are used to diagnose food allergies. Food exclusion, and blind and placebo-controlled oral food tests are also effective, but must be done under careful supervision.

Skin prick test

A medic pierces the patient's skin with tiny amounts of suspected allergens, producing localized allergic responses in the form of bumps and redness.

SWOLLEN LIPS

SWOLLEN THROAT

Treatment options

The main treatment for allergies is to avoid the trigger food, but this isn't always easy. In severe cases, even tiny amounts of the allergen can cause reactions. Medicines are used to prevent and alleviate the symptoms of allergic reactions. For mild allergies, such as hayfever, antihistamines can help by blocking receptors from binding to histamine chemicals.

AUTOINJECTOR

Emergency treatment

People with severe allergies may need to carry with them two autoinjectors (a spring-loaded syringe) of adrenaline for emergency treatment. Adrenaline narrows blood vessels, relieves blood pressure, and reduces swelling.

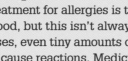

MAST CELL

Protein bound to antibody

4 **Proteins bind to antibodies**
On subsequent exposure, mast cells identify the protein allergen, which then binds to the antibodies on the mast cells. This activates a process called degranulation.

SYMPTOMS OCCUR

SWOLLEN HANDS

PEANUTS

ONLY IN EXTREME CASES

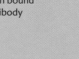

MAST CELL

Chemicals such as histamine released

Chemicals released over entire body

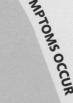

Body-wide allergic reaction

ABDOMINAL PAIN

5 **Mast cell releases chemicals**
As the mast cell degranulates it releases histamine and other chemicals into the bloodstream. It is the effect of these chemicals on the body that produces different allergic symptoms.

6 **Anaphylaxis**
In severe cases, known as anaphylaxis, the whole body is affected over a very short period, resulting in a combination of extreme symptoms that can include throat swelling, severe asthma, and a drop in blood pressure. Emergency treatment is necessary.

Intolerances

Intolerances occur when the body is unable to digest a component of food. They differ from allergies in that they do not aggravate the immune system. People can be intolerant to a range of foods—and either be born intolerant, or become sensitive later in life.

What causes intolerances?

Intolerance can occur when you don't have a particular digestive enzyme that helps break down nutrients. Sometimes, it is a part of the food that can cause intolerances, such as artificial additives, natural chemicals, or toxins. Symptoms often arise hours after eating and may continue for days. They vary from case to case, but commonly include nausea, bloating, cramps, and diarrhea. Rarely, temporary intolerances can arise after bouts of gastroenteritis or courses of antibiotics.

Diagnosis

Intolerances are difficult to diagnose as symptoms are delayed and more than one intolerance can coexist. Exclusion diets instruct a patient to cut a potentially problematic food out of their diet for a few weeks to see if symptoms improve. If symptoms recur once the food is reintroduced, an intolerance is diagnosed.

FOOD

| Exclusion period | Reintroduction period

SYMPTOMS

TOLERANCE

Time

Creating tolerance
Extended elimination (weeks to months) of the offending food can, in some cases, lead to a rise in tolerance. Reintroducing the food in small doses may be tolerated and symptoms may lessen with time.

Lactose intolerance
This type of intolerance is one of the most common. It occurs due to a lack of the enzyme lactase, which breaks down lactose sugar. Without this enzyme, the sugar is fermented by bacteria in the colon.

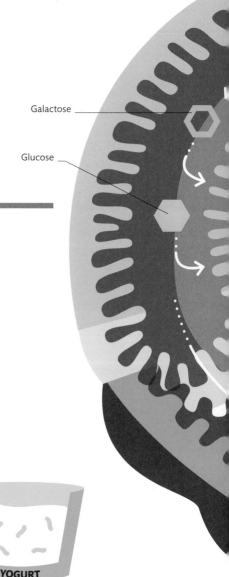

Galactose

Glucose

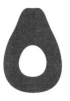

PEOPLE **INTOLERANT** TO **AVOCADOS** ARE SENSITIVE TO A **SUBSTANCE** IN THEM CALLED **TYRAMINE**

YOGURT

Live cultures
Research has shown that yogurts with live cultures (bacteria) can help relieve the symptoms of lactose intolerance, because the bacteria break down the lactose for you.

SMALL INTESTINE

Lactase enzyme

Lactose sugar

1 Lactose in small intestine
When the cells that line the walls of the small intestine encounter the sugar lactose, they start to produce the digestive enzyme lactase.

2 Lactose digested by lactase
Lactase breaks lactose into two smaller sugars—galactose and glucose.

3 Galactose and glucose absorbed
These two smaller sugars are then absorbed into the bloodstream by the small intestine.

1 Undigested lactose
Those who are lactose intolerant will not have the lactase enzyme, so lactose cannot be absorbed and instead passes into the large intestine.

WHY CAN LACTOSE INTOLERANCE DEVELOP LATER IN LIFE?

Lactase production decreases at varying rates with age, so your ability to digest dairy products may reduce as you get older.

WHAT IS CANDIDA?

Candida is a group of yeasts that live naturally in the body, most commonly in the mouth and vagina. The yeasts may also live in the gut, as part of the normal gut flora. It is often thought that overgrowth of *Candida* in the gut can cause irritable bowel syndrome, but research suggests that it may be the reverse – bouts of IBS can upset the balance in your gut and cause *Candida* to thrive. This may lead to symptoms akin to having IBS or even a persistent food intolerance: nausea, gas, diarrhea—leading to *Candida* being falsely blamed as the "cause" of these afflictions.

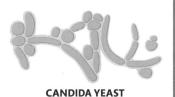

CANDIDA YEAST

Bacteria ferment lactose

2 Bacterial fermentation
Lactose is fermented by bacteria living in the large intestine, producing gas and acids in the process.

3 Disruption in the bowel
Acids draw water into the bowel, causing diarrhea, while the gas produced by fermentation causes bloating and discomfort.

Gas and acids released by bacteria

LARGE INTESTINE

Undigested lactose enters the large intestine

Exclusion diets

For people who suffer from a food allergy or intolerance, often the only treatment is to avoid the trigger food. Unfortunately, if they aren't careful, this can lead to deficiencies in certain nutrients.

Allergies and intolerances

The body's adverse immune response to proteins in certain foods can lead to a variety of allergic symptoms, from itching and rash, to nausea and anaphylactic shock. Food allergies affect more than 1 in 20 children but are less common in adults. In cases of food intolerance, symptoms arise from deficiency of certain digestive enzymes (as is the case with lactose intolerance), or the direct action of chemicals within foods.

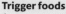 **FOOD ALLERGIES VARY REGIONALLY. IN ASIA, RICE ALLERGY IS ONE OF THE MOST COMMON**

Trigger foods
Any preprepared food or drink sold in Europe must clearly state on the label if it contains any of the ingredients shown here (right). However, in other parts of the world, different trigger foods are more common.

DAIRY NUTRIENTS	ALTERNATIVE SOURCES
Calcium	Leafy green vegetables, fortified milk alternatives
Zinc	Red meat, whole grains
Vitamin B2	Beef liver, lamb, almonds
Vitamin D	Sunlight, oily fish, fortified milk alternatives, fortified cereals

Dairy-free diet
Cutting out dairy means losing out on a valuable source of nutrients, but it is fairly easy to swap cow's milk products for alternatives made with soy, rice, and nut milks. There are plenty of alternatives to replace the calcium, zinc, and vitamins in dairy foods.

TREE NUTS
Tree nuts include cashews, brazil nuts, hazelnuts, walnuts, and almonds, but not peanuts, which are legumes. People with tree nut allergies are usually sensitive to most tree nuts.

EGGS
Egg is one of the most common food allergens, particularly in young children. Fortunately, most children grow out of egg allergy by the time they reach double digits.

MUSTARD
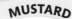
Although very rare, mustard allergy is thought to be more common in countries where mustard—including mustard seeds—plays a large part in the diet, such as France.

LUPIN
Lupin is a legume in the same family as peanuts, and like peanuts, its allergens can trigger anaphylaxis. Lupin flour and seeds are sometimes used in baking and pasta.

MOLLUSKS
Mollusks include scallops, mussels, clams, oysters, octopus, and squid. They have only quite recently been added to the EU list for mandatory labeling of allergens.

MILK
Milk from cows (or other animals) is one of the most common allergic triggers, particularly in children. It is distinct from lactose intolerance, which is nonallergic.

SOYBEANS
Soybeans are widely used in processed foods and in Asian sauces. Allergy to soybeans is quite common, especially in young children, but symptoms are typically mild.

PEANUTS

One of the most common food allergies, peanut allergy has been on the rise in children in the last few years. Exposure to even trace amounts can cause potentially fatal anaphylaxis.

GLUTEN

Intolerance to gluten, found in wheat, rye, and barley, is spreading around the world, probably due to the Westernization of diets, and the replacement of rice with wheat products.

NUTRIENTS IN GLUTEN-RICH FOODS	ALTERNATIVE SOURCES
Fiber	Beans, fruit, vegetables, nuts
B vitamins	Non-gluten-containing whole grains such as brown rice and quinoa
Vitamin D	Sunlight, oily fish, fortified milk products
Folic acid	Leafy green vegetables, beans
Iron	Meat, leafy green vegetables
Calcium	Dairy foods
Zinc	Red meat, dairy foods
Magnesium	Leafy green vegetables, nuts, and seeds

FISH

Fish including tuna, salmon, and halibut, can cause severe allergic reactions in some people. These should not be confused with our reaction to histamine released by *Vibrio* bacteria—that is food poisoning.

CRUSTACEANS

Thought to result in the greatest number of severe allergic reactions, the allergy to crabs, lobsters, and shrimp, usually appears during adulthood.

Gluten-free diets
A wide range of gluten-free foods is available, but a diet free of gluten can be short of nutrients. There are many natural and unprocessed foods that can help you to remedy any deficiencies in fiber, vitamins, and minerals.

Diet dangers

There is a risk that exclusion diets can lead to malnutrition, particularly in children. If a child doesn't receive the right balance of proteins, carbohydrates, and fats, as well as essential vitamins and minerals, their growth and development may be affected, and they are at risk of various illnesses. It is important that the parents of children with allergies understand how to replace any nutrients missing from their child's diet.

SESAME SEEDS

Sesame seeds are also eaten in the form of flour, oil, and paste. Although relatively uncommon, sesame allergy is more common in people allergic to other foods.

Stunted growth
Children with multiple food allergies have been shown to be shorter, on average, than others their age, suggesting diet-related growth problems.

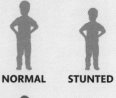

NORMAL   STUNTED

SULFITES

Sulfites are used as preservatives in products such as pickled and dried foods and alcoholic drinks. Although uncommon, intolerance can produce asthmalike symptoms.

CELERY

Exposure to celeriac and celery can trigger severe symptoms, including anaphylactic shock. It is most common in European countries.

Rickets
Cases of children developing rickets (osteomalacia) through inadequate calcium and vitamin D intake because of milk allergy have been seen.

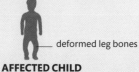

deformed leg bones

AFFECTED CHILD

Diet and blood pressure

Along with other lifestyle choices, what we eat and drink can have a direct effect on our blood pressure. High blood pressure—also known as hypertension—is a long-term medical condition that can lead to cardiovascular disease. However, this "silent killer" is both preventable and treatable.

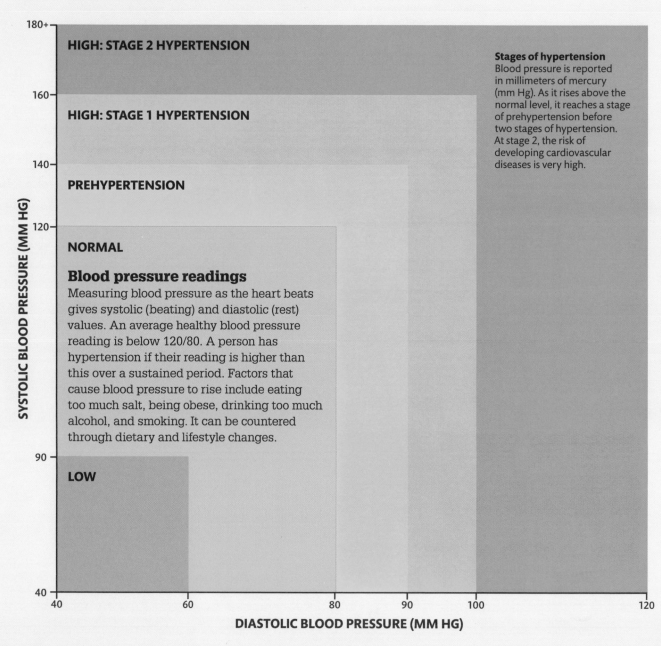

HIGH: STAGE 2 HYPERTENSION

HIGH: STAGE 1 HYPERTENSION

PREHYPERTENSION

NORMAL

Blood pressure readings
Measuring blood pressure as the heart beats gives systolic (beating) and diastolic (rest) values. An average healthy blood pressure reading is below 120/80. A person has hypertension if their reading is higher than this over a sustained period. Factors that cause blood pressure to rise include eating too much salt, being obese, drinking too much alcohol, and smoking. It can be countered through dietary and lifestyle changes.

LOW

Stages of hypertension
Blood pressure is reported in millimeters of mercury (mm Hg). As it rises above the normal level, it reaches a stage of prehypertension before two stages of hypertension. At stage 2, the risk of developing cardiovascular diseases is very high.

SYSTOLIC BLOOD PRESSURE (MM HG)

180+
160
140
120
90
40

40   60   80   90   100   120

DIASTOLIC BLOOD PRESSURE (MM HG)

Why is high blood pressure dangerous?

Although there are rarely any symptoms of high blood pressure, if it is left untreated the heart gradually becomes enlarged and less efficient. Slowly, the blood vessels, kidneys, eyes, and other parts of the body can become damaged. As blood pressure goes up, artery walls become thicker and stronger and arteries become narrower, threatening to slow or even stop blood flow. This increases the risk of heart attack, heart failure, and stroke.

WHAT IF I CAN'T GIVE UP SALT?

Alternatives to regular salt are available. These usually contain potassium rather than sodium. However, too much potassium can be dangerous for people with kidney problems.

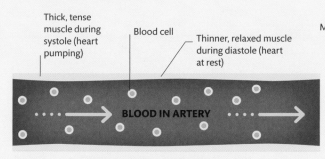

Thick, tense muscle during systole (heart pumping)

Blood cell

Thinner, relaxed muscle during diastole (heart at rest)

BLOOD IN ARTERY

Much-thickened muscle tenses during systole

Restricted blood flow

NORMAL BLOOD PRESSURE

CHRONIC HIGH BLOOD PRESSURE

Healthy arteries
A normal blood pressure changes from a high, as the heart pumps, to a low, when it relaxes. The muscles in our artery walls respond to these fluctuations by tensing and relaxing in rhythm.

Narrowing arteries
If your blood pressure is high, your arteries have to work harder to resist the pressure, so their walls become stronger and thicker. As your arteries get narrower, blood pressure rises further.

Dietary solutions

The best ways to reduce blood pressure are to reduce your salt intake and maintain a healthy weight. Sodium is the dangerous ingredient in salt, and switching to salt with low sodium can help. More broadly, the DASH (Dietary Approaches to Stop Hypertension) diet is an initiative in the US that focuses on eating more fruit, vegetables, and whole grains, as well as reducing salt, saturated fats, and alcohol. Although it wasn't designed for weight loss, it can easily be adapted by reducing portion sizes. The DASH diet has been shown to lower blood pressure, reduce cholesterol, and improve insulin sensitivity.

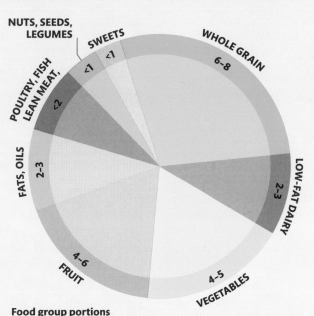

NUTS, SEEDS, LEGUMES

SWEETS

POULTRY, FISH LEAN MEAT,

WHOLE GRAIN
6–8

<1

<1

<2

LOW-FAT DAIRY
2–3

FATS, OILS
2–3

VEGETABLES
4–5

FRUIT
4–6

Food group portions
The DASH diet offers a guide to how many portions of each food group to eat each day. For nuts, seeds, and legumes, the advised dose is 4–5 portions a week; for sweets, 5 portions or fewer a week.

WORLDWIDE, THE **NUMBER OF PEOPLE WITH UNCONTROLLED HYPERTENSION EXCEEDS 1 BILLION**

HIGH LDL-, HIGH HDL-CHOLESTEROL

HIGH LDL-, LOW HDL-CHOLESTEROL

LOW LDL-, HIGH HDL-CHOLESTEROL

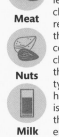

Meat

Nuts

Milk

Saturated fats

These fats tend to increase levels of both bad and good cholesterol in blood. Until recently, experts thought that the good cholesterol could compensate for the bad cholesterol, but now it is thought this isn't true. Some types of saturated fats are harmful in certain people so it is worth limiting intake to less than 7–10 percent of total energy intake.

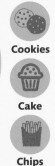

Cookies

Cake

Chips

Trans fats

Trans fats, which are created by hydrogenating vegetable oils, raise bad cholesterol levels and lower good cholesterol levels. People eat them in cakes, cookies, margarine, and deep-fried foods. They are so bad for you that some authorities can find no safe amount of trans fats to recommend in the diet, and some countries have gone as far as banning them altogether.

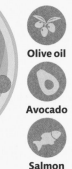

Olive oil

Avocado

Salmon

Unsaturated fats

Eating unsaturated fats can lower the level of bad cholesterol and raise levels of good cholesterol. This leads to a range of benefits such as lower blood pressure and a lower risk of heart disease. Olive oil is a good source of monounsaturated fat, and its beneficial effects on cholesterol levels may be key to the healthiness of the Mediterranean diet.

Fats and cholesterol

Although fat is an important part of our diet, some fats are healthier than others. Eating different types of fats affects the levels of the different types of cholesterol in our blood (see pp.30–31), with negative and positive effects. While "bad" cholesterol contributes to the build up of fatty deposits on our artery walls, "good" cholesterol transports cholesterol to the liver for removal.

Heart disease and stroke

Diet plays a major role in the development of heart disease—the leading cause of death in the developed world. By eating less of some types of foods and more of others, we can combat the key conditions that lead to heart disease and stroke, including high cholesterol levels, high blood pressure, and obesity.

IS HEART DISEASE REVERSIBLE?

By making radical diet and lifestyle changes some people have been known to halt the development of heart disease and achieve improved blood flow to the heart.

Cholesterol and heart disease

In people with a diet low in antioxidants (found in fruit and vegetables), too much cholesterol may lead to a buildup of fatty deposits (atheroma) on the walls of the arteries. The body reacts with an inflammatory response that swells and thickens the artery walls. This restricts blood flow, and tissues beyond that point are starved of oxygen. If this happens in the coronary arteries it can lead to the death of heart tissue. If enough dies, a heart attack or heart failure can result.

610,000
THE **NUMBER OF AMERICANS** WHO DIE EACH YEAR FROM **HEART DISEASE**

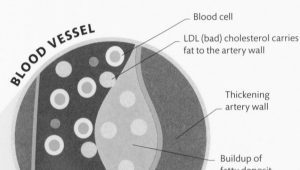

BLOOD VESSEL

Blood cell

LDL (bad) cholesterol carries fat to the artery wall

Thickening artery wall

Buildup of fatty deposit (atheroma)

HDL (good) cholesterol

Narrowed artery

HEART

Heart tissue starved of oxygen dies

Restricted blood flow
Bad cholesterol carries fats to the artery wall allowing fatty deposits to form, narrowing the artery. Fatty deposits may eventually rupture and cause blood clots that can completely block blood vessels. When this type of obstruction occurs in arteries supplying the brain, it results in a stroke.

FOOD FOR THE HEART AND BRAIN

Certain foods can have a beneficial effect on the heart by making the blood less viscous. Intake of omega-3 fatty acids reduces the "stickiness" of blood, reducing the risk of clotting. Garlic is thought to have the same effect. Other foods are able to make blood vessels widen (dilate), allowing more blood to pass. Leafy greens, which encourage the production of nitric oxide, are known to relax the blood vessels in this way. It may also be one mechanism by which moderate alcohol intake may lower the risk of heart disease and stroke (see p.165).

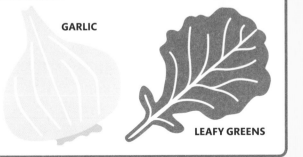

GARLIC

LEAFY GREENS

Diabetes

Insulin is a hormone that helps muscle and fat cells absorb glucose. Diabetes occurs when the pancreas can't produce insulin or cells become insensitive to it. If cells can't absorb glucose, blood sugar levels can become dangerously high.

Types 1 and 2

In type 1 diabetes, insulin-producing cells in the pancreas are damaged and produce little or no insulin. In type 2, the pancreas secretes insulin, but muscle and fat cells do not respond to it by absorbing glucose, and blood sugar levels become high. While type 1 usually starts early in life, type 2 tends to develop later, and is linked to obesity. Type 2 diabetes, which accounts for 90 percent of cases, is on the rise globally.

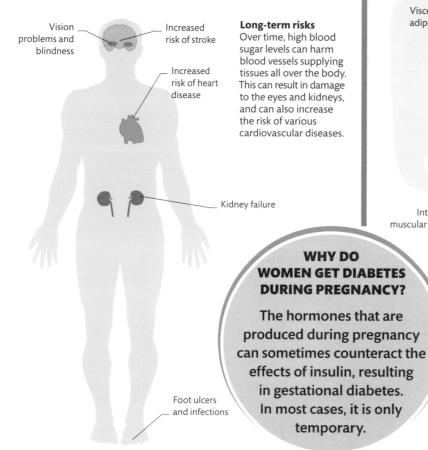

Vision problems and blindness

Increased risk of stroke

Increased risk of heart disease

Long-term risks
Over time, high blood sugar levels can harm blood vessels supplying tissues all over the body. This can result in damage to the eyes and kidneys, and can also increase the risk of various cardiovascular diseases.

Kidney failure

Foot ulcers and infections

WHY DO WOMEN GET DIABETES DURING PREGNANCY?

The hormones that are produced during pregnancy can sometimes counteract the effects of insulin, resulting in gestational diabetes. In most cases, it is only temporary.

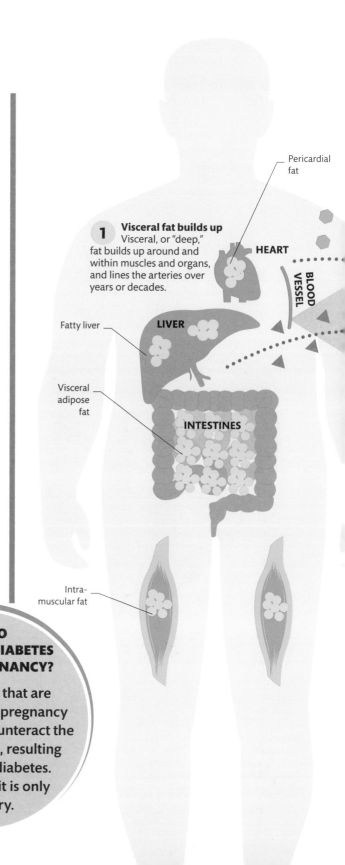

1 **Visceral fat builds up**
Visceral, or "deep," fat builds up around and within muscles and organs, and lines the arteries over years or decades.

Pericardial fat

HEART

BLOOD VESSEL

Fatty liver

LIVER

Visceral adipose fat

INTESTINES

Intra-muscular fat

2 Glucose enters system
Glucose enters the bloodstream through the digestion of carbohydrates in food. This triggers cells in the pancreas to secrete insulin into the blood.

3 How insulin should work
The pancreas produces insulin when blood glucose levels rise. Insulin triggers receptors on muscle and fat cells, opening channels in the cell membrane and letting glucose in.

Insulin molecule opens muscle cell

Glucose flows in through open channel

Glucose molecule

INSULIN WORKING

INSULIN RESISTANT

Buildup of fat causes insulin resistance

4 How insulin can fail
In muscle cells with a buildup of fat, the insulin receptors in the cell membranes become resistant and block them. The glucose channels do not open.

Buildup of glucose not absorbed by muscle cell

5 Insulin overload
As levels of glucose continue to rise, cells in the pancreas increase their production of insulin, resulting in insulin overload.

Flood of insulin in blood

Insulin molecule

Prevention and management

Losing weight is the single best thing you can do to prevent and control type 2 diabetes. There is evidence that a Mediterranean diet can help to stabilize blood sugar levels, and some research suggests low-carbohydrate, low-GI, and high-protein diets can also help.

DO	DON'T
Eat plenty of non-starchy fruit and vegetables daily	Eat too many processed foods that have hidden carbs and calories
Have an eating plan and become familiar with the glycemic index	Overeat, as this can cause spikes in blood sugar levels
Drink plenty of water, which helps to dilute the blood	Skip meals or eat at irregular times to avoid blood sugar dips
Watch out for hidden carbohydrates, especially in fruit drinks	Drink much alcohol, as this can keep blood sugar level elevated
Choose healthy fat and low-sugar food alternatives	Eat too much salt, as high blood pressure is common in diabetics

Obesity and insulin resistance

Obesity is the single best predictor of type 2 diabetes. The global rates of each have risen to an almost epidemic state. Most people who are obese not only have fat in the outwardly obvious fat stores, but also hidden throughout their bodies. This fat increases the resistance of muscle and fat cells to insulin, so that the cells fail to respond and do not absorb glucose, no matter how high insulin levels become. Sugar then builds up in the blood—so much so that it can make the blood thick, syrupy, and prone to infection.

THE WORLD HEALTH ORGANIZATION PREDICTS THAT DEATHS FROM DIABETES WILL RISE BY MORE THAN 50 PERCENT OVER THE NEXT DECADE

COUNTING CARBS

People with type 1 diabetes, and those taking medication for type 2 diabetes, may choose to count the carbohydrate content of each meal or snack they eat, so they know how much insulin to give themselves afterward. Overmedication can lead to a "hypo"—an episode of low blood sugar that can be very dangerous.

Cancer, osteoporosis, and anemia

What we choose to eat and drink directly affects our health and, ultimately, our longevity. By consuming more of some foods and drinks but restricting others, we can reduce the risks of developing diseases and conditions including cancer, osteoporosis, and anemia.

Cancer

There is a seemingly constant turnover of foods and drinks that make the headlines for either causing or curing cancer. However, interpretation of scientific findings can be subjective, and claims for "evidence" are often misleading. Cancer is a hugely diverse range of diseases, and the causes and treatment of one type may be very different from another. Nevertheless, there are a few dietary choices we can make that most experts believe will reduce our risk of developing a range of cancers and improve our general health.

EXPERTS BELIEVE THAT **1 IN 10** CANCER CASES COULD BE **PREVENTED** BY **HEALTHY DIETS**

WHERE DO THESE FINDINGS COME FROM?

Most of these findings come from the EPIC study, which has been following more than half a million people across Europe since the mid-1990s, looking at their diets and health.

Fish oils and omega-3 fats
Several studies have produced evidence to suggest that eating increased amounts of oily fish, which are rich in omega-3 fatty acids, decreases the risk of breast cancer in women.

Foods that hurt or heal
By having a healthy, balanced diet you can reasonably expect to reduce your risk of developing cancer. However, there is increasingly strong scientific evidence that certain foods and drinks can cause, or help to prevent, specific types of cancer.

Fruit and vegetables
High fruit intake lowers the risk of developing upper gastro-intestinal tract cancer, while both fruit and vegetables reduce the risk of developing bowel cancer.

Fiber
Increased fiber intake has been linked with a reduced chance of developing cancers including those of the bowel and liver. Fiber helps to keep your bowels moving, which may prevent the buildup of cancer-causing compounds.

MOUTH

ESOPHAGUS

LIVER

BOWEL

SMALL INTESTINE

Saturated fats
There is some evidence to suggest that increased saturated fat intake leads to an increased risk of certain types of breast cancer in women.

Cancer cells

BREAST

Alcohol
Even at moderate levels, alcohol increases the risk of several kinds of cancer. These include cancers of the mouth, larynx, esophagus, liver, breast, and bowel.

STOMACH

Salt
Salt intake has been linked to stomach cancer. This could be because it damages the stomach lining, or because it makes it more sensitive to other cancer-causing chemicals.

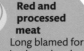

Red and processed meat
Long blamed for causing bowel and stomach cancers, the role of red meat in cancer has been cast into doubt by new studies. Nitrites in processed meat are still regarded as a risk factor.

Osteoporosis

If bones do not take up or retain enough calcium, they can become weak, with the increased risk of fractures—a condition called osteoporosis. Although it is more common in older people, the process can start much earlier. While hormone levels play a major role, a poor diet can be a contributing factor.

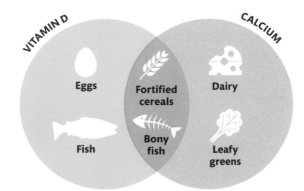

Foods for bone health
Osteoporosis can be prevented by eating a healthy diet containing foods rich in vitamin D and calcium. These include dairy products, fish, and leafy greens.

Anemia

Iron-deficiency anemia occurs when the body does not receive enough iron to produce enough red blood cells for healthy circulation. A lack of vitamin B12 or B9 (folic acid) can cause macrocytic anemia—a rarer form in which red blood cells are too large and don't work properly.

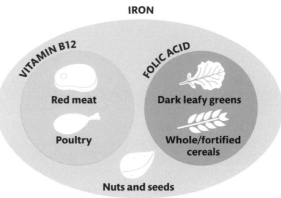

Preventing anemia
You can prevent the onset of anemia by including sufficient iron-rich food in your diet, as well as foods rich in vitamin B12 and B9.

What to eat during pregnancy

Diet plays an important part in the health of a woman and her baby during pregnancy. Eating well will help the fetus to develop healthily and ensure that its mother's body is in peak condition for the birth.

Food to enjoy

Eating the right balance of different food types is essential for a healthy pregnancy. To keep energy levels high, mothers-to-be can eat more unrefined starches, such as whole grains. Good sources of protein and calcium, including lean meats and dairy products, are vital for supporting the baby's growth and development. Eating at least five portions of fruit and vegetables a day helps mothers get enough vitamins and minerals to keep them and their growing babies in optimum health. A balanced diet will also help to ensure that weight gain during pregnancy remains within healthy limits.

Good for mother and child

Particular micronutrients present in different foods have specific health benefits for a mother and her unborn baby. In most cases these can be obtained naturally through eating sufficient amounts of certain foods, but for some vitamins and minerals—as in the case of folate (folic acid, or vitamin B9)—dietary supplements are recommended.

Manganese
A mineral found in many different foods, manganese aids the formation of bone, cartilage, and connective tissues in the growing fetus.

Magnesium
Magnesium aids fetal bone and muscle development, and can help prevent the uterus from contracting prematurely.

PLACENTA

Folate
Folic acid (vitamin B9) is essential for the development of an unborn baby. Deficiencies in the mother can increase the risk of her baby's spinal cord failing to form properly, leading to spina bifida.

BONES

SPINAL CORD

SPINE

BLOOD VESSEL

Copper
Copper plays an important role in the formation of a baby's heart, blood vessels, blood cells, and skeletal and nervous systems.

Iodine
Iodine is important for the growth and development of the brain and nervous system. Deficiency can cause cognitive and developmental problems.

KEY

Eggs	Mushrooms	Whole grains
Bread	Rice	Peanuts
Peas	Cashews	Milk
Broccoli	Avocados	Soybean
Bananas	Cheese	Fruit

Foods to avoid

Some foods that can usually be eaten as part of a healthy diet pose a risk during pregnancy, either because they carry a higher than average risk of food poisoning or because they contain specific organisms or toxins that can be passed on from the mother to the unborn baby and affect its development.

Caffeine
Consumption of caffeine should be limited as high levels have been linked to low birth weight and miscarriage.

Liver
Liver, and some sausages and patés, contain high levels of vitamin A, which can cause birth defects.

Alcohol
Alcohol is thought to be unsafe for the developing baby, so expectant mothers should avoid it completely.

Fish
High levels of pollutants mean that big predatory fish should be avoided and consumption of oily fish should be limited.

Soft and blue cheese
Exposure to pathogens like listeria from unpasteurized dairy products can cause miscarriage and stillbirth.

Undercooked meat
Eating undercooked meat can lead to bacterial or parasitic infections that can seriously harm a fetus.

Game meat
Game meat that has been killed with lead shot should be avoided due to the health risks posed by the lead.

Multivitamins
It's best to avoid multivitamins that contain high levels of vitamin A, since this can be toxic to an unborn baby.

GESTATIONAL DIABETES

Brought on by hormonal changes or simply the physical demands of pregnancy, gestational diabetes occurs when the effects of insulin are counteracted and blood-sugar levels become high. If left untreated, there are increased risks of the baby growing too large, premature birth, and abnormal labor. Treatment involves tracking blood sugar and making dietary changes.

WHAT CAUSES FOOD CRAVINGS?

Many women experience food cravings and aversions during pregnancy. These are thought to be caused by the extreme hormonal changes that can affect a mother's taste and smell.

PREGNANT WOMEN ARE MUCH MORE LIKELY TO CATCH **INFECTIONS**

Calcium
Calcium is an essential mineral in the formation of bones and teeth, so ensuring you have enough calcium in your diet is crucial during pregnancy.

Iron
Both the placenta and the growing fetus place heavy demands on the mother's supply of iron. Iron intake must increase to supply the placenta and to create the fetus's new blood cells.

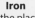

BRAIN

Choline
Only recently classified as an essential nutrient, choline is key in the development of the brain and spinal cord. Like folate, it is thought to reduce the risk of neural defects.

Babies and children

During the first years of life, nutrition is critical for healthy development. Infants' diets must provide the right balance of protein, fat, and carbohydrate, along with vitamins and minerals including calcium and vitamin D for bones and vitamin A for developing eyes.

DIETS MUST BE BROAD

Babies raised vegan or on other restricted diets must be carefully monitored to ensure they get all the essential nutrients. Even getting enough calories can be difficult because vegan or vegetarian diets have lower energy densities than diets that include meat and fish. Plenty of protein sources must be included, along with adequate vitamin B12, iron, and vitamin D. Supplements may be necessary.

Babies

For the first 6 months, babies get almost everything they need from breast milk or formula, although breast-fed babies may need extra vitamin D. After this, some of the milk should gradually be replaced with solid food. Puréed fruit and vegetables are good starting points, followed by chicken and other protein sources.

Cup of water offered at meal times

Pureed food introduced

KEY

○ Milk and dairy foods

● Other foods

Breast milk or formula still the major part of the diet

First solids

Babies often dislike a food the first time they taste it, so it is good to introduce new foods one at a time, repeating each one even if they react negatively. Offering food that is easy to hold helps babies learn to feed themselves.

Mother produces colostrum for a few days after giving birth, then breast milk

Meat, fish, and dairy should now form part of the diet

6–9 MONTHS

Liquid diet

Breast milk has the right balance of nutrients for newborns, helps boost their immune system, and establishes their gut bacteria (see p.25). Formula is usually made from cow's milk, but has higher whey content and less casein protein to make it more similar to breast milk and easier to digest.

Changing gut microbes

By the end of their first year, the types of bacteria in the baby's gut begin to look more like those in an adult's. Before this time, they vary dramatically between infants, depending on the bacteria their environment has exposed them to.

BIRTH–6 MONTHS

9–12 MONTHS

Young children

As the proportion of calories from milk is reduced, young children tend to be encouraged to try lots of different foods. But their diets should differ from adults' in some ways. Too much fiber, for example, can fill small stomachs quickly, preventing children from eating enough calories. Protein (including dairy) is important.

Fruit juice can be given with a meal, once a day

Breakfast cereal is a good way to combine grains and dairy in a meal

DO CHILDREN NEED SUPPLEMENTS?

Babies and young children often can't get all the vitamins they need from milk and food. Vitamins A, C, and D are usually recommended for children from 6 months to 5 years.

Growing needs

A healthy diet for a 2-to-5-year-old should include three to four servings of starchy foods, the same of fruit and veg, and two servings of protein. Skim milk or other dairy products (such as yogurt and cheese) can replace the whole milk. These are a good source of protein and calcium, needed for growing bones.

2–5 YEARS

Starchy food, such as butternut squash and grains should now be a part of meals

Diet continues to include protein, such as chicken

Infant can start drinking whole cow's milk

Milk alternatives

From 1 year old, the baby's intestines are able to digest the higher casein content of whole cow's milk. Fortified alternatives such as soy milk can be used instead, but growth should be monitored because they contain fewer calories than whole cow's milk.

1–2 YEARS

Low-fat (1 percent) milk can be introduced to replace skim milk

Grown-up foods

By 5 years, children's diets are, ideally, varied and similar to an adult's. Salt should not be added because of the potential harmful effect on kidneys. Low-fat or skim milk is now fine, since children will get enough calories from food.

5+ YEARS

PORTION SIZES

With childhood obesity rising, portion sizes are important. For a child under 3–4, a portion might be one slice of toast, ¹/₂oz (15g) of oats, half an apple, or one egg, but this depends on activity levels.

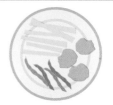

RICE MILK SHOULD NOT BE GIVEN TO CHILDREN UNDER 5 AS THE **ARSENIC** LEVELS ARE TOO HIGH

Eating disorders

Eating disorders are mental health conditions involving an unhealthy relationship with food and abnormal eating habits. They have a devastating impact on the day-to-day lives of millions of people and can cause a wide range of serious medical problems.

HOW LONG DO EATING DISORDERS USUALLY LAST?

Research carried out in Australia suggests that the average length of time that someone suffers with anorexia and bulimia is eight and five years respectively.

Three main types

People with anorexia believe themselves to be fat and starve themselves to keep their weight as low as possible. Bulimia involves some of the same attitudes as anorexia, but people alternate cycles of binge eating with purging—either vomiting or taking laxatives. Binge eating is compulsively eating vast quantities of food, often without feeling hungry.

 1 IN 100 FEMALES IN THE DEVELOPED WORLD WILL **DEVELOP ANOREXIA**

Causes

Eating disorders usually involve a degree of body dysmorphic disorder—a negative distortion of how an individual sees themselves. There may be a combination of factors that contribute to this.

LOW SELF-ESTEEM

People with low self-esteem often have a negative body image. As a result, they may either find it hard to value and take care of their body or feel the drastic need to change it.

GENETICS

Eating disorders run in families, so may be passed on genetically, or by learning attitudes toward food. People who have a close relative with an eating disorder are much more likely to develop one themselves.

CULTURE

An emphasis on thinness in the beauty stereotypes presented in the mass media has distorted the idea of an ideal body shape and encouraged people to base self-value on outward appearance.

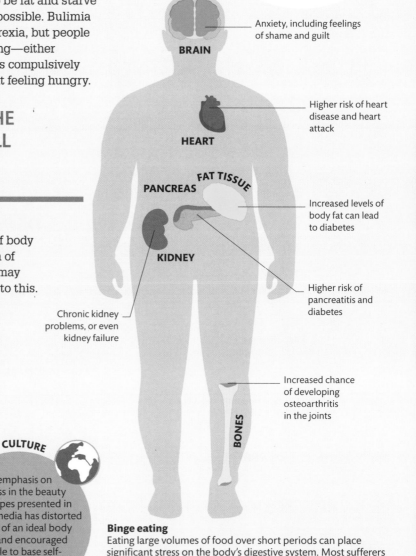

BRAIN

Anxiety, including feelings of shame and guilt

HEART

Higher risk of heart disease and heart attack

PANCREAS **FAT TISSUE**

Increased levels of body fat can lead to diabetes

KIDNEY

Chronic kidney problems, or even kidney failure

Higher risk of pancreatitis and diabetes

BONES

Increased chance of developing osteoarthritis in the joints

Binge eating

Eating large volumes of food over short periods can place significant stress on the body's digestive system. Most sufferers are likely to be overweight or obese, so suffer associated health problems, including cardiovascular disease and diabetes.

FEMALE BIAS

Eating disorders are much more common in women than in men. This may reflect that they are more sensitive to the cultural pressures that can lead to eating disorders. The proportion of men in cases of binge eating is more than twice as high as in anorexia.

20%
80%
BINGE EATING

8%
92%
ANOREXIA

KEY
Percentage of cases who are women

Percentage of cases who are men

Anorexia (left diagram)

Dizziness, depression, anxiety, and low self-esteem are common

HAIR
Hair becomes dry and brittle and may fall out

BRAIN

MUSCLES

Muscles become weak and wasted

HEART
Muscle protein of the heart itself can even begin to break down to be used as fuel, weakening the heart

BOWEL
Bloating and constipation are common

NAILS
Nails become dry and brittle

HORMONES
In women, uterus shrinks and periods stop; it becomes harder to conceive

SKIN
Skin becomes dry and scaly, and fine downy hair may appear

BONES
Increased risk of osteoporosis

Bulimia (right diagram)

High incidence of gum disease, sensitive teeth, tooth erosion, and decay

MOUTH

THROAT
Sore throat and inflammation of the esophagus are common

MUSCLES

HEART

STOMACH
Stomach pain, ulceration, and bloating are common

BOWEL
Constipation, diarrhea, and cramps may develop due to overuse of laxatives

NAILS

HORMONES

SKIN

BONES

Anorexia
Severe calorie restriction and a deficiency of essential dietary nutrients can have a traumatic effect on the body, causing serious health problems. Often these effects are irreversible, and if it continues for a sustained period, anorexia is life-threatening.

Bulimia
Although some people with bulimia may maintain a normal body weight, potentially they can suffer from all the health problems linked with anorexia. However, they may also have additional problems associated with frequent vomiting and laxative use.

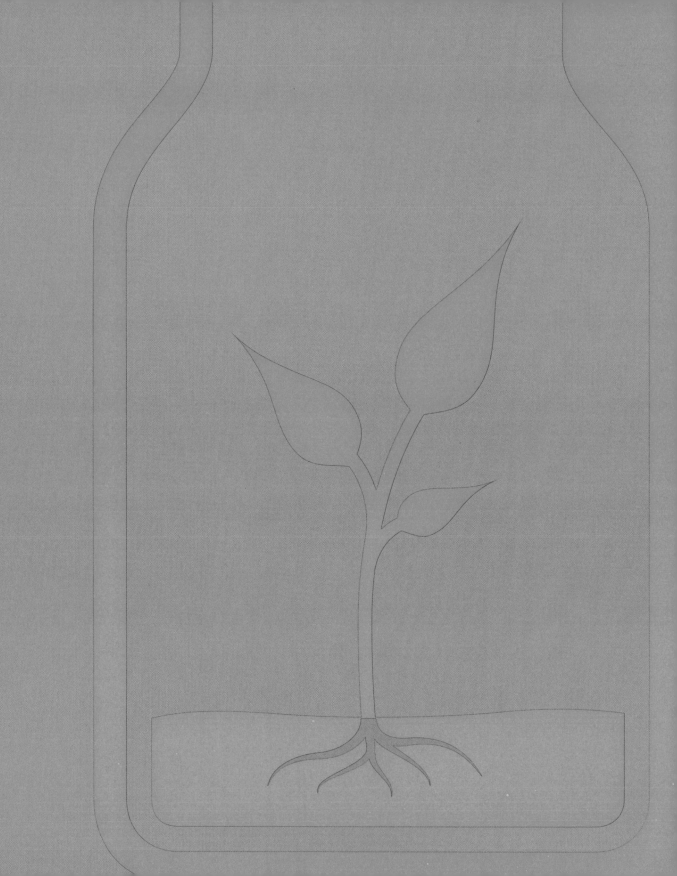

FOOD AND ENVIRONMENT

Feeding the world

The scale and efficiency of food production has improved over the past 60 years, due to technological advances, and in response to a growing population. Some people, however, still go hungry. Hunger will likely stay with us, as the more affluent people among the world's growing population increasingly gain a taste for meat. Eating meat takes up a disproportionate amount of Earth's resources.

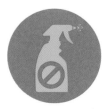

Biotechnologies
High-yield, drought-resistant hybrid crops and massive application of fertilizers, pesticides, herbicides, and other biochemicals dramatically increased yields.

Green revolution

In the 1960s and 70s there was widespread concern about a looming mismatch between food supply and demand on a global basis in the face of a skyrocketing global population. Books such as Stanford University professor Paul Ehrlich's 1968 best-seller, *The Population Bomb*, predicted a looming famine crisis. The success of the Green Revolution saw a radical increase in agricultural productivity. Improvements in agricultural machinery, biotechnological chemicals, and social collaboration were made that averted the crisis.

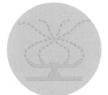

Mechanical improvements
Large scale mechanization of agriculture (such as irrigation machines) made intensive farming possible on a vast scale, boosting yields.

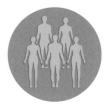

Social plans
Consolidation of small farms into giant ones, and small businesses into transnational agribusinesses, created economies of a global scale and improved yields.

Rise in meat consumption

Despite the Green Revolution, we still face food sustainability challenges—one of which is meat eating. Global demand for meat has increased five-fold in the last 50 years. While meat is stable at around 30 percent of the diet in the West, in some developing countries, the rate of meat consumption is skyrocketing. Farming livestock relies heavily on the availability of water, land, feed, fertilizer, fuel, and waste disposal capacity—and the pressure on these resources is climbing.

Global meat and cereal consumption
This graph shows a global rise in total consumption of meat and cereals to the present day and projected up to 2020.

KEY
- Meat consumption per capita
- Cereal consumption per capita

YEAR

2006   2008   2010   2012

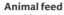

30%
FEEDS HUMANS

GRAIN PRODUCED IN DEVELOPED COUNTRIES

70%
FEEDS LIVESTOCK

Animal feed
Worldwide, animals (mainly cows) consume an estimated one-third or more of human grain production. In developed countries, the proportion is even higher, at around 70 percent of grain fed to livestock.

800 MILLION
THE NUMBER OF PEOPLE IN THE WORLD WHO DO NOT GET ENOUGH FOOD

WHAT IS THE MOST SUSTAINABLE TYPE OF FOOD?

Probably beans—they add nitrogen back into soil, reducing or eliminating the need for fossil fuel-based fertilizers, reducing carbon dioxide emissions.

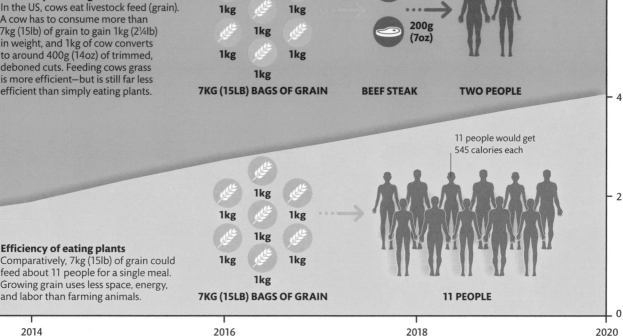

Efficiency of eating animals
In the US, cows eat livestock feed (grain). A cow has to consume more than 7kg (15lb) of grain to gain 1kg (2¼lb) in weight, and 1kg of cow converts to around 400g (14oz) of trimmed, deboned cuts. Feeding cows grass is more efficient—but is still far less efficient than simply eating plants.

1kg 1kg 1kg
1kg 1kg 1kg
1kg 1kg 1kg
1kg 1kg 1kg
1kg
7KG (15LB) BAGS OF GRAIN

400g (14oz) meat, or two large steaks

200g (7oz)
200g (7oz)
BEEF STEAK

1 meal, 545 calories each
TWO PEOPLE

Efficiency of eating plants
Comparatively, 7kg (15lb) of grain could feed about 11 people for a single meal. Growing grain uses less space, energy, and labor than farming animals.

1kg 1kg 1kg
1kg 1kg 1kg
1kg 1kg 1kg
1kg 1kg 1kg
1kg
7KG (15LB) BAGS OF GRAIN

11 people would get 545 calories each
11 PEOPLE

PERCENT CHANGE SINCE 2006

10

8

6

4

2

0

2014   2016   2018   2020

Intensive or organic?

Intensive farming on an industrial scale has helped to keep pace with a rapidly growing population, but at a cost to the natural environment. In response, the emergence of organic food appeals to our appetites, conscience, and health.

SUNLIGHT

Intensive farming

In the 1960s, the Green Revolution saw biochemical advances in agriculture (see p.228)—such as fertilizers that speed crop growth and pesticides that protect crops from pests—both of which help produce much higher yields. However, intensive farming has severe impacts on surrounding ecosystems—fertilizers and pesticides can leak into the water and soil and affect wild plants and animals. Not only that, but there is a concern that certain foods may contain pesticide residues— remnants of the toxic chemicals applied to crops.

Intensive farming
Farming large areas means farmers have to apply fertilizer and pesticide over entire fields and in large amounts to ensure that the target crop plants get enough.

KEY
- Pesticides
- Fertilizer

1 Fertilizer runoff
Excess fertilizer from industrial farms is flushed off fields by rain, and into rivers and lakes. This causes wild plants to overgrow.

2 Algal blooms
Fertilizer runoff can also stimulate overgrowth of algae, forming algal blooms. This dense vegetation can collect on a lake's surface. Algal blooms can kill off entire aquatic ecosystems by using all of the lake's oxygen, and also block sunlight from reaching the lake floor.

Plants on lake bank overgrow

FERTILIZER RUNOFF

CROPS

BEES

Pesticides can harm bees

ALGAL BLOOM

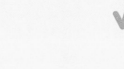

1 Pesticide runoff
Pesticides sit on the plants that we will eventually eat. These chemicals can kill the bees that pollinate many crops. Pesticide as runoff can even be carried by rain into lakes and ingested by invertebrates (such as worms) that live there.

PESTICIDE RUNOFF

WORMS

Plants at bottom of lake die without sunlight

SUNLIGHT BLOCKED

40 PERCENT OF THE WORLD'S POPULATION RELIES ON CROPS GROWN USING NITROGEN FERTILIZER

What is organic food?

Organic foods are crops that are grown without the help of artificial fertilizer and pesticides, and processed and stored without chemical fumigants. Instead of these, natural alternatives are used—manure is a natural fertilizer, and natural predators, such as ladybugs, can be used to control pests, such as crop-damaging aphids. Standards of what constitutes organic food can vary. Organic food is appealing for those concerned about their health, because they are likely to have much lower levels of pesticide residue.

NO ARTICIAL FERTILIZER

NO ARTIFICIAL PESTICIDES

CAN MEAT BE ORGANIC?

Meat can be organic, if livestock are fed on organically grown feed, allowed to go outside, not given growth hormones, and given antibiotics only if the animal is sick.

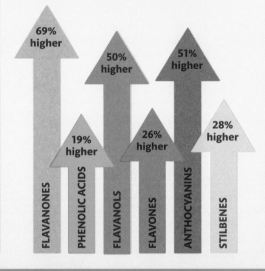

- 69% higher — FLAVANONES
- 19% higher — PHENOLIC ACIDS
- 50% higher — FLAVANOLS
- 26% higher — FLAVONES
- 51% higher — ANTHOCYANINS
- 28% higher — STILBENES

Nutritional difference
There is debate over whether organic food is actually nutritionally superior to nonorganic food, with several studies casting doubt on the claims. A review in 2014 found that the levels of six types of antioxidant (see pp.110–111), on average, were higher and pesticide residues lower in organic foods.

Pesticide in food can affect our health

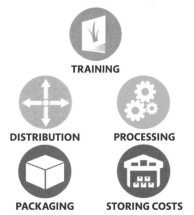

2 Up the food chain
Ingested pesticides are concentrated up the food chain. Worms may only contain tiny amounts, but if fish eat enough of them, then the fish can contain more pesticide. Animals or even humans at the top of the food chain can accumulate large amounts.

THE PRICE OF ORGANIC FOODS

Organic food is more expensive because yields are generally lower and overhead costs are higher. For instance, organic dairy yields are generally one-third lower than conventional ones—so organic food prices are raised in order to make a profit. Extra costs can include farmer training, the extra cost of processing and storing without chemical fumigants, a shorter shelf life of crops, and the costs associated with a higher instance of spoilage as a result.

TRAINING

DISTRIBUTION

PROCESSING

PACKAGING

STORING COSTS

Factory farmed or free-range?

Intensive livestock rearing methods make meat cheaper and more widely available, but there are ethical issues to consider. Intensive farming has consequences for animal welfare and can even influence food nutrition.

Ethics of intensive rearing

Intensive livestock agriculture on a large scale can be attributed to the explosive growth of confined animal feeding operations, or CAFOs. These factory farms have very high numbers and densities of animals, confined in small areas and fed grain with many enhancers and additives, such as antibiotics and hormones. CAFOs fuel the economy by producing large amounts of meat quickly, but at a great cost to animal welfare, nutritional value (see p.71), and the environment. Intensively farming animals causes them to suffer from stress for the majority of their lives and this ethical issue has influenced some changes in animal rearing to keep livestock happier and healthier.

Living space
A hen can be reared under various regimes (see opposite), and the amount of space that the animal can inhabit during its lifetime will vary depending on the country. These are average figures from a farm in Austin, Texas.

Free-range hens have an average of 11sq ft (1sq m) in which to roam and the option of going outside

DO HAPPIER ANIMALS PRODUCE BETTER MEAT?

Livestock such as cows and pigs that are allowed to roam outside are generally less stressed—but it is the natural diet of grasses and nuts they eat outside that makes their meat more nutritious.

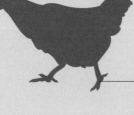

Pasture-raised hens have an average of 108sq ft (10sq m) in which to roam

Natural diet
Pigs fed on their natural diet of leaves and nuts generally have more healthy omega-3 fatty acids (see p.136) in their diet and this means that their meat has more omega-3 in it.

Factory diet
Factory-farmed pigs are fed mainly on corn, which is very high in unhealthy polyunsaturated omega-6 fatty acids (see p.136)—high levels of this fatty acid can also be found in their meat.

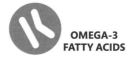

OMEGA-3 FATTY ACIDS

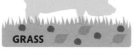

GRASS

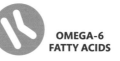

OMEGA-6 FATTY ACIDS

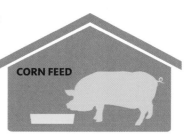

CORN FEED

PASTURE-RAISED

FREE-RANGE

Caged hens may live in spaces only ½sq ft (450sq cm) big and do not have the option to roam outside

CAGED

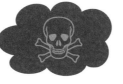

OVER 168 GASES
ARE RELEASED IN **CAFO WASTE,** SOME OF WHICH ARE **DANGEROUS CHEMICALS**

OVERUSE OF ANTIBIOTICS

Some farmers give antibiotics to uninfected animals as a precaution against disease organsims, which thrive in crowded conditions. Because growth is stunted while an animal is ill, precautionary antibiotics increase the rate of weight gain on average, leading to higher meat production. This indiscriminate overuse of antibiotics, however, contributes to the spread of antibiotic-resistant bacteria in both livestock and humans. These bacteria outcompete beneficial bacteria and can become "superbugs" for which we have no defense.

Types of animal rearing

There are a confusing number of terms that can be found on food. They describe farming practices, but many of them mean something different to what consumers may assume they mean. Even within one category there can be wide variations. Although free-range sounds idyllic, chickens may still live in high densities and stay cooped up inside for most of their lives since they only have the option to go outside for a small amount of time each day and some farmers never actively shepherd them onto pasture. There are voluntary farming practices that keep animals in good, healthy conditions, but producers must join a certified program set and checked by authorities to put welfare labels on their produce. The table below provides a guide to the most common labels found on beef or chicken.

TERMS	DEFINITION
Free-range	Free-range standards may simply include having access—no matter how remote—to outdoor space, but animals may never actually go outside. Chickens can live in high densities and can be debeaked (have their beaks removed) and cows can also live in high densities.
Barn-raised	Animals are not caged, but they are restricted indoors, kept at a high density, are usually debeaked (for chickens), and are not allowed to forage or eat grass.
Organic	This primarily refers to organic feed, and to the banning of antibiotics and hormones. Food that is organic usually includes higher welfare standards such as outdoor time and no debeaking in chickens.
Grass-fed	After weaning, animals are allowed to eat only grasses. Cows that eat their natural diet of grass produce meat and milk (see p.89) that is more nutritious.
Pasture-raised	This is similar to grass-fed, although some grain feed is allowed. Livestock are raised outdoors, eating a selection of nutrient-dense forage crops.

Fair trade

A tiny number of enormous global corporations dominate each stage of the complex chain that brings food from field to plate. Powerful businesses use their influence to maximize their share of profits, which keeps food producers, often in the developing world, in poverty. Fair trade can help farmers and businesses alike.

What is fair trade?

The principle of fair trade can always be applied when doing business. However, food can only be labeled as fairly traded if companies join a certification system that makes sure their supply chains follow strict guidelines. These include paying their farmers and workers fairly and providing farmers in the developing world the opportunity to sell their produce on the international market. Fair trade food gives consumers a chance to help farmers at the other end of the supply chain. Organizations that support fair trade work with millions of farmers around the world, especially those producing fruit, sugar, cocoa, tea, and coffee.

ARE THERE ANY ALTERNATIVES?

Some coffee roasters negotiate one-to-one with buyers (direct trade) as an alternative to fair trade—they do this for many reasons, including avoidance of fair trade certification fees.

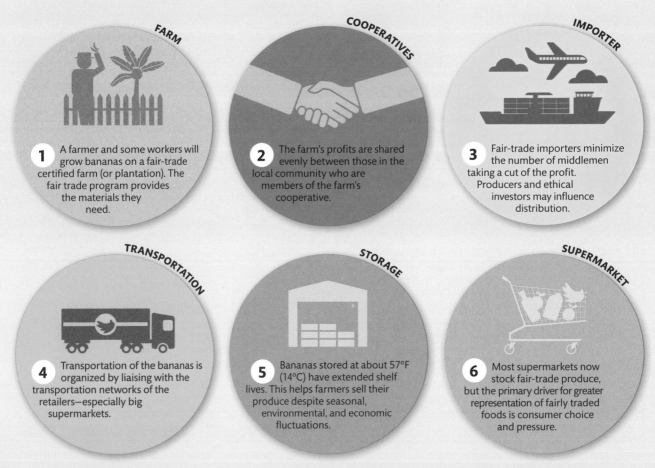

FARM

1 A farmer and some workers will grow bananas on a fair-trade certified farm (or plantation). The fair trade program provides the materials they need.

COOPERATIVES

2 The farm's profits are shared evenly between those in the local community who are members of the farm's cooperative.

IMPORTER

3 Fair-trade importers minimize the number of middlemen taking a cut of the profit. Producers and ethical investors may influence distribution.

TRANSPORTATION

4 Transportation of the bananas is organized by liaising with the transportation networks of the retailers—especially big supermarkets.

STORAGE

5 Bananas stored at about 57°F (14°C) have extended shelf lives. This helps farmers sell their produce despite seasonal, environmental, and economic fluctuations.

SUPERMARKET

6 Most supermarkets now stock fair-trade produce, but the primary driver for greater representation of fairly traded foods is consumer choice and pressure.

GLOBAL PRODUCERS

Much of the world's food supply is controlled by a few relatively large corporations. They oversee production, distribution, and gain most of the profit. This means they influence consumer tastes, and, hence, demand—creating a difficult-to-break cycle.

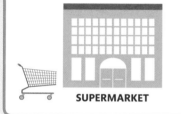

SUPERMARKET

BANANAS GROWN IN ECUADOR AND SOLD TO THE EU

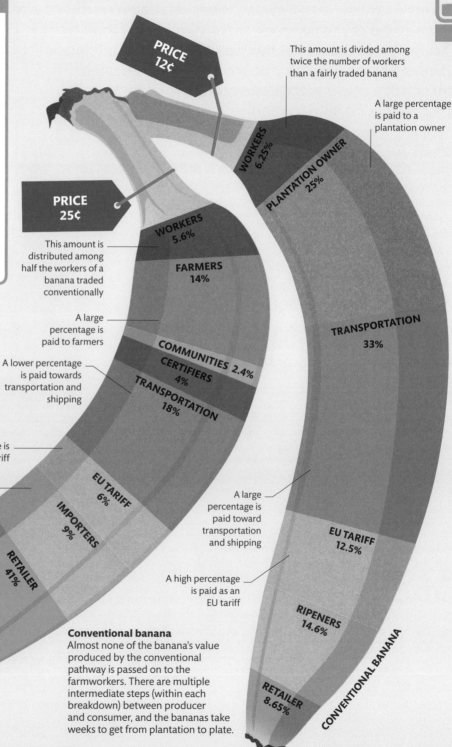

PRICE 12¢

This amount is divided among twice the number of workers than a fairly traded banana

A large percentage is paid to a plantation owner

PRICE 25¢

This amount is distributed among half the workers of a banana traded conventionally

WORKERS 6.25%

PLANTATION OWNER 25%

WORKERS 5.6%

FARMERS 14%

A large percentage is paid to farmers

A lower percentage is paid towards transportation and shipping

COMMUNITIES 2.4%

CERTIFIERS 4%

TRANSPORTATION 18%

TRANSPORTATION 33%

A lower percentage is paid as an EU tariff

A lower percentage is paid to importers

A large percentage is paid to the retailer

EU TARIFF 6%

IMPORTERS 9%

RETAILER 41%

A large percentage is paid toward transportation and shipping

EU TARIFF 12.5%

A high percentage is paid as an EU tariff

RIPENERS 14.6%

RETAILER 8.65%

Fairly traded banana

A larger proportion of the price of a fairly traded banana is paid to the farmer and workers, despite distributing a portion to the local community and reserving a cut for the fair-trade certifiers. The retailer benefits financially from a fairly traded banana so that they have the incentive to promote fair trade.

Conventional banana

Almost none of the banana's value produced by the conventional pathway is passed on to the farmworkers. There are multiple intermediate steps (within each breakdown) between producer and consumer, and the bananas take weeks to get from plantation to plate.

FAIRLY TRADED BANANA

CONVENTIONAL BANANA

Food fraud

Food products are always in demand, but where there's money to be made there's an incentive to cheat. Food fraud is perpetrated at a scale far beyond most people's imagination, with the risk of serious consequences for human health.

What is food fraud?

Food fraud can take many forms, including substitution, dilution, origin masking, artificial enhancement, mislabeling, theft and resale, brand counterfeiting, and intentional distribution of contaminated food. The scale of the problem is unprecedented, but the practice itself has been going on for centuries.

HORSE-MEAT SCANDAL

In 2013, DNA testing revealed that in several processed foods, such as hamburgers and preprepared lasagne meals, a substantial proportion of ground meat claimed to be beef was actually horse. Complex supply chains made it hard to verify the origins of meat.

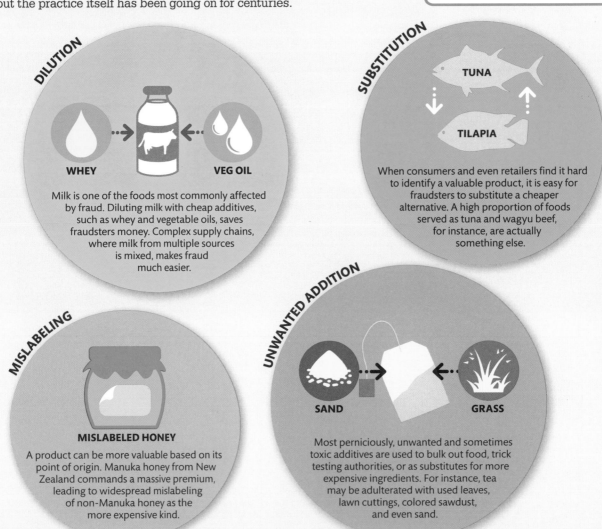

DILUTION

WHEY **VEG OIL**

Milk is one of the foods most commonly affected by fraud. Diluting milk with cheap additives, such as whey and vegetable oils, saves fraudsters money. Complex supply chains, where milk from multiple sources is mixed, makes fraud much easier.

SUBSTITUTION

TUNA

TILAPIA

When consumers and even retailers find it hard to identify a valuable product, it is easy for fraudsters to substitute a cheaper alternative. A high proportion of foods served as tuna and wagyu beef, for instance, are actually something else.

MISLABELING

MISLABELED HONEY

A product can be more valuable based on its point of origin. Manuka honey from New Zealand commands a massive premium, leading to widespread mislabeling of non-Manuka honey as the more expensive kind.

UNWANTED ADDITION

SAND **GRASS**

Most perniciously, unwanted and sometimes toxic additives are used to bulk out food, trick testing authorities, or as substitutes for more expensive ingredients. For instance, tea may be adulterated with used leaves, lawn cuttings, colored sawdust, and even sand.

1.7 TRILLION US DOLLARS
HOW MUCH **FOOD FRAUD COST** THE FOOD INDUSTRY WORLDWIDE IN 2015

Slippery business

In a survey in 2014–15, most of the olive oil consumed by Italians could not be accounted for by any known olive oil production, either domestic or international. The shortfall was most likely cheaper oil passed off as sought-after olive oil.

Italians consumed 14,000 tons of correctly labeled, domestically produced olive oil

14,000 TONS DOMESTIC CONSUMPTION

Italy imported 100,000 tons of correctly labeled, foreign olive oil

100,000 TONS IMPORTS

A supply gap of 407,000 tons is not accounted for by known olive oil sources

WHAT CAN PEOPLE DO TO AVOID FOOD FRAUD?

You can look into the supply chains of the food that you buy—but this may be time consuming if the supply chain is long. Buying from personally known suppliers that you trust may be the answer.

Olive oil fraud

When the figures don't add up, there can be circumstantial evidence of fraud. A case in point is olive oil in Italy. Italians are among the highest consumers of olive oil, but their domestic production does not come close to matching this demand, especially since the majority is exported. Even the 100,000 tons imported cannot account for the nearly half a million tons consumed. Analysis in 2014–15 showed that lower-quality oils had been mislabeled as extra-virgin olive oil. Fraudsters are known to be able to pull off this trick by adding colors and aromas.

407,000-TON SUPPLY GAP

FAKE FISH?

A 2013 survey by the Oceana ocean protection group studied samples of fish on sale around the US, using DNA analysis to reveal whether the species matched the label. They found that around one-third of samples were not what they claimed to be, with 28 different species being sold as red snapper, for instance.

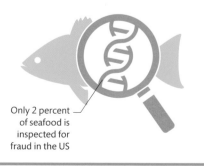

Only 2 percent of seafood is inspected for fraud in the US

Italians believe they consumed 521,000 tons of olive oil

521,000 TONS TOTAL CONSUMPTION

Food waste

The amount of food wasted worldwide could easily feed all of those going hungry on our planet today. Food waste costs money and damages the environment, and can happen at all stages of the food production process.

Effects of food waste

Food is wasted at every stage of the production and supply process, and this is a problem that affects both the developed and developing world. Food waste costs money and drives up food prices, and its environmental impact is severe—3.3 billion tons (3.3 billion metric tons) of greenhouse gases are released from food waste to the atmosphere every year. Water, energy, and space is wasted in producing and distributing food that will never get eaten—28 percent of the world's agricultural land is devoted to growing wasted food, while food garbage rots and gives off methane, a potent greenhouse gas.

GLOBALLY, ONE-THIRD OF ALL **FOOD PRODUCED** FOR HUMAN CONSUMPTION IS **WASTED**

HOW TO REDUCE WASTE

Even individuals can help minimize waste. Steps include: planning meals; preparing food in advance; freezing or reusing leftovers; shopping little and often; buying food that is near the end of its shelf life; buying produce loose rather than in multipacks; and buying oddly shaped fruit and vegetables (so supermarkets do not reject them).

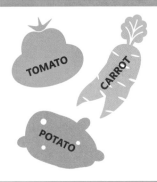

TOMATO

CARROT

POTATO

100%

When food is wasted
This graphic shows how much food produced on land is wasted at each stage. These are global figures; in developing countries there is more waste toward the start of the process due to a lack of cooling and storage capabilities so more food is spoiled, while in developed countries, most waste occurs toward the end of the process because people are more able to afford to purchase and waste food.

67%

–11.5%

5 **Consumption**
Much of food waste, especially in developed countries, occurs at the consumption stage, when food is thrown away after it is purchased or even after it is prepared.

–4%

78.5%

4 **Distribution and market**
Retailers throw away foods that are not bought by shoppers and even foods that are not aesthetically pleasing to consumers (such as strangely shaped vegetables).

1 Agriculture
Some farmers, especially those in developing countries, may possess limited agricultural resources, infrastructure, and knowledge—and this can lead to lower yields.

92%

–8%

CAN FOOD WASTE BE RECYCLED?

Food waste can be composted into soil conditioner or fermented using microbes to create fertilizer. The gas emitted during fermentation can be collected and used to generate electricity.

–8%

2 Postharvest and slaughter
Inappropriate storage techniques and poor chilling facilities may cause some food to go bad or spoil.

84%

–1.5%

3 Processing and packaging
Mistakes in the processing stage can lead to further waste. For example, milk that has been incorrectly pasteurized (see p.84) may be discarded.

82.5%

What food is wasted?

The biggest cause of waste is perishability. Foods with the shortest shelf lives, or that are the most easily damaged, are those that tend to get wasted the most. This means that the more easily damaged fruit and vegetables and roots and tubers are wasted the most, followed by fish and seafood that have short shelf lives. Less meat is lost, but it takes more land to produce meat, which destroys natural habitats—so the environmental impact of this waste is greater.

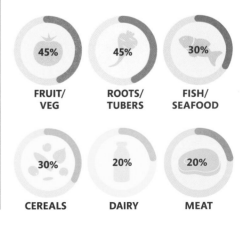

PERCENTAGE WASTED

FRUIT/VEG	ROOTS/TUBERS	FISH/SEAFOOD
45%	45%	30%

CEREALS	DAIRY	MEAT
30%	20%	20%

Food miles

Until recent years, diets were limited by seasonality and locality, but the pace of modern transportation means that a Western shopper can buy any food at any time—but at what cost to the environment?

Local versus global

The local food movement is based on the drive to reduce the environmental impact of industrial agriculture. One of its most obvious goals is to reduce pollution caused by transporting food long distances from source to market—hence, the concept of food miles. In fact, the true impact of food miles is hard to unpick; for instance, having local produce delivered to your doorstep by a local supplier might produce more emissions than walking to the supermarket to buy food bulk-transported from abroad.

MORE THAN **15 PERCENT** OF THE **FOODS** EATEN IN THE US ARE **IMPORTED**

The bull's-eye diet

Advocates of the local food movement have made this simple guide that prompts consumers to think about the zones of production they can support to reduce their environmental footprint. At the center is what you can grow in your own yard or even window box, while outer rings should contribute progressively less and less to your diet.

GLOBAL FOOD PRODUCERS
DOMESTIC FOOD PRODUCERS
LOCAL FARMERS
NEIGHBORHOOD
HOME

USA

Seasonality

A major driver of increased food miles in modern food consumption is the demand for food at all times of year, irrespective of whether it is in season. Fruits, for instance, naturally have limited seasonal availability in any one territory, but suppliers work around this natural constraint by importing foods from faraway sources, or by cold-storing fruit on a colossal scale (many "fresh" apples were actually picked many months ago).

British strawberries

UK strawberry growers have contrived to extend their domestic season greatly, but suppliers still turn to imports to keep shelves stocked for the other five months of the year.

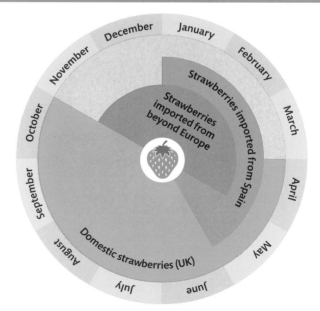

January
February
March
April
May
June
July
August
September
October
November
December

Strawberries imported from beyond Europe
Strawberries imported from Spain
Domestic strawberries (UK)

Sourcing ingredients for pork dumplings

One way to assess the cost of the transportation involved in producing a dish is to look at its "foodshed"—the equivalent of a watershed for a river—showing all the sources that contribute. A processed food such as siu mai (steamed pork dumplings) produced in Hong Kong can have a complex transnational foodshed.

KEY
Countries exporting the ingredients for siu mai (steamed pork dumplings) to Hong Kong

Pork

Shrimp

Rice

Wheat for dumplings outer case

Sesame oil

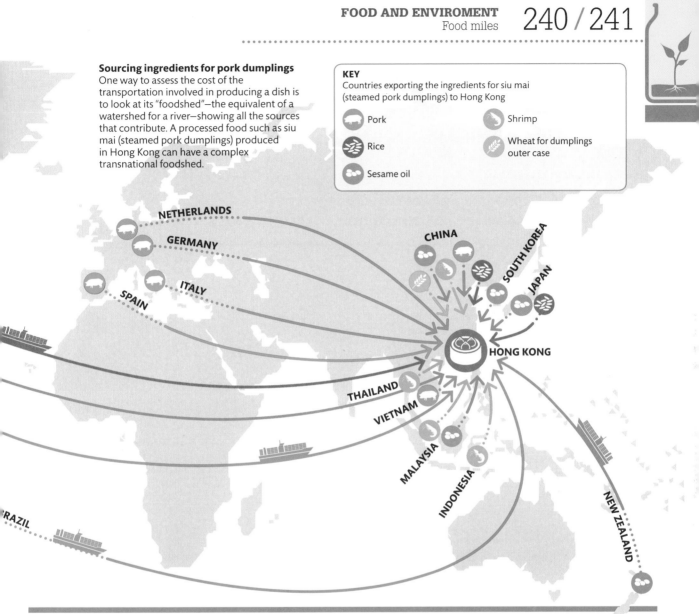

NETHERLANDS
GERMANY
ITALY
SPAIN
CHINA
SOUTH KOREA
JAPAN
HONG KONG
THAILAND
VIETNAM
MALAYSIA
INDONESIA
NEW ZEALAND
BRAZIL

Do food miles really matter?

Some experts doubt that food mileage is the most important part of food production. According to one estimate, transportation contributes just 3.6 percent to food-related energy use. The nature of your food makes a far bigger impact than where it comes from. Vegans have a carbon footprint dramatically lower than meat eaters, because meat takes so much more energy to produce. The local food movement in fact targets industrial agriculture rather than solely minimizing food miles.

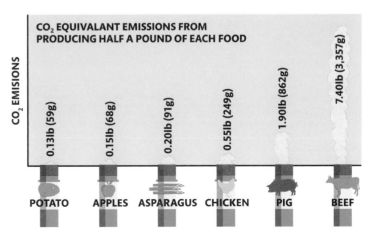

CO₂ EQUIVALANT EMISSIONS FROM PRODUCING HALF A POUND OF EACH FOOD

CO₂ EMISSIONS

POTATO	APPLES	ASPARAGUS	CHICKEN	PIG	BEEF
0.13lb (59g)	0.15lb (68g)	0.20lb (91g)	0.55lb (249g)	1.90lb (862g)	7.40lb (3,357g)

Genetically modified foods

The hype, discord, and intentionally misleading information surrounding genetically modified foods, or simply GM foods, obscures the reasoned debate necessary about the risks and rewards of this new frontier in food production and agriculture.

SHOULD GM FOODS BE LABELED?

This is subject to fierce debate. Advocates say it gives consumers more control and choice, but critics argue that consumers are not sufficiently informed to make rational choices.

What are GM foods?

Genetically modified foods are crops that have had specific genes altered or manipulated using techniques of genetic engineering. Traditional breeding mixes hundreds or thousands of genes at a time, but this happens over the course of generations. New technologies make it possible to target single genes and to transfer genes from one species to another unrelated organism, for instance, from bacterium to plant. Such changes cannot be achieved by conventional plant breeding.

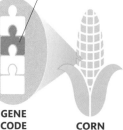

SUGAR BEET · CORN · SOY · COTTON · PAPAYA

GM foods
Eight types of GM foods are commercially available—corn, soybeans, cotton (for oil), canola (also a source of oil), squash, papaya, sugar beets (for sugar), and alfalfa (for animal feed).

Inserting genes
A desirable gene from one species is transplanted to a new species. Insecticide-producing genes from *Bacillus thuringiensis* have been inserted into the DNA of corn to produce a crop that makes its own insecticide.

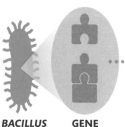

Insecticide-producing genes from bacteria inserted into corn

BACILLUS THURINGIENSIS · **GENE CODE** · **GENE CODE** · **CORN**

Suppressing genes
Alternatively, organisms can be modified by switching off genes so they don't express themselves. Some fruits, such as tomatoes, have softening genes turned off so they will last longer. This method is less common.

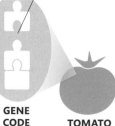

Gene switched off

GENE CODE · **TOMATO**

Why are they made?
GM foods are made so that more crops are resistant to pests and disease, and therefore survive to provide higher yields. Herbicide-resistant crops allow farmers to use herbicide more efficiently to kill weeds, and crops can even be genetically modified to enhance nutrition.

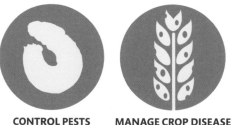

CONTROL PESTS · **MANAGE CROP DISEASE** · **MANAGE WEEDS** · **CHANGE NUTRITION**

The GM debate

Despite the flourishing culture of anti-GM food opinion and activism, there are no well-supported or scientifically respectable large-scale studies to support claims that GM foods pose a risk to human health. The rational counterargument is that GM foods comprise a colossal public health experiment without informed consent and with unknown long-term outcomes. The spread of new, altered genes into wild populations also has unknown effects on the environment. Meanwhile, the food industry has moved on without waiting for the debate to settle—GM foods are commonplace in countries such as the US.

ARGUMENTS FOR GM

Good or bad?
Supporters argue that there are real and potential benefits to GM foods, but there are biological, environmental, and economic concerns to consider. Here are just some of the arguments for and against.

Options for vegans
Plants could contain meat and dairy components (such as vitamin B12) if they had the genes for them. This could open up new dietary possibilities for vegans.

Fewer chemicals
Pest-resistant, fast-growing GM crops mean there is a reduced need for pesticides and fertilizers, which benefits the environment (see pp.230–31).

Global demand
Modifying crops that are adapted for difficult and changing conditions, with enhanced nutrition, will be necessary to meet the demands and changing needs of a growing population.

ARGUMENTS AGAINST GM

Risk of disease
Some GM crops are monocultures (genetically identical) and this genetic similarity means they all may be equally vulnerable to the same infectious disease.

More chemicals
If GM crops are bred to be resistant to weed-killer chemicals (herbicides), farmers are free to use more herbicide, which can kill natural plants living around the farm and cause wide environmental damage downstream.

Corporate power
GM foods are produced using genetically modified organisms (GMOs), and are generally patented and have to be bought anew each growing season. They are controlled by a handful of major multinationals.

90 PERCENT OF SOY, CORN, COTTON, CANOLA, AND SUGAR BEETS SOLD IN THE US HAVE BEEN GENETICALLY ENGINEERED

Overfishing and sustainable fishing

Fish are more popular than ever, partly due to the increasing awareness of their health benefits. But the world's insatiable appetite has almost drained the once apparently limitless resources of the ocean—often with catastrophic results to ecosystems. Fish farming and sustainable fishing may provide solutions to these problems.

Global hunger for fish

Around three billion people in the world, in order to obtain enough protein, rely on either wild-caught or farmed seafood, including fish. On average, each person eats four times as much seafood now than they did in 1950. To satisfy this great demand, global fisheries have already been pushed past their limits. When fish stocks (populations) fall steadily, they are being overfished—and this is unsustainable because these fish will, sooner or later, become too scarce to support a fishery—or worse, become extinct entirely. The United Nations Food and Agriculture Organization (UNFAO) says we will need another 40 million tons (36.3 million metric tons) of seafood worldwide per year by 2030 just to meet current consumption rates, based on current population projections.

IS IT OK TO EAT TUNA?

The once-abundant bluefin tuna is now critically endangered, and many other tuna species are decimated. They are large predators, and so like big cats or birds of prey, they are naturally scarce—so we can't eat them too much or too fast.

A rise in fishing

Since the 1950s, global fishing of wild populations (wild fisheries) has been rapidly increasing, along with aquaculture (fish farming). By the 1990s, fishing plateaued as fish stocks became depleted. In response, fish farming grew even more rapidly—and continues to grow.

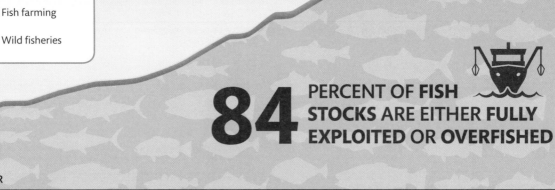

KEY

● Fish farming

● Wild fisheries

84 PERCENT OF **FISH STOCKS** ARE EITHER **FULLY EXPLOITED OR OVERFISHED**

YEAR

1950   1960   1970

How to fish sustainably

Sustainable fishing preserves fish populations and allows them to replenish themselves. It involves a mixture of good practice, such as: no-catch areas, where fishing is illegal; no bottom-trawling, to avoid damaging fragile ecosystems such as reefs; preventing fraud, in which fishers misreport catches; reducing bycatch by using nets that allow fry and other accidentally caught species to escape; buying other species of fish that are not overfished; and fishing using a line and pole, which targets individual fish rather than entire schools.

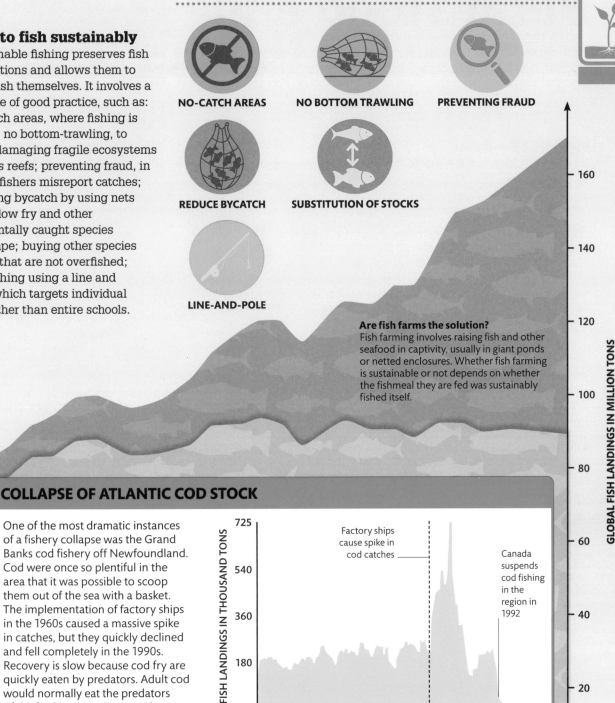

NO-CATCH AREAS

NO BOTTOM TRAWLING

PREVENTING FRAUD

REDUCE BYCATCH

SUBSTITUTION OF STOCKS

LINE-AND-POLE

Are fish farms the solution?
Fish farming involves raising fish and other seafood in captivity, usually in giant ponds or netted enclosures. Whether fish farming is sustainable or not depends on whether the fishmeal they are fed was sustainably fished itself.

GLOBAL FISH LANDINGS IN MILLION TONS

- 160
- 140
- 120
- 100
- 80
- 60
- 40
- 20

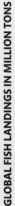

COLLAPSE OF ATLANTIC COD STOCK

One of the most dramatic instances of a fishery collapse was the Grand Banks cod fishery off Newfoundland. Cod were once so plentiful in the area that it was possible to scoop them out of the sea with a basket. The implementation of factory ships in the 1960s caused a massive spike in catches, but they quickly declined and fell completely in the 1990s. Recovery is slow because cod fry are quickly eaten by predators. Adult cod would normally eat the predators of the fry, but since they are absent very few cod ever grow up.

FISH LANDINGS IN THOUSAND TONS

725

540

360

180

0

Factory ships cause spike in cod catches

Canada suspends cod fishing in the region in 1992

1900   1925   1950   1975   2000

YEAR

1990   2000   2010

Future foods

The technology behind food production and agriculture continues to improve, bringing about more efficient, sustainable ways to produce food—on both large and local scales.

Farms of the future

Tomorrow's farms will have to feed a rapidly growing population that will demand more and better food. They will also have to cope with climate change, soil degradation, water shortages, non-native pests, and new diseases. To overcome these challenges and meet these needs, innovative solutions are already being explored, by retooling the agricultural wisdom of ancient cultures, or by creating entirely new, controlled systems.

Seawater greenhouses

For hot, arid seaside regions where crops are unable to grow, seawater greenhouses produce a hospitable growing climate and create freshwater with which to irrigate crops.

2 Sun's energy
Surface seawater runs through pipes along the greenhouse roof where it is heated by the sun. Solar panels harvest sunlight to generate the electricity to power the fans and pumps that move the seawater.

3 Air humidified
The hot seawater runs down another porous wall. The cool, moist air is drawn through this wall, and as it passes through it is heated and can pick up even more moisture.

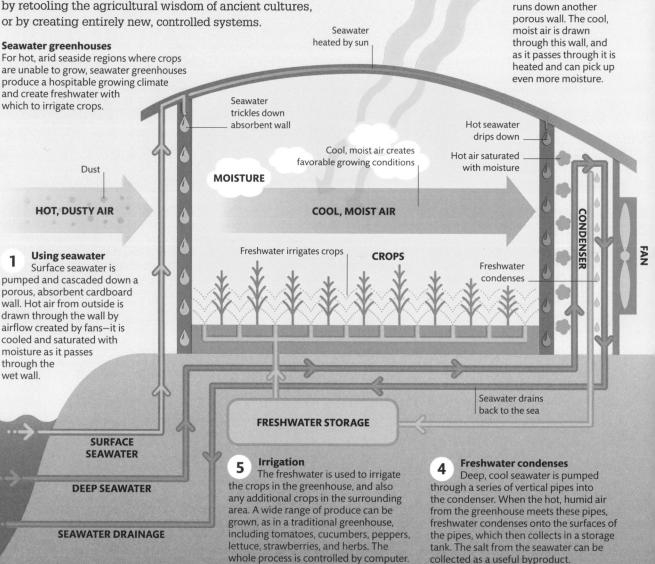

Seawater heated by sun

Seawater trickles down absorbent wall

Cool, moist air creates favorable growing conditions

Hot seawater drips down

Hot air saturated with moisture

MOISTURE

Dust

HOT, DUSTY AIR

COOL, MOIST AIR

CONDENSER

FAN

1 Using seawater
Surface seawater is pumped and cascaded down a porous, absorbent cardboard wall. Hot air from outside is drawn through the wall by airflow created by fans—it is cooled and saturated with moisture as it passes through the wet wall.

Freshwater irrigates crops

CROPS

Freshwater condenses

Seawater drains back to the sea

FRESHWATER STORAGE

SURFACE SEAWATER

DEEP SEAWATER

SEAWATER DRAINAGE

5 Irrigation
The freshwater is used to irrigate the crops in the greenhouse, and also any additional crops in the surrounding area. A wide range of produce can be grown, as in a traditional greenhouse, including tomatoes, cucumbers, peppers, lettuce, strawberries, and herbs. The whole process is controlled by computer.

4 Freshwater condenses
Deep, cool seawater is pumped through a series of vertical pipes into the condenser. When the hot, humid air from the greenhouse meets these pipes, freshwater condenses onto the surfaces of the pipes, which then collects in a storage tank. The salt from the seawater can be collected as a useful byproduct.

New sources of meat

The growing demand for meat around the world—and the inefficiency with which some countries raise their livestock (see pp.228–29)—means there is an urgent need for alternatives. Insects are already eaten by many (see p.148) and could be a more sustainable source of meat. Not only is 80 percent of a cricket's body edible, compared to only 40 percent of a cow's, there is actually more protein in 3½oz (100g) of cricket than in beef.

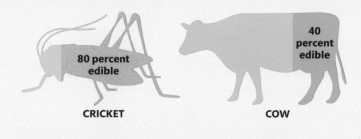

80 percent edible

CRICKET

40 percent edible

COW

GREENHOUSES ON MARS

Martian soil contains most of the nutrients needed to grow plants, but there is almost no atmosphere on Mars, freezing temperatures, no running water, and damaging radiation. Greenhouses have been proposed that might be able to concentrate the sun and trap gases to create growing conditions.

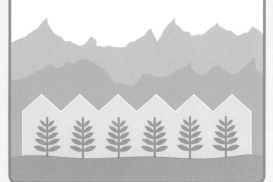

Reimagining ideas

Medieval Aztecs used to raise crops without soil whilst suspending them above lakes. Today, aquaponics does something similar. It is an agricultural system that combines fish farming and growing plants without soil. It functions independently—and therefore could be a more sustainable way to farm fish and raise crops.

SCIENTISTS IN JAPAN ARE WORKING ON A **KITCHEN THAT PROJECTS PREPARATION INSTRUCTIONS** ONTO **FOOD**

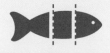

PLANTS

Natural fertilizer
Microbes and composting worms feed on the fish waste and turn it into a natural fertilizer for the suspended plants.

FISH WASTE

Food source
The waste the fish produce provides a food source for microbes and composting worms.

FISH

Cleansing
Plants are grown in the same water as the fish. They filter the water, which helps keep the fish healthy.

Index

Acknowledgments

DK would like to thank the following people for help in preparing this book: Marek Walisiewicz at Cobalt id, Sam Atkinson, Wendy Horobin, and Miezan van Zyl, for editorial assistance; Simon Murrell at Sands Design, Darren Bland and Paul Reid at Cobalt id, Clare Joyce, and Renata Latipova for design assistance; Harish Aggarwal, Priyanka Sharma, and Dhirendra Singh for jackets assistance, Helen Peters for indexing, and Ruth O'Rourke for proofreading.